Posterior Circulation Stroke

Jong S. Kim

Editor

Posterior Circulation Stroke

Advances in Understanding and Management

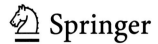 Springer

Editor
Jong S. Kim
Department of Neurology
Asan Medical Center
University of Ulsan
Seoul
South Korea

ISBN 978-981-15-6741-4   ISBN 978-981-15-6739-1   (eBook)
https://doi.org/10.1007/978-981-15-6739-1

This Springer imprint is published by the registered company Springer Nature Singapore Pte Ltd.
The registered company address is: 152 Beach Road, #21-01/04 Gateway East, Singapore
189721, Singapore

Preface

As a medical student, I was amazed to see my professors localize brainstem lesions merely through the evaluation of patients' eye movements and the sensory-motor system. Owing to its anatomical and functional complexity, a study of the human brainstem is complicated; however, this challenge itself motivated me to become a neurologist and has continued to intrigue me throughout my career.

During my career as a professor, however, I have realized that compared with anterior circulation strokes, posterior circulation strokes have not gained sufficient attention. Students, residents, and even some professors do not take their time enough to understand the clinical syndromes and pathogenetic mechanisms contributing to this disease entity. The same trend is observed among researchers; posterior circulation strokes have been neglected in large clinical trials that investigated the efficacy of thrombolysis and endovascular therapy, even if acute basilar artery occlusion results in extremely serious neurological conditions.

Thanks to thoughtful teaching imparted by pioneers such as Dr. Caplan, we can now better understand posterior circulation stroke. However, I strongly feel that more should be written in the literature. My own experience in this field and comparative studies of posterior and anterior circulation strokes in the literature show several similarities as well as differences between these anatomically different conditions. The former is more commonly associated with arterial diseases, whereas the latter is more closely associated with cardiac embolism. The ischemic lesions tend to be smaller, and the mode of onset is less abrupt in posterior circulation strokes. Although few trials have been reported, recanalization therapy for posterior circulation strokes appears to be effective if rapid diagnosis and prompt evaluation is made in this complex condition. Considering its characteristics, the therapeutic time window may even be longer in posterior than in anterior circulation strokes. Development of novel technologies to treat pathological conditions occurring in relatively small arteries has facilitated easier and better management of posterior circulation strokes.

This book aims to provide readers with comprehensive and up-to-date knowledge of posterior circulation strokes, including the vascular anatomy, pathology, epidemiology, pathogenesis, stroke syndromes including ocular/auditory disturbances, diagnostic modalities, and treatment strategies, such as antithrombotics, angioplasty/stenting, and surgical interventions. In addition, it presents an extensive discussion of non-atherosclerotic arterial diseases, such as dissection, vasculitis, and miscellaneous disorders; therefore, this book covers a wide scope of topics that range from academic subjects to practical guidelines. All chapters are written by leading international experts and established scientists. In my view, the interesting results of cutting-edge research such as the application of high-resolution magnetic resonance imaging or the development of interventional procedures will be of much interest to readers.

It must be acknowledged that despite extensive research and well-presented facts, much ambiguity persists in some areas. The optimal medical therapy, patient categories that would benefit most from angioplasty/stenting or bypass surgery, and the therapeutic time window for recanalization therapy are among the several questions that warrant further investigation. I hope that this book is informative, interesting, and stimulating for readers and serves as a useful guide in their clinical and research activities. Finally, I wish to sincerely thank all the contributors for their valuable time and efforts in preparing the excellent manuscript. I am also grateful to Springer for providing me the opportunity to communicate with readers worldwide.

Seoul, South Korea   Jong S. Kim

Contents

1 History of Vertebrobasilar Territory Stroke and TIA 1
Louis R. Caplan

2 Arterial Anatomy and Collaterals 15
Kunakorn Atchaneeyasakul and David S. Liebeskind

3 Epidemiology, Risk Factors, and Stroke Mechanisms 21
Philip B. Gorelick and Jong S. Kim

4 Brain Stem Infarction Syndromes 35
Jong S. Kim

**5 Thalamic and Other Posterior Cerebral Artery
Stroke Syndromes** 67
Stefania Nannoni and Patrik Michel

6 Cerebellar Infarction 85
Cristina Hobeanu, Elena Viedma-Guiard,
and Pierre Amarenco

7 Ocular, Vestibular, and Otologic Syndromes 101
Eun-Jae Lee, Hyo-Jung Kim, and Ji-Soo Kim

8 Hemorrhagic Strokes 121
Jong-Won Chung and Chin-Sang Chung

9 Imaging Diagnosis 135
Yunsun Song and Seung Chai Jung

10 Medical Treatment 165
Kazunori Toyoda and Jong S. Kim

11 Thrombolysis and Thrombectomy 177
Christine Hawkes, Kavit Shah, and Tudor G. Jovin

**12 Angioplasty and Stenting for Posterior
Circulation Stroke** 191
Hugh S. Markus

13 Surgical Therapy 199
Christopher J. Stapleton and Sepideh Amin-Hanjani

14 Non-atherosclerotic, Uncommon Diseases 213
     Jong S. Kim

15 Outcomes and Prognosis 231
     Nitish Kumar, Vamshi K. S. Balasetti, Farhan Siddiq,
     Brandi R. French, Camilo R. Gomez, and Adnan I. Qureshi

History of Vertebrobasilar Territory Stroke and TIA

Louis R. Caplan

Early Anatomical and Clinical–Pathological Studies

The first important attention to disease of the posterior circulation was likely by a Swiss pathologist and physician: Johan Jacob Wepfer. He followed the example of Vesalius and performed meticulous necropsy examinations. He described the results of his dissections in his magnum opus on apoplexy published in 1658 [1]. Wepfer distinguished two types of apoplexy: in one form, the supply of blood to the brain was obstructed or precluded, and in the other, animal spirits escaped and hemorrhage occurred. He described the appearance and the course of the intracranial arteries and recognized blockage of the carotid and vertebral arteries caused by disease of the arterial walls as a cause of apoplexy, the obstruction preventing entry of sufficient blood into a portion of the brain. He described the anatomy of the intracranial vertebral arteries as follows: "As regards the vertebral arteries, they emerge from the nearest foramen, that great orifice through which the spinal marrow descends. They advance to the sides of the medulla oblongata…. When they reach that place where the sixth pair of nerves (IX, X, XI, XII) arises, the right and left branches are joined and form a single channel (basilar artery) and remain united along the whole marrow tract."

The next attention to the posterior circulation was by clinicians and researchers in Europe during the second half of the nineteenth century and early twentieth century. These observers were mostly interested in brain and vascular anatomy and in anatomical–physiologic correlations. The so-called classic brainstem syndromes all eponymic and named after the original describers of the syndromes, were stimulated by a fascination of the authors with the anatomy and functions of the brainstem. Recognized still today are these various constellations of findings as the syndromes of Benedikt, Claude, Millard–Gubler, Babinski–Nageotte, Foville, and Wallenberg, among others [2]. Retrospective reviews of these reports showed that many lesions were not vascular in etiology; the underlying arterial lesions and vascular pathology were very seldom studied or commented upon. More modern studies of series of patients with brainstem and cerebellar ischemia indicate that all but Wallenberg's syndrome are rare. During that era, clinicians were mostly interested in how the brain and its nuclei and tracts worked. The brainstem with its dense, packed heterogeneous and complex anatomy was of particular interest. Focal lesions limited to one location in the midbrain, pons, or medulla provided great insight into the anatomy and physiology of the brainstem. Of special utility in localization were crossed syndromes in which cranial nerve abnormalities involved one side of

L. R. Caplan (✉)
Beth Israel Deaconess Medical Center, Harvard Medical School, Boston, MA, USA
e-mail: lcaplan@bidmc.harvard.edu

© Springer Nature Singapore Pte Ltd. 2021
J. S. Kim (ed.), *Posterior Circulation Stroke*, https://doi.org/10.1007/978-981-15-6739-1_1

the head while long tract motor or sensory or extrapyramidal-cerebellar abnormalities involved the limbs and trunk on the opposite side of the body. The Millard–Gubler syndrome of ipsilateral facial palsy and contralateral hemiparesis was an example. Since there was no way during that time to identify the causative vascular lesion during life, and no treatment was known or available even if the causes were known, there was no interest in stroke etiology or the mechanism of ischemia in patients with brainstem or cerebellar infarcts.

Posterior Circulation Ischemia

The first detailed study of the clinical, pathological, and etiological aspects of brainstem infarction was by a German physician Adolf Wallenberg. During a period of 27 years, Wallenberg published 4 reports on the topic of infarction of the lateral medulla: a detailed analysis of the clinical findings in one patient, the necropsy findings in that patient, a single case report of another patient, and the clinical and pathological findings in the 15th patient he had studied [3–6]. Wallenberg had first seen the original patient, a ropemaker in 1889, for appendicitis. In 1993, the patient developed severe vertigo, intense pain in the left eye, difficulty swallowing, and hoarseness. Wallenberg reported a detailed clinical neurological examination that showed horizontal and vertical nystagmus, loss of pain and temperature sensation in the left face and right face and body, weakness of the left palate, paralysis of the left vocal cord, and left limb ataxia. Wallenberg wrote, "We are dealing with an insult on the left side of the medulla. It begins just above the pyramidal decussation. It passes through the accessory olive and the inferior olive more rostrally. Laterally it destroys the entire medulla to the pia mater. Rostrally and medially it reaches the ascending lemniscus damages the restiform body and ultimately also the cerebellum."

Six years after the initial report, the patient had another acute stroke and died. Wallenberg

performed the autopsy himself and described and illustrated the location and extent of the medullary infarct. The vertebral arteries were severely diseased, and the left posterior inferior cerebellar artery was occluded.

Anatomists and researchers working during the early part of the twentieth century became interested in the blood vessels that supply the brain including the brainstem and cerebellum. Duret [7, 8] in France and Stopford [9] in England meticulously dissected the arteries that supply the brainstem. Particularly prolific in performing studies that clarified arterial anatomy was Charles Foix who worked in the clinics and pathology laboratories at the Salpetriere hospital in Paris [10]. Foix and his colleagues defined the distribution and localization of brain infarcts ("ramollissements") and the corresponding neurological abnormalities that they caused during life. They also sought to clarify the anatomical distribution of the arterial supply to these areas. During 4 short years, between 1923 and 1927, Foix and his colleagues defined the arterial distribution of the posterior cerebral artery including the branches to the thalamus, and the supply of the pons, and the medulla oblongata [11–15]. Most importantly, Foix noted the common pattern of irrigation of all parts of the brainstem by paramedian, short circumferential, and long circumferential arteries. This schema is illustrated in Fig. 1.1.

Probably the single most important and influential communication regarding posterior circulation ischemia was the report on basilar artery occlusion by Kubik and Adams published in 1946 [16]. This report was one of the most complete and most detailed clinical–pathological studies of any vascular syndrome. Kubik and Adams did not publish the very first report of occlusion of the basilar artery; there had been prior reports. Hayem had described the pathological findings in a necropsy specimen from a single patient with basilar artery occlusion but did not describe the clinical findings [17]. Leyden had reported 2 patients with syphilitic arteritis of the basilar artery [18]. Marburg wrote a review of pontine and medullary infarcts in 1911 [19]. Lhermitte and Trelles reported a number of

Fig. 1.1 Foix diagram of pontine supply. (a) Long circumferential artery, (b) short circumferential artery, (c) paramedian artery, (d) pons, (e) cerebellar vermis, and (f) lateral lobe of the cerebellum. (From Caplan, L.R. Charles Foix - The first modern stroke neurologist. Stroke 1990;21:348-356 with permission)

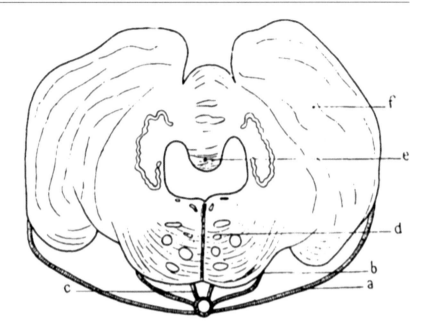

patients with pontine infarcts, some of whom had thrombosis within the basilar artery or its branches [20]. Pines and Gilinsky described a single patient with a likely embolic occlusion of the rostral basilar artery in which the brainstem had been serially sectioned and the infarcts well defined [21]. The report of Kubik and Adams was very important and influential because of the large size of the series (18 patients), the meticulous dissection and illustration of the brain lesions at the various brainstem levels, as well as delineation of the vascular occlusion (Figs. 1.1 and 1.2), and the details of the clinical findings.

At the time of their report, Kubik and Adams were both neuropathologists working in the necropsy laboratories at the Massachusetts General Hospital and the Boston City Hospital in Boston, as well as being active on the neurology wards of the hospitals. The authors examined some of the patients during life and later reviewed their clinical charts. The extent and location of the thrombosis correlated well with the areas of brainstem infarction, and usually, only a portion of the basilar artery was occluded. Figure 1.2 is a redrawing of a diagram of the location and extent of the basilar artery occlusion and the resultant infarcts in the pons. The infarcts were mostly confined to

the territories of the paramedian and short circumferential pontine arteries. The authors discussed the pathological distinctions between thrombosis that formed in situ and embolism and concluded that 7 of the 18 basilar artery occlusions were embolic. The symptoms in most patients began abruptly, and all cases were fatal (or else the patient would not have reached their laboratory in the morgue). Each patient was described in detail, and the brain and vascular lesions were diagrammed. The clinical symptoms and signs during life such as dizziness, altered consciousness, dysarthria, paresthesias, pseudobulbar palsy, hemiplegia or quadriplegia, pupillary and oculomotor abnormalities, facial paralysis, and visual loss correlated well with the brainstem and posterior hemispheral structures involved. The authors emphasized that recognition of these signs should allow for accurate antemortem diagnosis of basilar artery occlusion. In fact, at the conclusion of the article, the author reported the clinical findings that led them to suspect basilar artery thrombosis in 7 patients who were still alive. Unfortunately, with the limited technology available at the time, there was no safe way to document the nature of the vascular lesion.

Fig. 1.2 Cartoon showing the pons with an infarct caused by occlusion of the basilar artery. (**a**) midbrain, (**b**) upper pons, (**c**) lower pons, and (**d**) medulla. (From Caplan, L.R.: Caplan's Stroke: A Clinical Approach, 4th edition. Philadelphia: Elsevier, 2009 redrawn from Kubik C, Adams R. Occlusion of the basilar artery: a clinical and pathologic study. Brain 1946; 69:73-121)

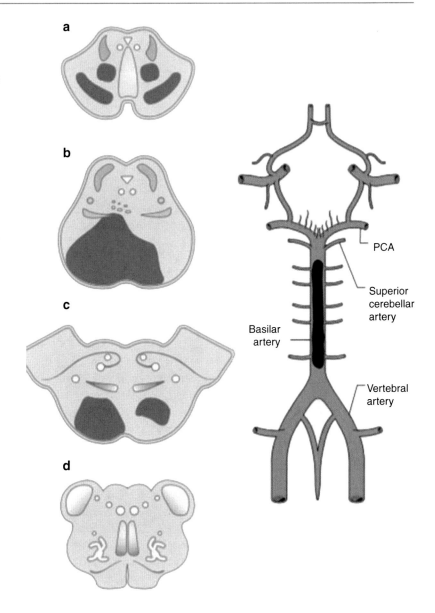

Early Clinical Studies

During the first half of the twentieth century and before that time, most brain infarcts were attributed to occlusion of intracranial arteries. In the report of Kubik and Adams, the occlusion involved the basilar artery, an important intracranial artery, and most anterior circulation infarcts were attributed to occlusion of the middle cerebral artery. As in Kubik and Adams's report, clinicians of that era thought that strokes generally came abruptly without warning but often progressed after the onset of ischemia.

Miller Fisher's reports on the clinical features of carotid artery disease appeared just 5 and 8 years after Kubik and Adams's report [22, 23]. Fisher made two key observations that had an important influence on the approach of clinicians to posterior circulation ischemia. Fisher's patients with carotid artery disease often had warning spells, TIAs, that preceded and warned of an impending stroke. The occlusive disease was in the neck where it was potentially reachable by surgery. This was the first emphasis on occlusive disease in the neck. Several years after Fisher's report, Hutchinson and Yates began to systematically dissect and examine the cervicocranial arteries in the neck [24]. They found a high frequency of occlusive disease in the cervical vertebral arteries near their origins from the subclavian arteries. Vertebral artery occlusive disease in the neck seemed to parallel carotid occlusive disease leading Hutchinson and Yates to coin the term "carotico-vertebral" stenosis [25]. Later, Miller Fisher also emphasized the importance of occlusive disease involving the vertebral arteries in the neck, which often involved these vessels bilaterally [26].

In the ensuing years, description of the so-called subclavian steal syndrome added more weight to the growing evidence that extracranial occlusive disease was common. The report by Reivich and colleagues called attention to patients with periodic attacks of dizziness and vertigo, sometimes precipitated by arm exercise, who had occlusive lesions involving the subclavian artery proximal to the vertebral artery origin [27, 28]. Angiography and blood flow studies showed that blood coursed from the contralateral subclavian artery up the vertebral artery to reach the cranium and then traveled retrograde down the vertebral artery ipsilateral to the subclavian artery stenosis or occlusion. Ultimately, the retrograde vertebral artery flow went into the ischemic arm. Later, Hennerici and colleagues showed that reversed vertebral artery flow was common in patients with subclavian artery occlusive disease but rarely produced important neurological symptoms or signs [29].

During the 1950s and 1960s, arteriography of the aortic arch and its cervicocranial branches became feasible. A great advance in angiography was made when Seldinger, in Sweden in 1953, introduced angiography by catheterization of the femoral artery, allowing selective catheterization of all the vessels to be studied [30]. During the 1970s, there were improvements in angiography performance, namely that trained experienced full-time neuroradiologists began to perform the procedure; newer safer dyes were developed and introduced; and biplane filming techniques were

perfected. These advances led to safer, more useful angiography. Impressed by the lesson from the subclavian steal syndrome that the occlusive lesion could be at a distance from the ischemia, physicians advocated full opacification of the aortic arch and all 4 main arteries supplying the brain. Routine "arch and 4" angiography was performed. Arch angiography, a cumbersome procedure necessitating lots of dye, was used in the very large Joint Study of Extracranial Arterial Occlusions begun in the middle years of the twentieth century. This study corroborated the high frequency of extracranial occlusive disease in the carotid, subclavian, and vertebral arteries in the neck [31].

During the 1950s, clinicians had become alerted to the presence of TIAs by Fisher [22, 23]. They had also become aware of the usual symptoms and signs in patients who were later proven to have fatal basilar artery occlusions by Kubik and Adams [16]. During the late 1950s and early 1960s, a series of articles written by American and British clinicians concerned patients with TIAs that indicated involvement of brain structures fed by posterior circulation arteries. When studied during life by angiography, there was a high frequency of severe vertebrobasilar occlusive lesions. The lesions involved mostly the basilar artery, but the cervical and intracranial portions of the vertebral arteries were also often stenosed or occluded. The syndrome of intermittent TIAs involving the posterior circulation was dubbed "vertebrobasilar insufficiency" (VBI) by neurologists at the Mayo Clinic in Rochester, Minnesota: Clark Millikan, Robert Siekert, and Jack Whisnant [32]. The so-called VBI was not at all rare; in fact, Bradshaw and McQuaid conclude their article on VBI by stating that "the syndrome is one of the most common causes of neurological illness [33]."

Influenced greatly by the report of Kubik and Adams on necropsy-proven cases of basilar artery occlusion, clinicians during the middle of the twentieth century widely believed that severe occlusive disease of the intracranial posterior circulation arteries was a very serious, often mortal disease. During this era, the popular drug that was being used for occlusive vascular disease was warfarin. Anticoagulation had been used in patients with thrombophlebitis and pulmonary embolism, myocardial infarction, and rheumatic valve disease with systemic and brain embolism. Warfarin seemed to be worth trying for occlusive vascular disease. Using this reasoning, Millikan, Siekert, and Shick from the Mayo Clinic published an important and very influential paper on the use of warfarin anticoagulation to treat patients with VBI [34]. Patients with the clinical symptoms and signs of VBI (angiography was not often used) were given warfarin in an uncontrolled observational study. Many patients stopped having attacks, and many had no or minimal strokes. Believing that the disease was usually fatal or disabling without treatment, the authors reasoned and believed that warfarin was clearly effective and indicated to treat patients with symptoms suggesting VBI.

By the middle of the 1960s, there was widespread belief in the medical and neurological community that posterior circulation TIAs and ischemic strokes could be readily diagnosed clinically; transient attacks and insufficiency states were explained by hemodynamic factors; and anticoagulation with heparin-warfarin therapy was an effective treatment. Angiography was generally considered not to be indicated although a few anecdotal studies later showed the ability of angiography to clarify the nature of the underlying vascular causes and prognosis in isolated instances. Patients with posterior circulation ischemia were usually given heparin and warfarin unless contraindicated. Little investigations were performed. This situation remained until modern brain and vascular imaging, including MRI, MRA, and CTA, became widely available during the last years of the twentieth century.

Many years later, in the Warfarin–Aspirin for Symptomatic Intracranial Disease (WASID) trial of patients with severe intracranial atherosclerosis, there was no significant difference in the prevention of new strokes between aspirin and warfarin [35]. The study drugs were initiated often weeks after the last ischemic event. Warfarin was difficult to control; patients maintained within the target therapeutic INR range of warfarin performed better than patients treated with

1300 mg aspirin per day. In those treated with warfarin whose INR levels were below the target range, more infarcts developed, and more hemorrhages developed in those above the target INR range. There were too few patients with severe (>80%) intracranial vertebral (107 patients) or basilar artery stenosis (112 patients) to render meaningful conclusions about the treatment of these specific occlusive lesions.

Although the mechanism of TIAs involving the anterior and posterior circulations was uncertain, opinion during the middle years of the twentieth century favored hemodynamic, general circulatory mechanisms. In a series of influential papers, Derek Denny-Brown put forth the hypothesis that intermittent spells of ischemia were explained by circulatory perturbations, and he called the temporarily inadequate blood flow "insufficiency." Denny-Brown hypothesized that carotid and vertebrobasilar insufficiency was a "physiological, potential hemodynamic state in which reversible hemodynamic crises could be elicited by any factor that impaired the collateral circulation." [36] Hemodynamic crises could be transient, or partially or completely reversible depending on the length and severity of the pathophysiological cause. Denny-Brown reviewed the anatomical, physiological, and experimental data that favored his hypothesis. However, his own tilt table experiments, performed with Dr. John Sterling Meyer, one of his chief assistants at that time, using EEG monitoring of patients with clinical "insufficiency," more often than not failed to provoke attacks or EEG changes.

Clinicopathologic and Clinical-Imaging Studies During the Second Half of the Twentieth Century

The advent of modern brain and vascular imaging (MRI, MRA, and CTA) facilitated the study of various clinical posterior circulation syndromes. Clinicians and researchers in the USA, Europe, and Asia studied and reported various clinical syndromes related to involvement of specific locations within the posterior circulation-supplied brain regions and caused by various stroke subtypes. These studies included reports about lateral medullary infarcts [37, 38]; medial medullary infarcts [39, 40]; cerebellar infarcts [41–45]; top of the basilar syndrome [46]; basilar artery occlusion [47]; thalamic infarcts [48–52]; pure motor hemiparesis, ataxic hemiparesis, and dysarthria-clumsy hand syndrome explained by pontine lacunar infarcts [53–56]; lateral tegmental pontine syndrome [57, 58]; basilar branch occlusion [59]; intracranial atheromatous branch disease [60]; midbrain infarcts [61]; and posterior cerebral artery territory infarcts [62, 63]. The distribution of brain and vascular lesions and clinical symptoms and signs and stroke outcomes were also studied in detail [64–67]. Nonatherosclerotic vascular lesions were also described [67, 68].

By the end of the first quarter of the twenty-first century, clinicians had become aware of the major stroke syndromes involving the posterior circulation and the frequency of various vascular lesions and various stroke subtypes.

Pathophysiology of infarction was also investigated. Clinicians and researchers began to question the importance of hypoperfusion alone in explaining most brain infarcts. Transcranial Doppler emboli monitoring of patients with vascular lesions showed the frequency and importance of intra-arterial emboli. Diffusion-weighted MRI scans documented small "rosary"-shaped arcs of tissue injury in border-zone regions related to microembolism. Stenotic vascular lesions generated fibrin-platelet and cholesterol crystal emboli, which often broke loose and traveled intracranially. When the donor vascular lesions became flow-reducing, the decreased perfusion inspired washout and clearance of these emboli. Hypoperfusion and embolism interacted and complemented each other to promote and enhance brain infarction in both the anterior and the posterior circulations [69–71].

Treatment of Patients with Posterior Circulation Ischemia

After publication of the NIHSS study of intravenous tPA thrombolytic study in 1995 [72], much data began to accumulate about the results of intravenous and intra-arterial administration of tPA and later tenecteplase. Most randomized trials involved either patients whose vascular lesion was not studied or included only patients with anterior circulation infarction. Anecdotal results showed that treatment with thrombolytics in patients with brainstem ischemia could be effective over a longer time window than in anterior circulation disease. Most posterior circulation patients in whom the vascular lesion was studied had basilar artery occlusions, and results were, in general, poor [73].

Angioplasty and stenting began to be applied in patients with posterior circulation occlusive lesions to prevent further infarction. In one major trial that studied stenting versus aggressive closely monitored medical treatment, stenting of intracranial arteries was less effective than medical treatment [74, 75]. Stenting of the basilar artery was often complicated by perforator territory brainstem infarcts, and hemorrhage was an important complication [74, 75].

Trained and experienced interventionalists also began to explore nonchemical means of opening blocked arteries. The strategies included aspirating the clot by creating a vacuum effect using a simple syringe, using a power-driven apparatus to create more of a vacuum to suck back the clot, and using a corkscrew-like device to try to hook the clot and then extract it. After these initial explorations, device-makers designed "stent retrievers" that proved more effective than previous devices in opening arteries. Interventionalists could manipulate these devices to and then through the occluding clots and, in doing so, quickly restore flow. The clot could be trapped within the stent and then pulled back down the catheter into a receptacle outside of the body. Randomized trials that used stent retrievers proved their effectiveness, even up to a full 24 h after stroke symptom onset [76, 77]. The randomized trials of mechanical clot retrieval included only patients with anterior circulation vascular disease, but mechanical vascular opening was also frequently applied to individuals with basilar artery occlusion. The success rates of mechanical manipulation were much higher than with chemical thrombolysis [78].

Vertebrobasilar Territory Brain Hemorrhages

The first recognition and description of a posterior circulation hemorrhage was contained in an influential treatise on apoplexy published in 1812 by an Irish physician John Cheyne [79]. Cheyne included in his treatise detailed clinical descriptions of patients, as they would be encountered socially in their usual attire, and the appearance of their brains at necropsy. Cheyne described brain softening and intracerebral and subarachnoid hemorrhages. In some patients who survived their apoplectic attack for some time, Cheyne found cavities filled with rusty yellowish serum within the brain at necropsy. Cheyne surmised that the cavities were lined by a membrane, which was able to absorb red blood cells, and that the lesion represented an old hemorrhage. One patient described by Cheyne had a pontine hematoma. Case 14 was a "carpenter, 35 years of age, phlegmatic, pale, muscular, not habitually intemperate." He had severe headaches and, after one such headache, he vomited and soon after "became insensible." About an hour later, his breathing became irregular, and he was deeply comatose and soon dead. Cheyne described this man's brain as follows: "In dissecting the base of the brain, there was discovered, formed by rupture in the substance of the pons varolii, a collection of dark clotted blood, in an irregular cavity, having a ragged surface and communicating with the fourth ventricle which was full of blood [79]."

Although accounting for only 8–10% of intracerebral hemorrhages, pontine hematomas attracted attention because the clinical findings were dramatic and distinctive. After Cheyne's description of a pontine hematoma, single case reports and series of cases were reported during the nineteenth century. In 1903, Charles Dana, then Professor of Neurology at Cornell University in New York, reviewed prior reports and his own personal experience and summarized the clinical aspects of pontine hemorrhages and infarcts [80]. Dana reviewed the brain and vascular anatomy of the pons. Among 2288 hematomas found at necropsy, 205 (9%) were pontine [80]. Dana described the typical patient: "Some prodromal

headache and malaise for a few days … then he falls suddenly as if by a lightning stroke, into a coma, usually very profound. There are twitching of the face or of the limbs or both … the pupils are contracted to a pinpoint … there is convergent strabismus or conjugate deviation of the eyes. The limbs are at first stiff but tone may be reduced later and the reflexes increased. The patient can not be aroused but can be made to vomit … the patient dies in 6 to 20 hours usually with paralysis of respiration [80]." Dana listed the "syndrome of the pons" as (1) headache, malaise, vomiting; (2) sudden profound coma; (3) face and limb twitching; (4) small pupils, convergent strabismus, or conjugate eye deviation; (5) slow irregular respirations; (6) irregular pulse; (7) dysphagia; (8) paralysis of all limbs, or crossed paralysis; (9) gradual rise of temperature; and (10) death within 24 h.

Gowers, in his 1892 textbook of Neurology, described the location of pontine hematomas [81]. The bleeding usually involved the tegmento-basal junction near the rostral end of the pons. Hematomas often spread rostrally but rarely spread caudally to the medulla; often, the hematomas dissected into the fourth ventricle [81].

Oppenheim, in his popular Neurology textbook, first published in 1892, included a review of the clinical signs in patients with pontine hemorrhages [82]. Occasionally a hemiplegia or asymmetric bulbar paralysis was present, but more often, there was bilateral limb weakness and bilateral paralysis of the mouth, palate, pharynx, and larynx. The pupils were small but could be dilated. Eye movements were often lost. Coma, trismus, and high fever were common. Oppenheim emphasized that the disorder was invariably fatal [82].

Some pontine hematomas described in the nineteenth century were accompanied by supratentorial hemorrhages. Separation of primary pontine hematomas from secondary, pressure-related lesions did not occur until the twentieth century. Duret produced brainstem hemorrhages experimentally by injecting fluids into the supratentorial tissues of dogs [83, 84]. Duret noted that humans with fatal head trauma often had hematomas in the midbrain and pons

[83]. Attwater, in 1911, separated more definitively primary pontine hematomas from secondary brainstem hemorrhages [85]. Attwater reviewed 77 pontine hematomas examined at necropsy at Guys hospital in London. Some patients, especially those with head trauma, had supratentorial bleeding as well as brainstem hemorrhages. Attwater posited that some pontine hemorrhages were due to "an increase in intracranial tension produced by the rapid entry of blood into the cranial cavity [85]." Duret, in later research, showed that the secondary hemorrhages in the midbrain and pons, now referred to as Duret hemorrhages, were caused by sudden intracranial supratentorial pressure that distorted and compressed the brainstem and its vessels causing the latter to stretch and tear [86].

Although most authors continued to emphasize the abrupt onset of symptoms, Kornyey, in a remarkable single case report, described the gradual inexorable progression of symptoms and signs in a young man whose pontine hematoma occurred and developed under observation [87]. The patient was a 39-year-old man sent to the hospital in Hungary where Kornyey practiced for treatment of severe malignant hypertension. While his history was being taken, the patient reported numbness and tingling of the hands followed by restlessness, dysphagia, and loss of hearing. His blood pressure was found to be 245/170 mm Hg. While being observed, he developed bilateral sixth nerve palsies, dysarthria, deafness, and left hemiparesis. Then, small pupils, quadriplegia, and coma developed. Within 2 h after walking into the clinic, he had died of a pontine hematoma [87]. Not until 2 decades later did Miller Fisher emphasize the gradual evolution of signs and hematoma growth [88, 89].

In 1951, Steegman reported 17 patients with primary pontine hemorrhages and summarized the literature up to that time [90]. The hematomas in his 17 patients usually involved the center of the pons, and in 10, the blood ruptured into the 4th ventricle; 3 had asymmetrical lesions affecting the tegmentum and base more on one side. Most patients were quadriplegic, but 2 had hemiplegia, 1 with crossed face and limb weakness. Steegman opined that the shivering, shaking,

twisting, and trembling were due to abnormalities of motor function and were likely not convulsive as had been previously thought [90]. Steegman emphasized abnormal respirations, which were often slow, labored, and gasping. Death was seldom instantaneous but usually occurred in 24–72 h.

CT and later MRI allowed for detection of smaller pontine hemorrhages that were previously not identified. The classic large central pontine hematomas were the result of the rupture of the large paramedian pontine artery penetrators. The next syndrome that was recognized was lateral tegmental hematomas, which arose from rupture of arteries penetrating into the lateral tegmentum as branches of long circumferential arteries, especially the superior cerebellar arteries [91–93]. These lesions cause a contralateral hemisensory loss due to the involvement of the sensory lemniscus formed in the pons from the merging of the lateral spinothalamic tract and the medial lemniscus. Ataxia and oculomotor abnormalities often were also present, but paresis was usually absent or minimal. Later smaller lateral tegmental hematomas were described that caused only contralateral sensory abnormalities. Small basal hematomas arising from small paramedian arteries and short circumferential penetrators could cause pure motor hemiparesis, or ataxic hemiparesis causing similar signs as patients with lacunar infarcts.

Another common region of posterior circulation bleeding is in the cerebellum. The first cases of cerebellar hemorrhage were those of Morgagni and Lieutard, which were cited in a paper describing a fatal cerebellar hemorrhage written by Sedillot in 1813 [94]. Childs in 1858 reported the first American patient, a 19-year-old woman who developed a cerebellar hemorrhage while shaking her head vigorously to amuse a child [95]. Carion, in a doctoral thesis in 1875, reported 7 patients who had cerebellar hemorrhages [96]. Michael, in 1932, described 10 of his own patients and reviewed the literature up to that time [97]. He noted that headache, vertigo, and weakness developed very quickly and wrote that "in fulminating cases antemortem localization is practically impossible [97]." In 1942, Mitchell and Angrist reported 15 of their own patients with spontaneous cerebellar hemorrhage and also reviewed the 109 cases reported to that time [98]. "Coma as a prominent symptom far overshadowed all other findings" and was present in 64 of the 124 patients (52%). The next most common symptoms were vomiting and headaches. Dizziness was present in only 16 patients (13%) and ataxia in 11 (9%) [98]. They concluded, as had Michael, that there was no consistent pattern of symptoms and signs in patients with cerebellar hemorrhage.

In 1960, Wylie McKissock and his London colleagues reported 34 patients with cerebellar hemorrhage who had been under the care of one surgeon (Mr. McKissock) [99]. Hypertension was the commonest cause, but 6 patients in the series had angiomas and 2 had aneurysms. In 18, the hematomas were confined to the cerebellum while in 10 hematomas spread into the brainstem and in 6 they ruptured into the 4th ventricle. All patients had some form of surgery except for 6 who died before surgery was possible; in 14, only ventriculography or ventricular drainage was performed [99]. The outcome was very poor since 19 of the 28 surgically treated patients died. The authors were pessimistic about the clinical recognition of cerebellar hemorrhage. "The neurological signs presented by these patients were in the main singularly unhelpful. Localizing signs could not be elicited in those patients who were unconscious except that most of them had constricted and non-reactive pupils and periodic respirations. In the conscious patients, signs of cerebellar dysfunction were present in less than half [99]."

Miller Fisher and colleagues, in a very important benchmark paper published in 1965, emphasized clinical findings that they thought would improve clinical recognition of cerebellar hemorrhage [100]. They described only 3 patients in detail. In an addendum, added after the paper had been accepted, the authors mentioned that they had since seen 8 other patients in whom the rules derived from the original 3 patients and outlined in the paper had allowed the diagnosis of cerebellar hematomas, which were confirmed at surgery [100]. Fisher and colleagues emphasized the importance of several clinical findings: *vomiting* was a very constant feature; inability to stand or walk especially unaided was a reliable and very consistent sign; ipsilateral 6th nerve palsy and *conjugate gaze palsy* were very common; and hemiparesis or hemiplegia was not observed, but often there was bilateral increased deep tendon reflexes and Babinski signs [100]. Headache, neck stiffness, limb ataxia, dysarthria, and dizziness were variable findings. The authors urged surgical exploration when the clinical signs were typical. Later, several large clinical series of patients with cerebellar hemorrhages corroborated the frequency of the symptoms and signs reported by Fisher et al. [101, 102].

More recently, CT and MRI have allowed for the diagnosis of smaller cerebellar hematomas. Most involve the cerebellar hemispheres, especially the white matter in the region of the dentate nucleus in the territory of the superior cerebellar arteries. Some also arise more caudally from PICA territory branches. Occasionally, hemorrhages arise in the vermis and compress the 4th ventricle and the medullary and pontine tegmentum, but the clinical findings in these patients with vermian cerebellar hematomas have not been fully clarified.

Although bleeding into the thalamus is another common site of posterior circulation hemorrhage, separation of the clinical symptoms and signs from those found in patients with putaminal and basal ganglionic hemorrhages did not occur until Fisher's discussion during a 1959 meeting of the Houston Neurological Society [88]. Fisher commented during his presentation, "The clinical and laboratory features of hemorrhage at most sites within the brain have been described in the past, but bleeding into the thalamus and subthalamus is rarely alluded to, and a comprehensive report on the subject has never been made [88]." Fisher emphasized the presence of vertical gaze paralysis, position of the eyes downward at rest as if the patient is peering at the tip of the nose, constricted pupils, and sensory signs on the contralateral limbs greater than hemiparesis. The thalamic hemorrhages that Fisher was able to diagnose clinically were large, and all were accompanied by blood in the CSF.

Smaller hemorrhages in the thalamus were not recognized until the advent of CT and later MRI scanning. Chung and colleagues in 1996 reviewed the findings in patients with thalamic hemorrhages in various loci in the thalamus according to the distribution of the bleeding artery: tuberothalamic, thalamo-geniculate, thalamic-subthalamic, and posterior choroidal [103]. Similarly, midbrain and medullary hemorrhages were not separated from ischemic lesions in those sites until the advent of CT and later MRI.

References

1. Wepfer JJ. Observationes anatomicae ex cadaveribus eorum, quos sustulit apoplexia, cum exercitatione de ejus loco affecto. Schaffhausen: Joh Caspari Suteri; 1658.
2. Wolf JK. The classical brain stem syndromes. Springfield Ill: Charles C Thomas Publ; 1971.
3. Wallenberg A. Acute bulbaraffection (Embolie der art. cerebellar post. inf.sinistr.?). Arch Psychiatr Nervenkr. 1895;27:504–40.
4. Wallenberg A. Anatomischer befund in einem als "acute bulbar affection (embolie der art. cerebellar post. inf. sinistra?)" beschreibenen falle. Arch Psychiatr Nervenkr. 1901;34:923–59.
5. Wallenberg A. Verschluss der arteria cerebelli inferior posterior sinistra. Neurol Zentralblatt. 1915;34:236–47.
6. Wallenberg A. Verschluss der arteria cerebelli inferior posterior dextra (mit sektionbefund). Deutsche Zeitschrift f Nervenheilk. 1922;73:189–212.
7. Duret H. Sur la distribution des arteres nouricierres du bulb rachidien. Arch Physiol Norm Path. 1873;5:97–113.
8. Duret H. Reserches anatomiques sur la circulation de l'encephale. Arch Physiol Norm Pathol. 1874;3:60–91, 316-353,664-693, 919-957
9. Stopford JSB. The arteries of the pons and medulla oblongata. J Anat Physiol. 1916;50:131–63. 255–280
10. Caplan LR. Charles Foix, the first modern stroke neurologist. Stroke. 1990;21:348–56.
11. Foix C, Hillemand P. Irrigation de la protuberance. C R Soc Biol (Paris). 1925;92:35–6.
12. Foix C, Hillemand P. Les syndromes de la region thalamique. Presse Med. 1925;33:113–7.
13. Foix C, Hillemand P, Schalit I. Sur le syndrome lateral du bulbe et I'irrigation du bulbe superieur. Rev Neurol (Paris). 1925;41:160–79.
14. Foix C, Hillemand P. Les arteres de I'axe encephalique jusqu'au diencephale inclusivemenl. Rev Neurol (Paris). 1925;41:705–39.
15. Foix C, Masson A. Le syndrome de I' artere cerebrale posterieure. Presse Med. 1923;31:361–5.
16. Kubik C, Adams R. Occlusion of the basilar artery: a clinical and pathologic study. Brain. 1946;69:73–121.
17. Hayem MG. Sur la thrombose par arterite du tronc basilaire Comme cause du mort rapide. Archiv Physiol Norm Path. 1868;1:270–89.
18. Marburg O. Uber die neuren fortscritte in der topischen diagnostik des ponsund der oblongata. Deutsche Zeitschrift f Nervebheilk. 1911;41:41–91.
19. Leyden E. Ueber die thrombose der basilar arterie. Zeitschr Klein Med. 1882;5:165–85.
20. Lhermitte J, Trelles JO. L'arteriosclerose du tronc basilaire et ses consequences anatomo-clinques. Jahrbucher f Psychiatrie Neurologie. 1934;51:91–107.
21. Pines L, Gilinsky E. Uber die thrombose der arteria basilaires und uber die vascularisation der brucke. Archiv f Psychiatrie Nervenkrank. 1932;97:380–7.
22. Fisher CM. Occlusion of the internal carotid artery. Arch Neurol Psychiatr. 1951;65:346–77.
23. Fisher M. Occlusion of the carotid arteries. Arch Neurol Psychiatr. 1954;72:187–204.
24. Hutchinson EC, Yates PO. The cervical portion of the vertebral artery, a clinic=pathological study. Brain. 1956;79:319–31.
25. Yates PO, Hutchinson EC. Carotico-vertebral stenosis. Lancet. 1957;1:2–8.
26. Fisher CM. Occlusion of the vertebral arteries. Arch Neurol. 1970;22:13–9.
27. Reivich M, Holling E, Roberts B, Toole JF. Reversal of blood flow through the vertebral artery and its effect on cerebral circulation. N Engl J Med. 1961;265:878–85.
28. Caplan LR. Dissections of brain-supplying arteries. Nat Clin Pract Neurol. 2008;4(1):34–42.
29. Hennerici M, Klemm C, Rautenberg W. The subclavian steal phenomenon; a common vascular disorder with rare neurological deficits. Neurology. 1988;88:669–73.
30. Seldinger SI. Catheter replacement of the needle in percutaneous arteriography. Acta Radiol. 1953;39:368–76.
31. Hass WK, Fields WS, North R, et al. Joint study of extracranial arterial occlusion. II. Arteriography, techniques, sites, and complications. JAMA. 1968;203:961–8.
32. Millikan C, Siekert R. Studies in cerebrovascular disease. The syndrome of intermittent insufficiency of the basilar arterial system. Mayo Clin Proc. 1955;30:61–8.
33. Bradshaw P, McQuaid P. The syndrome of Veretebrobasilar insufficiency. Q J Med. 1963;32:279–96.
34. Millikan C, Siekert R, Shick R. Studies in cerebrovascular disease: the use of anticoagulant drugs in the treatment of insufficiency or thrombosis within the basilar arterial system. Mayo Clin Proc. 1955;30:116–26.
35. Chimowitz M, Lynn MJ, Howlett-Smith H, et al. For the warfarin-aspirin symptomatic intracranial disease trial investigators. Comparison of warfarin and

aspirin for symptomatic intracranial arterial stenosis. N Engl J Med. 2005;352:1305–16.

36. Denny-Brown D. Basilar artery syndromes. Bull N Engl Med Center. 1953;15:53–60.

37. Fisher CM, Karnes W, Kubik C. Lateral medullary infarction: the pattern of vascular occlusion. J Neuropathol Exp Neurol. 1961;20:323–79.

38. Kim J. Pure lateral medullary infarction: clinical-radiological correlation of 130 acute, consecutive patients. Brain. 2003;126:1864–72.

39. Kim JS, Kim HG, Chung CS. Medial medullary syndrome: report of 18 new patients and a review of the literature. Stroke. 1995;26:1548–52.

40. Kim JS, Han YS. Medial medullary infarction clinical, imaging, and outcome study in 86 consecutive patients. Stroke. 2009;40:3221–5.

41. Amarenco P, Caplan LR. Vertebrobasilar occlusive disease, review of selected aspects: 3. Mechanisms of cerebellar infarctions. Cerebrovasc Dis. 1993;3:66–73.

42. Caplan LR. Cerebellar infarcts: key features. Rev Neurol Dis. 2005;2:51–60.

43. Amarenco P, Rosengart A, DeWitt LD, Pessin MS, Caplan LR. Anterior inferior cerebellar artery territory infarcts: mechanisms and clinical features. Arch Neurol. 1993;50:154–61.

44. Chaves CJ, Caplan LR, Chung C-S, Tapia J, Amarenco P, Wityk R, Estol C, Tettenborn B, Rosengart A, Vemmos K, DeWitt LD, Pessin MS. Cerebellar infarcts in the New England Medical Center Posterior Circulation Registry. Neurology. 1994;44:1385–90.

45. Amarenco P, Kase CS, Rosengart A, Pessin MS, Bousser M-G, Caplan LR. Very small (border-zone) cerebellar infarcts. Brain. 1993;116:161–86.

46. Caplan LR. Top of the basilar syndrome: selected clinical aspects. Neurology. 1980;30:72–9.

47. Voetsch B, DeWitt LD, Pessin MS, Caplan LR. Basilar artery occlusive disease in the New England Medical Center Posterior Circulation Registry. Arch Neurol. 2004;61:496–504.

48. Caplan LR, DeWitt LD, Pessin MS, Gorelick PB, Adelman LS. Lateral thalamic infarcts. Arch Neurol. 1988;45:959–64.

49. Graff-Radford NR, Damasio H, Yamada T, et al. Non haemorrhagic thalamic infarction. Brain. 1985;108:495–516.

50. Bogousslavsky J, Regli F, Assal G. The syndrome of tuberothalamic artery territory infarction. Stroke. 1986;17:434–41.

51. Bogousslavsky J, Regli F, Uske A. Thalamic infarcts: clinical syndromes, etiology, and prognosis. Neurology. 1988;38:837–48.

52. Fisher CM. Pure sensory stroke and allied conditions. Stroke. 1982;13:434–47.

53. Fisher CM. Pure motor hemiplegia of vascular origin. Arch Neurol. 1965;13:30–44.

54. Fisher CM. Ataxic hemiparesis. Arch Neurol. 1978;35:126–8.

55. Kim JS, Lee JH, Im JH, Lee MC. Syndromes of pontine base infarction, a clinical-radiological correlation study. Stroke. 1995;26:950–5.

56. Fisher CM. A lacunar stroke. The dysarthria-clumsy hand syndrome. Neurology. 1967;17:614–7.

57. Caplan L, Goodwin J. Lateral brainstem tegmental hemorrhage. Neurology. 1982;32:252–60.

58. Helgason CM, Wilbur AC. Basilar branch pontine infarctions with prominent sensory signs. Stroke. 1991;22:1129–36.

59. Fisher CM, Caplan LR. Basilar artery branch occlusion: a cause of pontine infarction. Neurology. 1971;21:900–5.

60. Caplan LR. Intracranial branch atheromatous disease. Neurology. 1989;39:1246–50.

61. Martin PJ, Chang H-M, Wityk R, Caplan LR. Midbrain infarction: associations and etiologies in the New England Medical Center Posterior Circulation Registry. J Neurol Neurosurg Psychiatry. 1998;64:392–5.

62. Pessin MS, Lathi E, Cohen MB, Kwan ES, Hedges TR, Caplan LR. Clinical features and mechanisms of occipital infarction in the posterior cerebral artery territory. Ann Neurol. 1987;21:290–9.

63. Yamamoto Y, Georgiadis AL, Chang H-M, Caplan LR. Posterior cerebral artery territory infarcts in the New England Medical Center Posterior Circulation Registry. Arch Neurol. 1999;56:824–32.

64. Caplan LR, Chung C-S, Wityk RJ, et al. New England Medical Center posterior circulation stroke registry: I. Methods, data base, distribution of brain lesions, stroke mechanisms, and outcomes. J Clin Neurol. 2005;1:14–30.

65. Caplan LR, Wityk RJ, Pazdera L, et al. New England Medical Center posterior circulation stroke registry: II Vascular lesions. J Clin Neurol. 2005;1:31–49.

66. Glass TA, Hennessey PM, Pazdera L, Chang H-M, Wityk RJ, DeWitt LD, Pessin MD, Caplan LR. Outcome at 30 days in the New England Medical Center Posterior Circulation Registry. Arch Neurol. 2002;59(3):369–76.

67. Searls DE, Pazdera L, Korbel E, Vysata O, Caplan LR. Symptoms and signs of posterior circulation ischemia in the New England Medical Center Posterior Circulation Registry. Arch Neurol. 2012;69(3):346–51.

68. Lou M, Caplan LR. Vertebrobasilar dilatative arteriopathy (dolichoectasia). In: the year in neurology, 2. Ann N Y Acad Sci. 2010;1184:121–33.

69. Caplan LR, Hennerici M. Impaired clearance of emboli (washout) is an important link between hypoperfusion, embolism, and ischemic stroke. Arch Neurol. 1998;55:1475–82.

70. Sedlaczek O, Caplan L, Hennerici M. Impaired washout – embolism and ischemic stroke: further examples and proof of concept. Cerebrovasc Dis. 2005;19:396–401.

71. Amin-Hanjani S, Du X, Rose-Finnell L, et al. On behalf of the VERITAS group. Hemodynamic

features of Vertebrobasilar disease. Stroke. 2015;46:1850–6.

72. The National Institute of Neurological Disorders and Stroke rt-PA Study Group. Tissue plasminogen activator for acute ischemic stroke. N Engl J Med. 1995;333:1581–7.

73. Schonewille WJ, Wijman CA, Michel P, et al. Treatment and outcomes of acute basilar artery occlusion in the basilar artery international cooperation study (BASICS): a prospective registry study. Lancet Neurol. 2009;8:724–30.

74. Chimowitz MI, Lynn MJ, Derdeyn CP, Turan TN, Fiorella D, Lane BF, et al.; For the SAMMPRIS Trial Investigators. Stenting versus aggressive medical therapy for intracranial arterial stenosis. N Engl J Med. 2011;365:993–1003.

75. Derdeyn CP, Chimowitz MI, Lynn MJ, Fiorella D, Turan TN, Janis LS, et al. Aggressive medical treatment with or without stenting in high-risk patients with intracranial artery stenosis (SAMMPRIS): the final results of a randomised trial. Lancet. 2014;383:333–41.

76. Albers G, Marks MP, Kemp S, et al.; for the DEFUSE 3 Investigators. Thrombectomy for stroke at 6 to 16 hours with selection by perfusion imaging. N Engl J Med. 2018;378:708–18.

77. Nogueira RG, Jadhav AP, Haussen DC, et al.; for the DAWN Trial Investigators. Thrombectomy 6 to 24 hours after stroke with a mismatch between deficit and infarct. N Engl J Med. 2018;378:11–21.

78. Kumar G, Shahripour RB, Alexandrov AV. Recanalization of acute basilar artery occlusion improves outcomes: a meta-analysis. J Neurointerv Surg. 2015;7:868–74.

79. Cheyne J. Cases of apoplexy and lethargy with observations upon the comatose diseases. London: J Moyes printer; 1812.

80. Dana CL. Acute bulbar paralysis due to hemorrhage and softening of the pons and medulla with reports of cases and autopsies. Med Rec. 1903;64:361–74.

81. Gowers WR. A manual of diseases of the nervous system. London: J and A Churchill; 1893.

82. Oppenheim H. Lehrbuch der Nervenkrankheiten. 7th ed. Basel: Verlag S Karger; 1923. p. 1216–45.

83. Duret H. Etudes experimentales et cliniques sur les traumatismes cerebraux. Paris: V. Adrien Delahayes; 1878.

84. Thompson RK, Salcman M. Brain stem hemorrhages: historical perspective. Neurosurgery. 1988;22:623–8.

85. Attwater H. Pontine hemorrhage. Guys Hosp Rep. 1911;65:339–89.

86. Duret H. Traumatismes craniocerebraux. Paris: Librairee Felix Alcan; 1919.

87. Kornyey S. Rapidly fatal pontine hemorrhage: clinical and anatomical report. Arch Neurol Psychiatr. 1939;41:793–9.

88. Fisher CM. In: Fields WS, editor. Clinical syndromes in cerebral hemorrhage in pathogenesis and treatment of cerebrovascular disease. Springfield, IL: Charles Thomas Publ; 1961. p. 318–42.

89. Fisher CM. Pathological observations in hypertensive cerebral hemorrhage. J Neuropathol Exp Neurol. 1971;30:536–50.

90. Steegman AT. Primary pontine hemorrhage. J Nerv Ment Dis. 1951;114:35–65.

91. Caplan LR, Goodwin J. Lateral tegmental brainstem hemorrhage. Neurology. 1982;32:252–60.

92. Tyler HR, Johnson P. Case records of the Massachusetts General Hospital. N Engl J Med. 1982;287:506–12.

93. Kase CS, Maulsby G, Mohr JP. Partial pontine hematomas. Neurology. 1981;30:652–5.

94. Sedillot J. Epanchement de sang dans le lobe droit du cervelet suivi de la mort. J Gen de Med Chir et Pharm. 1813;47:375–9.

95. Childs T. A case of apoplexy of the cerebellum. Am Med Month. 1858;9:1–3.

96. Carion F. Contribution a l'etude symptomatique st diagnostique de l'hemorrhagie cerebelleuse. Paris: Adrien Delhaye; 1875.

97. Michael JC. Cerebellar apoplexy. Am J Med Sci. 1932;183:687–95.

98. Mitchell N, Angrist A. Spontaneous cerebellar hemorrhage: report of fifteen cases. Am J Path. 1942;18:935–53.

99. McKissock W, Richardson A, Walsh L. Spontaneous cerebellar hemorrhage. Brain. 1960;83:1–9.

100. Fisher CM, Picard EH, Polak A, Dalal P, Ojemann R. Acute hypertensive cerebellar hemorrhage: diagnosis and surgical treatment. J Nerv Ment Dis. 1965;140:38–57.

101. Ott K, Kase C, Ojemann R, et al. Cerebellar hemorrhage: diagnosis and treatment. Arch Neurol. 1974;31:160–7.

102. Brennan R, Berglund R. Acute cerebellar hemorrhage. Analysis of clinical findings and outcome in 12 cases. Neurology. 1977;27:527–32.

103. Chung C-S, Caplan LR, Han W, Pessin MS, Lee K-H, Kim S-M. Thalamic haemorrhage. Brain. 1996;119:1873–86.

Arterial Anatomy and Collaterals

2

Kunakorn Atchaneeyasakul
and David S. Liebeskind

Embryology

The embryologic origin of the cerebral vasculatures is from mesenchymal elements, forming channels to cover the surface of the neural tube [1]. Around Day 24 of embryonic life, the internal carotid arteries appear from the joining of the third brachial arch arteries and distal segments of the paired dorsal aortae [2]. Around Day 28 of embryonic life, the hindbrain is supplied by the paired longitudinal neural arteries, which obtained their blood supply from carotid-vertebrobasilar anastomoses. The key anastomoses are formed by the trigeminal artery, otic artery, hypoglossal artery, and proatlantal artery, respectively, cranially to caudally. Around Day 29 of embryonic life, the paired longitudinal neural arteries fuse in the midline forming the basilar artery. The posterior communicating arteries then develop to connect the distal basilar artery with the distal internal carotid arteries while the trigeminal, otic, hypoglossal, and proatlantal arteries regress [3]. The vertebral arteries are formed by the fusion of cervical level longitudinal anastomotic arteries, from the proatlantal to C6 level arteries [3]. Around Days 30–35 of embryonic life onwards, the basilar artery and vertebral arteries assume similar distributions and connections as in the adult.

Anatomy

The posterior cerebral circulation provides blood supply to the posterior parts of the brain, which include the posterior portion of the cerebral cortex, cerebellum, and brainstem. The anatomy of the posterior circulation and the anastomosis with the circle of Willis greatly varies in each person. The major arteries of the posterior circulation include vertebral arteries, basilar artery, and posterior cerebral arteries.

Vertebral Artery

There are typically two vertebral arteries in each individual. The vertebral arteries are divided into four segments. The first segment is from the origin of the first branch of the subclavian artery until the entry to the transverse foramina of the cervical vertebra. The second segment is from the entry at transverse foramina at C5 or C6 to exiting at C2. The third segment is from the C2 transverse foramina exit point, sweeping laterally to pass into the C1 transverse foramina, eventually piercing the dura. The fourth segment is from the entry into the foramen magnum joining with the contralateral vertebral artery to form the basilar artery.

K. Atchaneeyasakul
University of California, Los Angeles, CA, USA

D. S. Liebeskind (✉)
Department of Neurology, Neurovascular Imaging Research Core, UCLA Comprehensive Stroke Center, University of California, Los Angeles, CA, USA

© Springer Nature Singapore Pte Ltd. 2021
J. S. Kim (ed.), *Posterior Circulation Stroke*, https://doi.org/10.1007/978-981-15-6739-1_2

Vertebral arteries vary in diameter from 1.5 to 5.0 mm, and hypoplasia is generally defined as a vessel with a diameter of less than 2 mm [4]. On the basis of multiple reports, vertebral artery hypoplasia has been reported with a frequency of 1.9% to as high as 35.2% [5, 6]. Atherosclerotic vertebral artery segment and hypoplasia need to be differentiated with caution. The left vertebral artery is more often the predominant side. Other variations include different vertebral artery origins (aortic arch, innominate artery).

Branches

Anterior Spinal Artery

The single anterior spinal artery arises from the fourth segment of the vertebral artery (intracranial portion) at the level of the medulla. A series showed 65.3% of anterior spinal artery arise from bilateral vertebral arteries [7]. The anterior spinal artery supplies the anterior surface of the medulla and the anterior surface of the spinal cord and descends within the anterior median fissure. Variations include duplication of the anterior spinal artery.

Posterior Inferior Cerebellar Artery

Posterior inferior cerebellar artery (PICA) is the largest branch of the vertebral artery, originating from the intracranial portion of the vertebral artery 10–20 mm before the vertebrobasilar junction, but the origins are highly variable and may arise from the basilar artery, extracranial portion of the vertebral artery, or ascending pharyngeal artery, or alternatively, be completely absent [8]. In the 20–24 mm embryologic stage, the PICA is clearly evident as an artery extending posteriorly from the hindbrain. Other variations include the termination of the vertebral artery at the PICA origin, in which the contralateral vertebral artery is generally larger. Duplication of the PICA and PICA–anterior inferior cerebellar artery (AICA) connections may be seen [9]. The size of the PICA also varies and is often inversely related to the size of the AICA, likely due to the fact that both arteries provide arterial supply to the inferior cerebellum [8, 10]. The PICA separates into two major trunks, the anterior and lateral trunks.

The PICA can also be segmented into an anterior medullary segment, lateral medullary segment, tonsillomedullary segment, telovelotonsillar segment, and cortical segments. The anterior and lateral medullary segments lie in front of the medulla and lateral to the medullar, respectively. The tonsillomedullary segment lies next to the lower half of the cerebellar tonsil. The telovelotonsillar segment lies between the inferior medullary velum and the superior pole of the cerebellar tonsil. The cortical segments lie over the inferior cerebellar surface. The brain territory that PICA supplies also varies based on the size of the AICA and PICA. Generally, the supplied territories include lower medulla, posteroinferior cerebellar hempishere, and inferior vermis.

Basilar Artery

The basilar artery extends cranially in the basilar groove of the pons from the joining of the two vertebral arteries at the pontomedullary junction. The basilar artery was formed from the fusion of the paired hindbrain vessels during the embryologic period; the irregularity in this formation can lead to variations of the basilar artery. The basilar artery ends at the upper border of the pons to form the two posterior cerebral arteries. The diameter of the basilar artery is usually 3–4 mm and can taper slightly in the distal portion [11]. The length of the basilar artery is 25–35 mm [12]. Multiple basilar artery variations have been documented, including persistent carotid-basilar anastomosis (persistent trigeminal artery, see Fig. 14.11 in Chap. 14), fenestrated basilar artery (Fig. 2.1), and hypoplastic basilar artery that can end in SCA [13].

Branches

Penetrator Branches

The anatomy of the basilar artery perforators is usually less than 1 mm in diameter and can be separated into three groups: rostral, middle, and caudal [14]. The rostral perforators mostly originate from the distal portion of the basilar artery as well as the SCA. The middle perforators

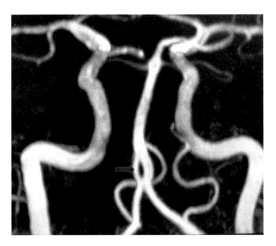

Fig. 2.1 MR angiography showing fenestrated basilar artery variant (red arrow)

originate from the middle portion of the basilar artery and can give rise to anterolateral, pontomedullary, and long pontine arteries. The caudal perforators originate from the proximal portion of the basilar artery.

Superior Cerebellar Artery

The superior cerebellar artery (SCA) originates from the rostral BA prior to the formation of the two posterior cerebral arteries. Each SCA separates into medial and lateral trunks to supply the medial and lateral parts of the cerebellar cortex, respectively [15]. The branches originating from the SCA include perforating branches, precerebellar branches supplying the connecting part of the cerebellum and the brainstem, and the cortical branches supplying the rostral half of the cerebellar hemisphere [15]. Variations documented include duplication of the SCA (most common), SCA originating from the PCA, and SCA originating from the ICA [16].

Anterior Inferior Cerebellar Artery

The anterior inferior cerebellar artery (AICA) mostly originates from the proximal third of the basilar artery and less commonly the middle third [17]. The vertebrobasilar junction is the origin in 9% of the cases. The average of the surgical anatomic diameter of the AICA is 1 mm [18, 19]. The territory that AICA supplies varies but usually includes lateral pons, anterior inferior por-

tion of the cerebellum, and the middle cerebellar peduncle. Each AICA separates into superior and inferior trunks at the pontomedullary junction. The AICA can be divided into four segments from the origin, including the anterior pontine segment ending at the axis that crosses inferior olive, lateral pontine segment ending at the floccule, flocculonodular segment ending at the middle cerebellar peduncle, and the cortical segment running to the petrosal surface of the cerebellum [17, 20]. The labyrinthine artery supplying the cochlear and labyrinth usually arises from the lateral pontine segment of the AICA. Other variations include AICA originating from the vertebral artery or the PICA. Less commonly seen is the duplication of AICA.

Posterior Cerebral Artery

The PCAs arise from the termination of the basilar artery in 70% of patients [21]. The PCA arises from the posterior communicating artery in 20% of the patients [21] (Fig. 2.2). The anatomy of the PCA can be divided into four segments, from P1 to P4 [22]. The P1 segment is from the PCA origin at the termination of the basilar artery to the connection with the posterior communicating artery. The average diameter of the P1 segment is

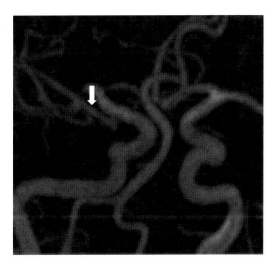

Fig. 2.2 MR angiography showing a fetal variant of posterior cerebral artery originating from the internal carotid artery (white arrow)

2.6 mm. The P2 segment is from the posterior communicating artery to the posterior margin of the midbrain. The average diameter of the P2 segment is 2.9 mm. The P3 segment, within the quadrigeminal cistern, is from the posterior midbrain to the anterior limit of the calcarine fissure. The P4 segment is the superficial cortical segments distal to the P3 segment.

Branches

The origin of each PCA branch and the supplying area varies greatly. Thalamoperforating branches arise from the P1 and the posterior communicating artery and supply the medial surface of the thalamus. Thalamogeniculate arteries most commonly arise from the P2 segment and supply the ventrolateral portion of the thalamus. The medial posterior choroidal artery most commonly arises from the P2 segment and supplies the posterior thalamus, geniculate bodies, pulvinar, pineal, midbrain, and the choroid plexus of the third ventricle. The lateral posterior choroidal artery most commonly arises from either the P2 segment or the cortical PCA branches and supplies the choroid plexus of the lateral ventricle. The tuberothalamic artery (polar artery) arises from the posterior communicating artery or is absent in up to 40% of population and supplies the reticular nucleus, ventral anterior nucleus, anterior nuclei, and part of the ventral lateral nucleus and dorsomedial nucleus of the thalamus [23]. The cerebral branches include inferior temporal arteries (hippocampal, anterior temporal, middle temporal, posterior temporal, common temporal), parieto-occipital arteries, calcarine arteries, and splenial arteries.

Collateral Circulation

The circle of Willis provides primary collateral pathways to the anterior and posterior circulation. The anatomy of the posterior circulation and the anastomosis with the circle of Willis greatly varies by each individual. The posterior communicating arteries may supply blood flow anteriorly to the anterior circulation vessels or posteriorly to the posterior circulation vessels [24]. Absence or

hypoplasia of the posterior communicating artery occurs in up to 30% [25, 26]. The size of the posterior communicating arteries also varies greatly from less than 1 mm to greater than 2 mm. The anterior choroidal artery, which arises from the posterior aspect of the internal carotid artery, anastomoses with the lateral branches of the posterior choroidal artery and posterior cerebral artery [27, 28]. Leptomeningeal collaterals are connections of small distal cerebral arteries, including the ACA/MCA/PCA, which may be present and highly variable individually as secondary collateral support [29]. The common anastomoses include the MCA to PCA via the anterior temporal artery and posterior temporal artery, and ACA to PCA via the pericallosal artery [24]. The collateral capacity may be enhanced in the setting of flow limitation in either of the major cerebral arteries [30]. Distal branches of the SCA, AICA, and PICA anastomose to form collateral supply between the basilar artery and the vertebral artery, limiting the infarct size after a basilar artery or vertebral artery occlusion [24, 31] (Fig. 2.3). Studies have developed posterior circulation collateral score involving the presence of posterior communicating arteries, SCA, AICA, and PICA

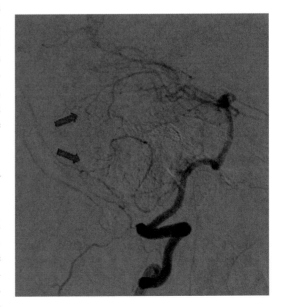

Fig. 2.3 Digital subtraction angiography showing anastomoses between the superior, anterior inferior, and posterior inferior cerebellar arteries (red arrows)

that predicts poorer outcome after basilar artery occlusion [32, 33]. The tectal plexus may be seen connecting the supratentorial and infratentorial blood supply via the PCA and SCA connection [34]. Less commonly seen (<1%) are persistent primitive connections from the ICA, including the trigeminal, otic, hypoglossal, and proatlantal arteries, providing collateral supply from the anterior circulation [35–37].

References

1. Raybaud C. Normal and abnormal embryology and development of the intracranial vascular system. Neurosurg Clin N Am. 2010;21(3):399–426.
2. Menshawi K, Mohr JP, Gutierrez J. A functional perspective on the embryology and anatomy of the cerebral blood supply. J Stroke. 2015;17(2):144–58.
3. Luh GY, Dean BL, Tomsick TA, Wallace RC. The persistent fetal carotid-vertebrobasilar anastomoses. AJR Am J Roentgenol. 1999;172(5):1427–32.
4. Szarazova AS, Bartels E, Bartels S, Turcani P. Possible morphological pathomechanisms of ischemic stroke in the posterior circulation of patients with vertebral artery hypoplasia. J Neuroimaging. 2015;25(3):408–14.
5. Delcker A, Diener HC. Various ultrasound methods for studying the vertebral artery—a comparative evaluation. Ultraschall Med. 1992;13(5):213–20.
6. Park JH, Kim JM, Roh JK. Hypoplastic vertebral artery: frequency and associations with ischaemic stroke territory. J Neurol Neurosurg Psychiatry. 2007;78(9):954–8.
7. Ballesteros L, Forero P, Quintero I. Morphological expression of the anterior spinal artery and the intracranial segment of the vertebral artery: a direct anatomic study. Rom J Morphol Embryol. 2013;54(3):513–8.
8. Lister JR, Rhoton AL Jr, Matsushima T, Peace DA. Microsurgical anatomy of the posterior inferior cerebellar artery. Neurosurgery. 1982;10(2):170–99.
9. Lesley WS, Dalsania HJ. Double origin of the posterior inferior cerebellar artery. AJNR Am J Neuroradiol. 2004;25(3):425–7.
10. Baskaya MK, Coscarella E, Jea A, Morcos JJ. Aneurysm of the anterior inferior cerebellar artery-posterior inferior cerebellar artery variant: case report with anatomical description in the cadaver. Neurosurgery. 2006;58(2):E388; discussion E.
11. Caplan LR. Primer on cerebrovascular diseases. London: Elsevier, Academic Press; 2017. Available from: http://VB3LK7EB4T.search.serialssolutions.com/?V=1.0&L=VB3LK7EB4T&S=JCs&C=TC000 1818395&T=marc.
12. Brassier G, Morandi X, Riffaud L, Mercier P. Basilar artery anatomy. J Neurosurg. 2000;93(2):368–9.
13. Adigun OO, Sevensma K. Anatomy, head and neck, basilar artery. Treasure Island, FL: StatPearls; 2019.
14. Marinkovic SV, Gibo H. The surgical anatomy of the perforating branches of the basilar artery. Neurosurgery. 1993;33(1):80–7.
15. Hardy DG, Peace DA, Rhoton AL Jr. Microsurgical anatomy of the superior cerebellar artery. Neurosurgery. 1980;6(1):10–28.
16. Uchino A, Sawada A, Takase Y, Kudo S. Variations of the superior cerebellar artery: MR angiographic demonstration. Radiat Med. 2003;21(6):235–8.
17. Fogwe DT, Mesfin FB. Neuroanatomy, anterior inferior cerebellar arteries. Treasure Island, FL: StatPearls; 2019.
18. Shrontz C, Dujovny M, Ausman JI, Diaz FG, Pearce JE, Berman SK, et al. Surgical anatomy of the arteries of the posterior fossa. J Neurosurg. 1986;65(4):540–4.
19. Pai BS, Varma RG, Kulkarni RN, Nirmala S, Manjunath LC, Rakshith S. Microsurgical anatomy of the posterior circulation. Neurol India. 2007;55(1):31–41.
20. Naidich TP, Kricheff II, George AE, Lin JP. The normal anterior inferior cerebellar artery. Anatomic-radiographic correlation with emphasis on the lateral projection. Radiology 1976;119(2):355–373.
21. Cereda C, Carrera E. Posterior cerebral artery territory infarctions. Front Neurol Neurosci. 2012;30:128–31.
22. Zeal AA, Rhoton AL Jr. Microsurgical anatomy of the posterior cerebral artery. J Neurosurg. 1978;48(4):534–59.
23. Bogousslavsky J, Regli F, Assal G. The syndrome of unilateral tuberothalamic artery territory infarction. Stroke. 1986;17(3):434–41.
24. Liebeskind DS. Collateral circulation. Stroke. 2003;34(9):2279–84.
25. Lippert H, Pabst R. Arterial variations in man : classification and frequency. München: J.F. Bergmann; 1985, 121 pp
26. Alpers BJ, Berry RG, Paddison RM. Anatomical studies of the circle of Willis in normal brain. AMA Arch Neurol Psychiatry. 1959;81(4):409–18.
27. Takahashi S, Suga T, Kawata Y, Sakamoto K. Anterior choroidal artery: angiographic analysis of variations and anomalies. AJNR Am J Neuroradiol. 1990;11(4):719–29.
28. Morandi X, Brassier G, Darnault P, Mercier P, Scarabin JM, Duval JM. Microsurgical anatomy of the anterior choroidal artery. Surg Radiol Anat. 1996;18(4):275–80.
29. Brozici M, van der Zwan A, Hillen B. Anatomy and functionality of leptomeningeal anastomoses: a review. Stroke. 2003;34(11):2750–62.
30. Tariq N, Khatri R. Leptomeningeal collaterals in acute ischemic stroke. J Vasc Interv Neurol. 2008;1(4):91–5.
31. Rhoton AL Jr. The cerebellar arteries. Neurosurgery. 2000;47(3 Suppl):S29–68.
32. van der Hoeven EJ, McVerry F, Vos JA, Algra A, Puetz V, Kappelle LJ, et al. Collateral flow predicts outcome after basilar artery occlusion: the posterior circulation collateral score. Int J Stroke. 2016;11(7):768–75.

33. Goyal N, Tsivgoulis G, Nickele C, Doss VT, Hoit D, Alexandrov AV, et al. Posterior circulation CT angiography collaterals predict outcome of endovascular acute ischemic stroke therapy for basilar artery occlusion. J Neurointerv Surg. 2016;8(8):783–6.

34. Romero JR, Pikula A, Nguyen TN, Nien YL, Norbash A, Babikian VL. Cerebral collateral circulation in carotid artery disease. Curr Cardiol Rev. 2009;5(4):279–88.

35. Suttner N, Mura J, Tedeschi H, Ferreira MA, Wen HT, de Oliveira E, et al. Persistent trigeminal artery: a unique anatomic specimen—analysis and therapeutic implications. Neurosurgery. 2000;47(2):428–33; discussion 33-4

36. Pinkerton JA Jr, Davidson KC, Hibbard BZ. Primitive hypoglossal artery and carotid endarterectomy. Stroke. 1980;11(6):658–60.

37. Obayashi T, Furuse M. The proatlantal intersegmental artery: a case report and review of the literature. Arch Neurol. 1980;37(6):387–9.

Epidemiology, Risk Factors, and Stroke Mechanisms

Philip B. Gorelick and Jong S. Kim

Prevalence of Posterior Circulation Stroke

Based on previous registry data using admitted stroke patients, posterior circulation stroke (PCS) was reported to account for 20–30% of stroke [1, 2]. However, the prevalence may vary depending on (1) the frequency of using MRI in the initial diagnosis of stroke and (2) the policy or criteria of each center for patient admission. For example, centers where MRI is frequently used for symptoms such as dizziness, small PCS will be more often detected. Some tertiary centers of South Korea have reported that PCS accounted for about 40% of admitted patients with ischemic stroke [3, 4].

In the studies that compared between ACS and PCS, [5–10] PCS accounts for 16–51%. (Table 3.1). Thus, almost all the studies showed that PCS is less common than ACS, although its portion varies. As discussed later, atrial fibrillation is a more important cause of ACS than PCS. This may explain why PCS is relatively more prevalent in Asian countries [6, 8], where atrial fibrillation is less common than in Caucasians [5, 9]. Patients with PCS were generally younger and more often males than those with ACS, although one study from China did not show such a trend [8]. This demographic difference seems to be in line with the more widespread presence of atrial fibrillation in ACS than in PCS patients.

In a multicenter registry study from South Korea, authors enrolled patients with ischemic stroke or transient ischemic attack (TIA) associated with cerebral atherosclerosis. They found that the proportion of PCS was 26%. In this study, the locations of symptomatic cerebral atherosclerosis were middle cerebral artery (MCA) (34%), internal carotid artery (29%: proximal 23%, distal 6%), vertebral artery (10%: proximal 4%, distal 6%), basilar artery (8%), posterior cerebral artery (6%), and anterior cerebral artery (5%) [11]. Between ACS and PCS, there were no differences in age and sex, probably because strokes associated with atrial fibrillation were excluded.

P. B. Gorelick
Davee Department of Neurology, Northwestern University Feinberg School of Medicine, Chicago, IL, USA

Population Health Research Institute, Faculty of McMaster University Health Sciences and Hamilton University Health Science, Hamilton, ON, Canada

Department of Translational Science and Molecular Medicine, Michigan State University College of Human Medicine, Grand Rapids, MI, USA

Department of Neurology and Rehabilitation, University of Illinois College of Medicine at Chicago, Chicago, IL, USA

Thorek Memorial Hospital, Chicago, IL, USA
e-mail: pgorelic@thorek.org

J. S. Kim (✉)
Department of Neurology, Asan Medical Center, University of Ulsan, Seoul, South Korea
e-mail: jongskim@amc.seoul.kr

© Springer Nature Singapore Pte Ltd. 2021
J. S. Kim (ed.), *Posterior Circulation Stroke*, https://doi.org/10.1007/978-981-15-6739-1_3

Table 3.1 Studies that compared characteristics between PCS and ACS

Author	Subramanian	Miyamoto	Zeng	Li	Sommer	Zurcher	Toyoda	Kim	Kim#
Published (year)	2009	2010	2015	2017	2018	2019	(unpublished)	(unpublished)	2012
Region	Canada	Japan	China	China	Austria	Switzerland	Japan	South Korea	South Korea
Study design	Multicenter	Retrograde	Retrograde	Retrospective	Nationwide	Single center	NCVC Stroke Registry	AMC registry	Multicenter
	Registry	Single center	Single center	Single center	Stroke unit registry	Registry		Stroke unit registry	Registry
Number (ACS/PCS) (%, PCS)	5844/2645 (26)	1089/430 (39)	1763/482 (21)	364/187 (51)	23,447/4604 (16)	983/466 (32)	2301/662 (22)	2773/833 (23)	736/264 (26)
Mean age (ACS/PCS, year)	74/70*	69/66*	63/62	61/66	49/40	70/67*	42/32*	67/65*	67/67
Sex (ACS/PCS, % female)	51/44*	36/27*	41/33*	39/34	49/40	46/39	75/73*	39/33*	35/36
Risk factors (%, ACS/PCS)									
Hypertension	69/67	50/57*	48/48	67/69*	81/78	66/64	76/82*	65/66	69/82*
Diabetes	24/27*	25/33*	14/21*	20/20	25/25	15/12	32/31*	29/37*	32/45*
Dyslipidemia	34/36	21/20	7/6	6/4	54/57	61/67*	50/53	29/35*	48/49
Smoking	37/39	18/33	33/38*	37/31	ND	23/20	18/18	32/39*	36/29*
Atrial fibrillation	20/16*	27/17*	8/3*	ND	29/22	31/16*	38/26*	15/16	
Past history of stroke	35/32	7/8	ND	22/9*	23/21	26/28	31/34	ND	26/22
Stroke subtype (%, ACS/PCS)	ND	*	*	ND			*	*	
LAD		20/34*	27/29		13/12	15/10	14/15	33/28*	
SVD		36/32	37/38		23/21	5/21	16/21	23/34*	
CE		31/20*	13/5*		29/24	41/25	38/23	27/20*	
NIHSS (at admission, ACS/PCS)	ND	ND	6.4/5.2*	4.3/3.2*	5/3	10.6/5.9*	5/3*	6.0/3.7*	

PCA posterior circulation stroke, *ACS* anterior circulation stroke, *LAD* large artery disease, *SVD* small artery disease, *CE* cardiac embolism, *ND* not described

#This study enrolled patients with atherosclerotic strokes only

*Data with statistical difference

Table 3.2 Ten factors accounting for approximately 90% of stroke attribution

Hypertension
Current smoking
Waist-to-hip ratio
Diet risk score
Exercise
Diabetes mellitus
Alcohol (consumption >30/month or binges)
Psychosocial stress and depression
Cardiac causes
Ratio of apolipoprotein B to A1

Table 3.3 Stroke risks by category according to the American Heart Association/American Stroke Association

Generally nonmodifiable risks
Age
Low birth weight
Race (e.g., blacks and some Hispanic/Latino Americans)
Genetic factors
Well-documented and modifiable risks
Physical inactivity
Dyslipidemia
Diet and nutrition
High blood pressure
Obesity and body fat distribution
Diabetes mellitus
Cigarette smoking
Atrial fibrillation
Other cardiac conditions
Asymptomatic carotid artery stenosis
Sickle cell disease
Less well-documented or potentially modifiable risks
Migraine
Metabolic syndrome
Alcohol consumption
Drug abuse
Sleep-disordered breathing
Hyperhomocysteinemia
Elevated lipoprotein (a)
Hypercoagulability
Inflammation and infection

Risk Factors

General Risk Factors

Stroke is not an accident as the traditional term "cerebrovascular accident (CVA)" would imply. Instead, there are well-documented modifiable risk factors for stroke and other risks that are part of the causal web leading to stroke. Based on a large-scale international case–control study, it has been estimated that 90% of ischemic stroke may be attributed to ten factors: hypertension, current smoking, waist-to-hip ratio, diet risk score, exercise, diabetes mellitus, alcohol consumption >30/month or alcohol binges, psychosocial stress and depression, cardiac causes, and the ratio of apolipoprotein B to A1 [12]. Table 3.2 lists the aforementioned factors. General stroke risk factors may be categorized according to the following scheme: generally nonmodifiable risks, well-documented and modifiable risks, and less well-documented or potentially modifiable risks [13]. Table 3.3 lists stroke risks in general by category according to the American Heart Association/American Stroke Association (AHA/ASA) [13].

Differences in the Risk Factors Between Posterior Circulation and Anterior Circulation Stroke

There have been studies that compared risk factors between ACS and PCS (Table 3.1). Overall, atrial fibrillation is more often associated with ACS than with PCS. Atherosclerotic risk factors such as diabetes and hypertension appear to be more prevalent in PCS than in ACS. This difference may be attributed to the fact that cardiac embolism is less frequent in PCS. However, in the study that enrolled only the patients with symptomatic cerebral atherosclerosis, atherosclerotic risk factors such as diabetes mellitus and hypertension were still more closely associated with PCS than with ACS [11]. This result suggests that the impact of each atherosclerotic risk factor may be different between anterior and posterior circulation. An alternative explanation would be that nonatherosclerotic diseases (e.g., moyamoya disease) may have been misdiagnosed as anterior circulation (e.g., MCA) atherosclerosis in certain cases, especially in Asia [14].

Finally, the genetic variant, ring finger protein 213 (RNF213) c.14576G>A (rs112735431), which was originally identified as a susceptibility genetic variant for moyamoya disease, is shown to be present in patients with intracranial cerebral atherosclerosis. In a study from Japan, RNF213 heterozygotes were present in 10 of 43 patients in patients with the anterior intracranial atherosclerosis, but none in the patients with PCS [15]. In another study from South Korea, RNF 213 heterozygotes were found in 13 of the 240 large artery disease (LAA) patients (5.4%), but none of the patients with PCS had this polymorphism [16]. Thus, this genetic variant may be one of the determinants for the location of cerebral atherosclerosis.

Stroke Mechanisms

As in ACS, PCS is caused by large artery disease, small artery disease, cardiogenic embolism, and other mechanisms.

Large Artery Disease

The main pathology of large artery disease consists of thrombosis superimposed on atherosclerosis. The pathologic features of PCS are not fundamentally different from those of ACS [17, 18]. In the posterior circulation, atherosclerosis is prone to occur in the proximal extracranial vertebral artery (VA), distal intracranial VA, lower-middle portion of the basilar artery (BA), and proximal posterior cerebral artery (PCA) [11, 19] (Fig. 3.1, left image). In the stenotic atherosclerotic vessel, thrombus may be superimposed. Thrombus formed within the intracranial VA often extends into the proximal BA [20]. Within the BA, atherosclerotic stenosis is common in the proximal 2 cm, more often seen on the ventral than in the dorsal side [17, 20]. Thrombi within the BA tend to have limited propagation [21], occasionally extending only to the orifice of the next long circumferential cerebellar artery such as anterior inferior cerebellar artery (AICA) or superior cerebellar artery (SCA).

Mechanisms of Stroke in Large Artery Disease

Detailed stroke mechanisms of large artery disease include artery-to-artery embolism, in situ thrombotic occlusion, branch occlusion, hypoperfusion, and their combinations.

Artery-to-Artery Embolism

A thrombus may occur in stenosed atherosclerotic vessels, especially when atherosclerotic plaques are eroded or ulcerated [22, 23]. The thrombus arising from the proximal vessels (e.g., extracranial VA) can be detached and can travel all the way to the distal arteries such as the PCA, SCA, PICA, and distal BA (embolization) [24] (Fig. 3.1, right image). This phenomenon has been described as "artery-to-artery embolism." Stenoses in the intracranial arteries such as intracranial VA, BA, or proximal PCA also produce embolism, although they may also produce infarction through other mechanisms such as branch occlusion [25, 26]. Embolism seems to occur more frequently in the setting of posterior fossa hypoperfusion associated with significant bilateral VA occlusive disease, due in part to ineffective washout of emboli in hypoperfused areas [27] (Fig. 3.2). Although uncommon, arterial embolisms may develop from more proximal arteries, such as the subclavian artery, the ascending aorta, and aortic arch [28].

In Situ Thrombotic Occlusion

In patients with intracranial artery atherosclerosis, thrombus formation in areas of plaque can result in total arterial occlusion, leading to an infarction in the relevant territory. In the posterior circulation, in situ thrombotic occlusion is often observed in the territories of PCA, and BA branches such as AICA or PICA [11, 29]. In situ thrombotic occlusion produces relatively large territorial infarction. However, unlike cardiogenic embolism, it less often produces massive "malignant" infarction because of relatively well-developed collateral circulation in the setting of

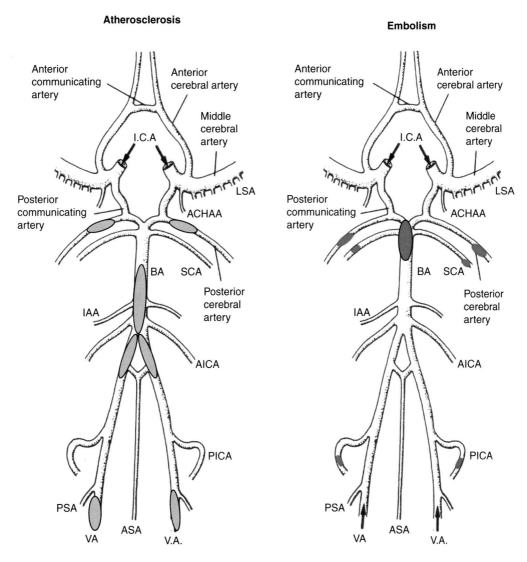

Fig. 3.1 Left image: Frequent location of atherosclerosis in the posterior circulation. Right image: Frequent site of embolic occlusion

the chronic atherosclerotic process [30]. With persistent occlusion, however, the initial infarct frequently grows, leading to progressive neurological worsening. Thus, the ultimate infarct volume varies according to the size of the occluded vessel, the speed of arterial occlusion, and the status of the collateral circulation. Patients with this mechanism more often experience transient ischemic attacks (TIAs) preceding main infarction (Fig. 3.3) than in those with cardiogenic embolism.

Branch Occlusion

Atherosclerotic plaques in an intracranial artery can occlude the orifice of one or several perforators, causing infarcts limited to the perforator territory [31] (Fig. 3.4A). Pathological features of this "atheromatous branch occlusion" were described [32, 33]. It seems that branch occlusion is more often observed in PCS than ACS; one study showed that this was the mechanism of stroke in 16% of symptomatic MCA atherosclerosis, whereas it occurred in 64% of the BA

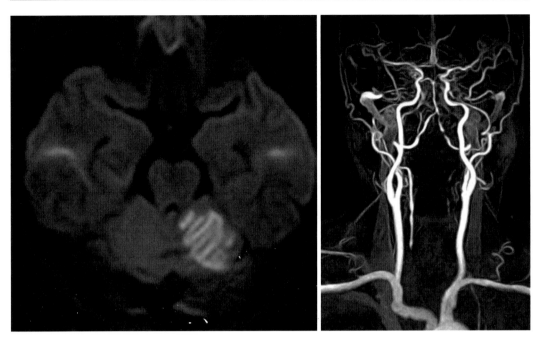

Fig. 3.2 A 64-year-old hypertensive man suddenly developed dysarthria and gait difficulty. Neurological examination showed dysarthria and limb ataxia on the left side. Diffusion-weighted MRI showed an infarction in the left superior cerebellar artery territory (left image). MRA showed bilateral proximal atherosclerotic occlusion of the vertebral arteries (right image). The probable stroke mechanism was artery-to-artery embolism

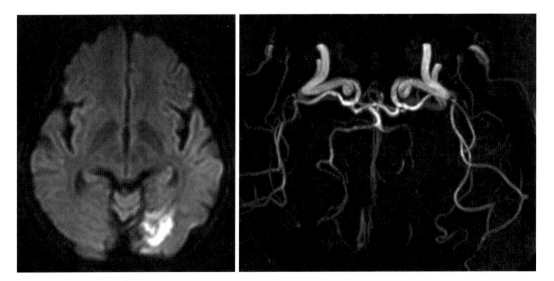

Fig. 3.3 A 72-year-old hypertensive and diabetic woman developed visual dimness on the right side, which was preceded by recurrent episodes of right limb tingling sensation that lasted approximately 10 min. Neurological examination showed normal findings except for right upper quadrantanopia. Diffusion-weighted MRI showed an infarction in the left occipital lobe (left image). MRA showed left posterior cerebral artery (PCA) occlusion (right image), which was not recanalized on follow-up MRA 5 days later. Cardiac examination and Holter monitoring findings were normal. The presumed stroke mechanism was in situ atherothrombotic occlusion of the left PCA

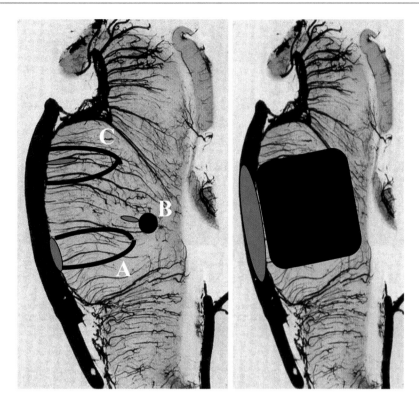

Fig. 3.4 Schematic drawing of the mechanism of brainstem infarction. Left image; A. atherothrombosis occurring in the basilar artery obliterates the orifice of the perforator. B. lipohyalinotic distal small artery occlusion. C. Atherosclerotic occlusion of the proximal portion of the perforator. A and C are referred to as "branch atheromatous disease." They produce infarcts abutting on the basal surface, whereas B (lypohyalinotic disease) produces an island-like deep infarction. Right image; Extensive atherosclerotic occlusion (or plaque rupture) producing multiple, bilateral branch occlusions leading to a large brainstem infarction. An embolic occlusion can also produce this syndrome. Single (or a few) branch occlusion (A, C in the left image). Extensive branch occlusion (right image)

atherosclerosis [11]. Thus, branch occlusion is the major mechanism of the isolated brainstem (e.g., pontine and medullary) (Fig. 3.5, upper panel) infarctions [25, 26, 34–36].

Brainstem infarcts associated with branch occlusion tend to extend to the basal surface (Figs. 3.4A and 3.5), whereas those caused by small artery lipohyalinotic disease (see below) produce a deep, island-like infarction within the parenchyma (Fig. 3.4B). The former is more often associated with atherosclerotic characteristics, [37] larger lesion volume, and an unstable and unfavorable clinical course than the latter [26, 38, 39] (Fig. 3.6).

Occasionally, the proximal small vessel disease also harbors characteristics of atherosclerosis, and the resultant brainstem infarction looks similar to that of branch occlusion due to BA atherosclerosis (Fig. 3.4C). Thus, this condition has been included in the category of atherosclerotic branch occlusion [31], although this is classified as small vessel disease in our clinical practice given that there is no large, atherosclerotic parenteral artery disease. Nevertheless, atheromatous branch occlusion cannot be ruled out in patients with normal-looking parenteral arteries on an angiogram. Nowadays, high-resolution vessel wall MRI (HR-MRI) can identify the small plaque that occludes the perforator, even in patients with apparently normal MRA findings [40, 41] (Fig. 3.5, lower panel; see also Chap. 9).

Compared with atherosclerotic lesions producing embolism or in situ thrombotic occlusion, branch occlusion is associated with less severe arterial stenosis [42]. However, the stenosis degree may be severe in occasional cases.

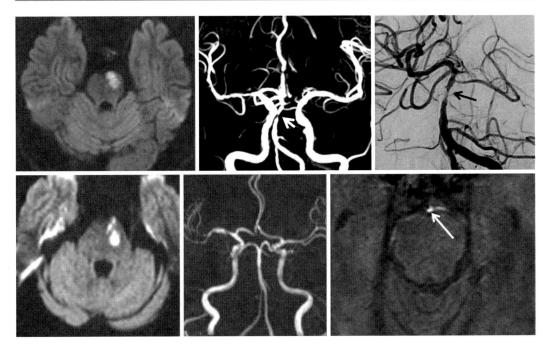

Fig. 3.5 Examples of atheromatous branch occlusion producing unilateral pontine infarction. Upper panel; Diffusion-weighted MRI shows a left pontine infarction (left image) caused by branch occlusion associated with basilar artery stenosis identified by MRA (middle image, arrow) and conventional angiogram (right image, arrow). Lower panel; Diffusion-weighted MRI shows a left pon- tine infarction (left image). Although MRA did not show significant basilar artery disease (middle image), high-resolution vessel wall MRI shows thickened, enhanced vessel wall in the dorsal portion of the basilar artery (arrow) that probably obliterated a perforator (right image)

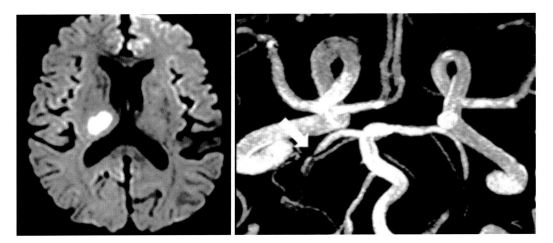

Fig. 3.6 A hypertensive 64-year-old man developed sud- den numb sensation in the left limb. The next day, he addi- tionally experienced left limb weakness and ataxia. Diffusion-weighted MRI showed an infarction in the right thalamus (left image). MRA showed focal stenosis in the P2 portion of the right posterior cerebral artery (right image) that probably occluded the orifice of the thalamic perforators

Sudden, extensive BA thrombotic occlusion due to either atherosclerotic rupture or embolization from proximal sources may produce extensive brainstem infarction by way of multiple, bilateral branch occlusions (Fig. 3.4, right image).

Hypoperfusion

In patients with severe vascular stenosis/occlusion and insufficient collaterals, hemodynamic TIAs can occur. Typically, symptoms such as dizziness, diplopia, and visual disturbances occur briefly and stereotypically in patients who are dehydrated or fatigued. When stroke develops, the symptoms may fluctuate widely according to the degree of hydration, blood pressure, and the position of the patient's head. Improving perfusion with hydration or induced hypertension may be of help in such patients [43, 44]. Although the efficacy has not yet been proven, [45] revascularization therapies, such as angioplasty/stenting or bypass surgeries (see Chap. 13), may relieve these symptoms.

Unlike ACS, MRI lesion patterns of hemodynamic infarction are not clearly established in the PCS, due in part to considerable normal variations and collateral patterns that influence perfusion. Small infarcts occurring in the cerebellar border zone (areas bordering PICA, AICA, and SCA) may be attributed to hypoperfusion associated with cardiac arrest or severe VA or BA occlusive disease (see Chap. 6). However, infarcts of the similar pattern are also produced by embolism to small arteries within the border zone areas [46]. Thus, the MRI imaging alone is not a reliable sign predicting hypoperfusion.

The stroke mechanism is often difficult to assess partly because severe vertebrobasilar atherosclerosis can induce both hemodynamic and embolic strokes and partly because the territory of each cerebellar artery often overlaps. PCS solely attributable to hemodynamic failure seems to be distinctly uncommon. More often, hypoperfusion plays an additive role in the development or progression of stroke, together with other major stroke mechanisms, e.g., small embolic infarcts in the border zone areas, progressive enlargement of infarction in patients with in situ thrombotic occlusion (see above).

Location of Large Artery Disease

Extracranial Vertebral Artery

The most frequent location of extracranial VA atherosclerotic disease is at the origin from the subclavian arteries. Atheroma may originate in the subclavian artery and spread to the proximal VA. Despite the high incidence of extracranial VA atherosclerosis, serious PCSs are relatively uncommon in this condition [47]. When stroke develops, it is almost always related to embolism from thrombi formed in the proximal VA [9, 31, 48–50]. Compared to unilateral VA lesions, bilateral steno-occlusive lesions (or unilateral disease with contralateral hypoplasia) generate embolism more often, probably related to hypoperfusion in the posterior fossa, which may promote thrombus generation and inefficient washout of emboli (Fig. 3.2). Hypoperfusion, in turn, is related to the effective development of collateral circulation, especially when the VA occlusion occurs gradually. Important sources of collaterals include occipital branches of the external carotid artery, the ascending cervical and transverse cervical branches of the thyrocervical trunk, and retrograde flow from the contralateral VA or from the posterior communicating system.

Intracranial Vertebral Artery

Generally, intracranial VA occlusive disease is more often symptomatic than extracranial VA disease. Unilateral intracranial VA disease may produce medullary (either lateral or medial) infarction through occlusion of the medullary perforators (branch occlusion, Fig. 4.4 in Chap. 4) or PICA. Cerebellar infarction with or without medullary involvement may also occur through the occlusion of the ostium of the PICA. Thrombi within the stenosed intracranial VA may also generate emboli that occlude distal vessels (artery-to-artery embolism). Bilateral intracranial VA occlusion is less well tolerated and often leads to TIAs or cerebellar and brainstem infarction [51–53] (Fig. 11.2 in Chap. 11), although some patients who have adequate collateral circulation may survive without the development of major infarction [53].

Basilar Artery

Pathologically [54] and angiographically [55] documented BA occlusion often leads to catastrophic bilateral pontine infarction (Fig. 3.4, right image), but some patients have only limited or transient deficits [48–50, 56]. The variable outcome depends on the extensiveness of the thrombus and the status of collateral circulation (e.g., backward flow from the well-developed posterior communicating artery or SCA). The collateral status may, in turn, be influenced by the extent of the atherothrombotic diseases in individuals. For example, collateral circulation through the PICA would be poor when the intracranial VA is also obstructed. When thrombus propagates to the distal BA, collateral circulation from the SCAs and the posterior communicating arteries becomes limited. The speed of BA occlusion also matters; BA embolism and dissection tend to result in sudden coma and quadriparesis, while progression of brainstem ischemia related to atherothrombosis is slow and progressive and earns time for collateral development. Early plaques associated with mild stenosis generally produce unilateral pontine infarcts through the mechanism of branch occlusion (Fig. 3.5).

Small Artery (Penetrating Artery) Disease

A single subcortical or brainstem infarct usually results from disease of penetrating arteries [57] (Fig. 3.4B). Its pathological hallmarks include irregular cavities, less than 15–20 mm in size, located in subcortical, brainstem, and cerebellar areas. Penetrating arteries associated with these lesions have disorganized vessel walls, fibrinoid material deposition, and hemorrhagic extravasation through arterial walls, first called "segmental arterial disorganization" and then lipohyalinosis by Fisher [33, 57–63]. These vascular changes develop in arteries or arterioles 40–400 μm in diameter and frequently affect the perforating arteries from the PCA or BA. Penetrating artery disease is the main mechanism of brainstem infarction, although brainstem infarctions may also be caused by atheromatous branch occlusion [31], as discussed before.

Cardiac Embolism

Given the fact that blood flow to the posterior circulation is only 1/5–1/4 of the anterior circulation, we can understand that a thrombus arising in the heart more often travels to the anterior circulation than to the posterior circulation system. Nevertheless, previous studies showed that about 1/5–1/4 of PCS result from cardiogenic embolism (Table 3.1). These emboli commonly occlude the PCA, rostral BA, SCA, and PICA (Fig. 3.1, right image). Infarcts are typically larger than those associated with large artery atherosclerotic disease, partly because the clots are larger and partly because of the insufficiently developed collateral circulation [64]. The onset is usually abrupt. Additional infarcts may be seen in the anterior circulation as well. The occluded artery is often spontaneously recanalized, and hemorrhagic transformation of an infarct is common, which may cause worsening headache or neurological deterioration.

It has been recognized that patent foramen ovale (PFO) with a large amount of shunt is an etiology of embolic infarcts (paradoxical embolism), especially in young patients without vascular risk factors [65, 66]. The posterior circulation seems to be a predilection site for embolism in patients with PFOs as compared to the anterior circulation [67, 68]. A recent study showed that embolic infarctions associated with PFO more often occurred in the posterior circulation than those associated with atrial fibrillation (44.4% versus 22.9%) [68]. Relatively poor adrenergic innervation in the vertebrobasilar circulation and inefficient response to sympathetic stimuli at the time of Valsalva maneuvers may explain the increased chance of blood clot to travel to the vertebrobasilar system. Given the evidence that PFO closure is effective in the prevention of PFO-related stroke in patients with a large amount of shunt, [69] PFO has been increasingly recognized as a treatable cause of stroke, especially in young patients. Identification of PFO through extensive cardiac workup (e.g., transesophageal echocardiogram) is important given the fact that lifelong administration of antithrombotics may be not needed if closure procedure is successfully performed (Fig. 3.7).

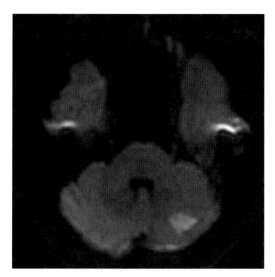

Fig. 3.7 A 36-year-old woman without any vascular risk factors suddenly developed dizziness and gait ataxia. Diffusion-weighted MRI showed a left cerebellar infarction. MRA showed normal findings. Holter examination was normal. Transesophageal echocardiography showed patent foramen ovale (PFO) with a large amount of right-to-left shunt. The probable stroke mechanism was paradoxical embolism due to PFO. PFO closure was performed by a cardiologist

Embolic infarction associated with cardiac catheterization also occurs preferentially in the posterior circulation [70, 71].

Differences in Stroke Mechanisms Between ACS and PCS

Stroke mechanisms differ from ACS and PCS; in most of the registry studies, CE is more common in ACS than in PCS (Table 3.1). LAD and SVD are relatively more prevalent in PCS.

In addition, detailed mechanisms appear to be different even in patients with "atherosclerotic" stroke. When the stroke mechanisms were compared between ACS and PCS patients who had atherosclerosis, the prevalence of artery-to-artery embolism, in situ thrombotic occlusion, local branch occlusion, and hemodynamic mechanism were 53 vs. 34, 21 vs. 14, 12 vs. 40 and 5 vs.0 [11]. Thus, branch occlusion is more important, and artery-to-artery embolism is less important mechanism in PCS than in ACS patients. This is in part due to the location of the

symptomatic atherosclerosis. Atherosclerosis of the proximal internal carotid artery accounted for 34% of ACS atherosclerosis, whereas proximal VA atherosclerosis accounted for only 14% of PCS atherosclerosis. In other words, compared with atherosclerosis in ACS, atherosclerosis in PCS patients is more often located in the intracranial artery. Nevertheless, even in patients with intracranial atherosclerosis, stroke mechanisms may still differ between ACS and PCS. For example, while MCA atherosclerosis often produces artery-to-artery embolism, BA atherosclerosis is more often associated with branch occlusion [11]. Although the reason remains unclear, shorter perforating arteries arising from the BA or VA may be more vulnerable for occlusion in the presence of parental artery disease compared with the relatively longer lenticulostriate arteries arising from the MCA.

Less Common Causes

Less common causes include arterial dissections, fibromuscular dysplasia, moyamoya disease, vasospasm, and infectious or immunologic vasculitis. Details are discussed in Chap. 14.

When large arteries are involved, the stroke mechanisms in patients with uncommon diseases are identical with what was discussed so far, i.e., artery-to-artery embolism, branch occlusion, hemodynamic insufficiency, and their combination. However, the importance of each mechanism differs among various diseases.

References

1. Bogousslavsky J, Van Melle G, Regli F. The Lausanne Stroke Registry: analysis of 1,000 consecutive patients with first stroke. Stroke. 1988;19(9):1083–92.
2. Moulin T, Tatu L, Crepin-Leblond T, Chavot D, Berges S, Rumbach T. The Besancon Stroke Registry: an acute stroke registry of 2,500 consecutive patients. Eur Neurol. 1997;38(1):10–20.
3. Lee BI, Nam HS, Heo JH, Kim DI. Yonsei Stroke Registry. Analysis of 1,000 patients with acute cerebral infarctions. Cerebrovasc Dis. 2001;12(3):145–51.
4. Lee JH, Han SJ, Yun YH, Choi HC, Jung S, Cho SJ, et al. Posterior circulation ischemic stroke in Korean population. Eur J Neurol. 2006;13(7):742–8.

5. Subramanian G, Silva J, Silver FL, Fang J, Kapral MK, Oczkowski W, et al. Risk factors for posterior compared to anterior ischemic stroke: an observational study of the Registry of the Canadian Stroke Network. Neuroepidemiology. 2009;33(1):12–6.

6. Miyamoto N, Tanaka Y, Ueno Y, Tanaka R, Hattori N, Urabe T. Comparison of clinical backgrounds with anterior versus posterior circulation infarcts. J Stroke Cerebrovasc Dis. 2010;19(5):393–7.

7. Zeng Q, Tao W, Lei C, Dong W, Liu M. Etiology and risk factors of posterior circulation infarction compared with anterior circulation infarction. J Stroke Cerebrovasc Dis. 2015;24(7):1614–20.

8. Li Y, Cai Y, Zhao M, Sun J. Risk factors between intracranial-extracranial atherosclerosis and anterior-posterior circulation stroke in ischaemic stroke. Neurol Res. 2017;39(1):30–5.

9. Sommer P, Posekany A, Serles W, Marko M, Scharer S, Fertl E, et al. Is functional outcome different in posterior and anterior circulation stroke? Stroke. 2018;49(11):2728–32.

10. Zurcher E, Richoz B, Faouzi M, Michel P. Differences in ischemic anterior and posterior circulation strokes: a clinico-radiological and outcome analysis. J Stroke Cerebrovasc Dis. 2019;28(3):710–8.

11. Kim JS, Nah HW, Park SM, Kim SK, Cho KH, Lee J, et al. Risk factors and stroke mechanisms in atherosclerotic stroke: intracranial compared with extracranial and anterior compared with posterior circulation disease. Stroke. 2012;43(12):3313–8.

12. O'Donnell MJ, Xavier D, Liu L, Zhang H, Chin SL, Rao-Melacini P, et al. Risk factors for ischaemic and intracerebral haemorrhagic stroke in 22 countries (the INTERSTROKE study): a case-control study. Lancet. 2010;376(9735):112–23.

13. Meschia JF, Bushnell C, Boden-Albala B, Braun LT, Bravata DM, Chaturvedi S, et al. Guidelines for the primary prevention of stroke: a statement for healthcare professionals from the American Heart Association/American Stroke Association. Stroke. 2014;45(12):3754–832.

14. Kim JS, Bonovich D. Research on intracranial atherosclerosis from the East and west: why are the results different? J Stroke. 2014;16(3):105–13.

15. Shinya Y, Miyawaki S, Imai H, Hongo H, Ono H, Takenobu A, et al. Genetic analysis of ring finger protein 213 (RNF213) c.14576G>A in intracranial atherosclerosis of the anterior and posterior circulations. J Stroke Cerebrovasc Dis. 2017;26(11):2638–44.

16. Kim YJ, Kim BJ, Lee MH, Lee H-B, Lee JS, Chang D-i, et al. Are Genetic Variants Associated with the Location of Cerebral Arterial Lesions in Stroke Patients?. Cerebrovascular Diseases. 2020;49(3):262–68.

17. Cornhill JF, Akins D, Hutson M, Chandler AB. Localization of atherosclerotic lesions in the human basilar artery. Atherosclerosis. 1980;35(1):77–86.

18. Schwartz CJ, Mitchell JR. Atheroma of the carotid and vertebral arterial systems. Br Med J. 1961;2(5259):1057–63.

19. Ueda K, Toole JF, McHenry LC Jr. Carotid and vertebrobasilar transient ischemic attacks: clinical and angiographic correlation. Neurology. 1979;29(8):1094–101.

20. Castaigne P, Lhermitte F, Gautier JC, Escourolle R, Derouesne C, Der Agopian P, et al. Arterial occlusions in the vertebro-basilar system. A study of 44 patients with post-mortem data. Brain. 1973;96(1):133–54.

21. Castaigne P, Lhermitte F, Buge A, Escourolle R, Hauw JJ, Lyon-Caen O. Paramedian thalamic and midbrain infarct: clinical and neuropathological study. Ann Neurol. 1981;10(2):127–48.

22. Fisher M, Paganini-Hill A, Martin A, Cosgrove M, Toole JF, Barnett HJ, et al. Carotid plaque pathology: thrombosis, ulceration, and stroke pathogenesis. Stroke. 2005;36(2):253–7.

23. Fuster V, Badimon L, Badimon JJ, Chesebro JH. The pathogenesis of coronary artery disease and the acute coronary syndromes (2). N Engl J Med. 1992;326(5):310–8.

24. Caplan LR, Amarenco P, Rosengart A, Lafranchise EF, Teal PA, Belkin M, et al. Embolism from vertebral artery origin occlusive disease. Neurology. 1992;42(8):1505–12.

25. Kim JS. Pure lateral medullary infarction: clinical-radiological correlation of 130 acute, consecutive patients. Brain. 2003;126(Pt 8):1864–72.

26. Kim JS, Cho KH, Kang DW, Kwon SU, Suh DC. Basilar artery atherosclerotic disease is related to subacute lesion volume increase in pontine base infarction. Acta Neurol Scand. 2009;120(2):88–93.

27. Caplan LR, Hennerici M. Impaired clearance of emboli (washout) is an important link between hypoperfusion, embolism, and ischemic stroke. Arch Neurol. 1998;55(11):1475–82.

28. Amarenco P, Cohen A, Tzourio C, Bertrand B, Hommel M, Besson G, et al. Atherosclerotic disease of the aortic arch and the risk of ischemic stroke. N Engl J Med. 1994;331(22):1474–9.

29. Lee E, Kang DW, Kwon SU, Kim JS. Posterior cerebral artery infarction: diffusion-weighted MRI analysis of 205 patients. Cerebrovasc Dis. 2009;28(3):298–305.

30. Wong KSCL, Kim JS. Stroke mechanisms. In: Kim JS, Caplan LR, Wong KS, editors. Intracranial atherosclerosis. Chichester, West Sussex: Blackwell; 2008. p. 57–68.

31. Caplan LR. Intracranial branch atheromatous disease: a neglected, understudied, and underused concept. Neurology. 1989;39(9):1246–50.

32. Lhermitte F, Gautier JC, Derouesne C. Nature of occlusions of the middle cerebral artery. Neurology. 1970;20(1):82–8.

33. Fisher CM, Caplan LR. Basilar artery branch occlusion: a cause of pontine infarction. Neurology. 1971;21(9):900–5.

34. Kim JS, Kim J. Pure midbrain infarction: clinical, radiologic, and pathophysiologic findings. Neurology. 2005;64(7):1227–32.

35. Park JY, Chun MH, Kang SH, Lee JA, Kim BR, Shin MJ. Functional outcome in poststroke patients with or without fatigue. Am J Phys Med Rehabil. 2009;88(7):554–8.

36. Kim JS, Yoon Y. Single subcortical infarction associated with parental arterial disease: important yet neglected sub-type of atherothrombotic stroke. Int J Stroke. 2013;8(3):197–203.

37. Nah HW, Kang DW, Kwon SU, Kim JS. Diversity of single small subcortical infarctions according to infarct location and parent artery disease: analysis of indicators for small vessel disease and atherosclerosis. Stroke. 2010;41(12):2822–7.

38. Bang OY, Joo SY, Lee PH, Joo US, Lee JH, Joo IS, et al. The course of patients with lacunar infarcts and a parent arterial lesion: similarities to large artery vs small artery disease. Arch Neurol. 2004;61(4):514–9.

39. Kwon JY, Kwon SU, Kang DW, Suh DC, Kim JS. Isolated lateral thalamic infarction: the role of posterior cerebral artery disease. Eur J Neurol. 2012;19(2):265–70.

40. Klein IF, Lavallee PC, Schouman-Claeys E, Amarenco P. High-resolution MRI identifies basilar artery plaques in paramedian pontine infarct. Neurology. 2005;64(3):551–2.

41. Swartz RH, Bhuta SS, Farb RI, Agid R, Willinsky RA, Terbrugge KG, et al. Intracranial arterial wall imaging using high-resolution 3-tesla contrast-enhanced MRI. Neurology. 2009;72(7):627–34.

42. Lee DK, Kim JS, Kwon SU, Yoo SH, Kang DW. Lesion patterns and stroke mechanism in atherosclerotic middle cerebral artery disease: early diffusion-weighted imaging study. Stroke. 2005;36(12):2583–8.

43. Lee MH, Kim JG, Jeon SB, Kang DW, Kwon SU, Kim JS. Pharmacologically induced hypertension therapy for acute stroke patients. J Stroke. 2019;21(2):228–30.

44. Bang OY, Chung JW, Kim SK, Kim SJ, Lee MJ, Hwang J, et al. Therapeutic-induced hypertension in patients with noncardioembolic acute stroke. Neurology. 2019;93(21):e1955–e63.

45. Markus HS, Harshfield EL, Compter A, Kuker W, Kappelle LJ, Clifton A, et al. Stenting for symptomatic vertebral artery stenosis: a preplanned pooled individual patient data analysis. Lancet Neurol. 2019;18(7):666–73.

46. Amarenco P, Kase CS, Rosengart A, Pessin MS, Bousser MG, Caplan LR. Very small (border zone) cerebellar infarcts. Distribution, causes, mechanisms and clinical features. Brain. 1993;116(Pt 1):161–86.

47. Fisher CM. Occlusion of the vertebral arteries. Causing transient basilar symptoms. Arch Neurol. 1970;22(1):13–9.

48. Fields WS, Ratinov G, Weibel J, Campos RJ. Survival following basilar artery occlusion. Arch Neurol. 1966;15(5):463–71.

49. Moscow NP, Newton TH. Angiographic implications in diagnosis and prognosis of basilar artery occlusion. Am J Roentgenol Radium Therapy, Nucl Med. 1973;119(3):597–604.

50. Pochaczevsky R, Uygar Z, Berman AJ. Basilar artery occlusion. J Can Assoc Radiol. 1971;22(4):261–3.

51. Caplan LR. Bilateral distal vertebral artery occlusion. Neurology. 1983;33(5):552–8.

52. Shin HK, Yoo KM, Chang HM, Caplan LR. Bilateral intracranial vertebral artery disease in the New England Medical Center, Posterior Circulation Registry. Arch Neurol. 1999;56(11):1353–8.

53. Bogousslavsky J, Gates PC, Fox AJ, Barnett HJ. Bilateral occlusion of vertebral artery: clinical patterns and long-term prognosis. Neurology. 1986;36(10):1309–15.

54. Kubik CS, Adams RD. Occlusion of the basilar artery; a clinical and pathological study. Brain. 1946;69(2):73–121.

55. Archer CR, Horenstein S. Basilar artery occlusion: clinical and radiological correlation. Stroke. 1977;8(3):383–90.

56. Caplan LR. Occlusion of the vertebral or basilar artery. Follow up analysis of some patients with benign outcome. Stroke. 1979;10(3):277–82.

57. Fisher CM. Lacunes: small, deep cerebral infarcts. Neurology. 1965;15:774–84.

58. Fisher CM. A lacunar stroke. The dysarthria-clumsy hand syndrome. Neurology. 1967;17(6):614–7.

59. Fisher CM. Lacunar strokes and infarcts: a review. Neurology. 1982;32(8):871–6.

60. Fisher CM. Ataxic hemiparesis. A pathologic study. Arch Neurol. 1978;35(3):126–8.

61. Fisher CM, Curry HB. Pure motor hemiplegia. Trans Am Neurol Assoc. 1964;89:94–7.

62. Fisher CM, Cole M. Homolateral ataxia and crural paresis: a vascular syndrome. J Neurol Neurosurg Psychiatry. 1965;28:48–55.

63. Fisher CM. Pure sensory stroke involving face, arm, and leg. Neurology. 1965;15:76–80.

64. Kim HJ, Yun SC, Cho KH, Cho AH, Kwon SU, Kim JS, et al. Differential patterns of evolution in acute middle cerebral artery infarction with perfusion-diffusion mismatch: atherosclerotic vs. cardioembolic occlusion. J Neurol Sci. 2008;273(1–2):93–8.

65. Mas JL, Arquizan C, Lamy C, Zuber M, Cabanes L, Derumeaux G, et al. Recurrent cerebrovascular events associated with patent foramen ovale, atrial septal aneurysm, or both. N Engl J Med. 2001;345(24):1740–6.

66. Lamy C, Giannesini C, Zuber M, Arquizan C, Meder JF, Trystram D, et al. Clinical and imaging findings in cryptogenic stroke patients with and without patent foramen ovale: the PFO-ASA Study. Atrial Septal Aneurysm. Stroke. 2002;33(3):706–11.

67. Venketasubramanian N, Sacco RL, Di Tullio M, Sherman D, Homma S, Mohr JP. Vascular distribution of paradoxical emboli by transcranial Doppler. Neurology. 1993;43(8):1533–5.

68. Kim BJ, Sohn H, Sun BJ, Song JK, Kang DW, Kim JS, et al. Imaging characteristics of ischemic strokes related to patent foramen ovale. Stroke. 2013;44(12):3350–6.

69. Abdelghani M, El-Shedoudy SAO, Nassif M, Bouma BJ, de Winter RJ. Management of patients with patent foramen ovale and cryptogenic stroke: an update. Cardiology. 2019;143(1):62–72.

70. Dawson DM, Fischer EG. Neurologic complications of cardiac catheterization. Neurology. 1977;27(5):496–7.

71. Keilson GR, Schwartz WJ, Recht LD. The preponderance of posterior circulatory events is independent of the route of cardiac catheterization. Stroke. 1992;23(9):1358–9.

Brain Stem Infarction Syndromes

4

Jong S. Kim

Medullary Infarction

The medulla is mainly supplied by a number of penetrating arteries arising from the intracranial vertebral arteries (Vas). The dorsal tegmental area is also supplied by branches arising from the medial posterior inferior cerebellar artery (PICA) and posterior spinal artery. The most rostral part can be supplied by branches from the basilar artery (BA) or anterior inferior cerebellar artery (AICA). The caudal part of the anterior medulla is supplied by penetrating arteries arising from the anterior spinal artery (ASA).

Lateral Medullary Infarction

Since the first description of Wallenberg's syndrome more than 100 years ago [1], clinical [2–5] and pathological [6] findings of lateral medullary infarction (LMI) have been reported. Recent studies using MRI [7–11] have rapidly expanded our understanding of LMI syndromes. One study reported that LMI represents 1.9% of all admitted acute stroke [2]. It is likely that institutes frequently using MRI may find more cases than previously reported.

J. S. Kim (✉)
Department of Neurology, Asan Medical Center,
University of Ulsan, Seoul, South Korea
e-mail: jongskim@amc.seoul.kr

Clinical Manifestations

Symptoms/signs of LMI are summarized in Table 4.1. The onset may be sudden, but in more than half of the patients, symptoms/signs develop progressively or stutteringly. While headache, vertigo, nausea/vomiting, or gait instability are usually the early symptoms/signs, hiccup tends to occur later [10]. Some of the symptoms/signs may appear days or even weeks after the onset. The progressive onset is usually associated with enlargement of the ischemic area detected by follow-up MRI, associated with persistent or progressive thrombosis. Thus, progressive addition of symptoms seems to be equivalent to the early neurological deterioration in patients with internal capsular infarction.

Dizziness, Vertigo, and Ataxia

A dizzy sensation and gait instability are the most common symptoms occurring in more than 90% of patients. Whirling vertigo, a symptom attributed to involvement of vestibular nuclei and their connections, occurs in approximately 60% [10]. Vertigo is an early sign that usually improves within days or weeks, although dizziness and gait instability last longer. Vertigo is usually accompanied by nystagmus and vomiting. Gait instability and dizziness can be attributed to either the dysfunctional vestibular or cerebellar system. In the acute stage, approximately 60% of patients are unable to stand or walk. Gait ataxia is usually more common and severe than limb incoordination [10, 12]. Lateropulsion (forced to sway when

© Springer Nature Singapore Pte Ltd. 2021
J. S. Kim (ed.), *Posterior Circulation Stroke*, https://doi.org/10.1007/978-981-15-6739-1_4

Table 4.1 Neurologic symptoms and signs published in the largest series (In, Kim, Pure lateral medullary infarction: clinical-radiological correlation of 130 acute, consecutive patients. Brain 2003;126:1864–72)

Items	N = 130
Sensory symptoms/signs	125 (96)
Ipsilateral trigeminal	34 (26)
Contralateral trigeminal	32 (25)
Bilateral trigeminal	18 (14)
Isolated limb/body	27 (21)
Isolated trigeminal	13 (10)
Gait ataxia	120 (92)
Severe gait ataxia[a]	79 (61)
Dizziness	119 (92)
Horner sign	114 (88)
Hoarseness	82 (63)
Dysphagia	84 (65)
Severe dysphagia[b]	52 (40)
Dysarthria	28 (22)
Vertigo	74 (57)
Nystagmus	73 (56)
Limb ataxia	72 (55)
Nausea/vomiting	67 (52)
Headache	67 (52)
Neck pain	9 (7)
Skew deviation of eyes	53 (41)
Diplopia	41 (32)
Hiccup	33 (25)
Facial palsy	27 (21)
Forced gaze deviation	8 (6)

Data are expressed as number (%)
[a]Unable to stand or walk alone
[b]Requires nasogastric feed for feeding

patients stand or sit) seems to be attributed to lesions affecting the vestibular nuclei and vestibulospinal projections [13], while limb and gait ataxia are related to damage to the inferior cerebellar peduncle, spinocerebellar fibers, or the cerebellum itself [12, 14]. Occasionally, patients fall to any direction [14]. Limb ataxia may be described as "weakness" or "clumsiness" by the patient.

Nystagmus and Ocular Motor Abnormality
Involvement of the vestibular nuclei and their connections lead to nystagmus. The nystagmus is mostly horizontal or horizontal-rotational to the side opposite to the lesions [5, 6]. Although forced conjugate eyeball deviation to the lesion side (ocular lateropulsion) [15] is uncommon,

milder degree of eyeball deviation is frequently observed when patients are ordered to close and then open the eyes, when correctional eyeball movements occur. Skew deviation, with the ipsilateral eye going down, and ocular tilt reaction occur [13]. Patients describe the symptoms as blurred vision, diplopia, oscillopsia, or tilting of visual images [5, 13]. Detailed mechanisms are described in Chap. 7.

Nausea/Vomiting
Nausea/vomiting is usually an initial and transient symptom closely associated with vertigo [10] and is probably caused by involvement of vestibular nuclei and their connections. It may also be caused by involvement of a putative vomiting center near the nucleus ambiguus [5, 12].

Horner Sign
Elements of the Horner sign are frequent (about 90%), caused by involvement of the descending sympathetic fibers in the lateral reticular substance. A constricted pupil with ipsilateral palpebral fissure narrowing is more frequently observed than facial anhidrosis.

Dysphagia, Dysarthria, and Hoarseness
Involvement of the nucleus ambiguus results in paralysis of the ipsilateral palate, pharynx, and larynx producing dysphagia, dysarthria, and hoarseness. Dysarthria may also be attributed to the concomitant involvement of the cerebellum. Dysphagia is present in approximately 2/3 of LMI patients, among whom about 60% require a nasogastric tube for feeding [10, 12]. Swallowing difficulty usually improves within days or months, but rare patients require persistent assistance in feeding. Dysphagia in LMI is more often associated with problems in the range of, than the timing of, hyolaryngeal excursion [16]. Hoarseness is equally common, while dysarthria is less common, occurring in about 1/4 of patients with pure LMI patients [10]. Some patients may show paralysis of the ipsilateral vocal cord.

Hiccup
Approximately 1/4 of patients develop hiccup [10, 12], often days after stroke onset. Hiccup

usually goes away within a few days but can persist for weeks or even months when it becomes an annoying symptom. Involvement of the dorsal motor nucleus of the vagus, solitary tract, and neurons related to expiration and inspiration in the reticular formation near the nucleus ambiguus may be responsible for hiccup [5, 10].

Sensory Symptoms/Signs

Sensory symptoms/signs are one of the most common manifestations of LMI. In the largest series, sensory function was intact in only 4% of patients [10]. Sensory symptoms/signs occur more frequently in the contralateral body/limbs (in approximately 85%) than in the face (58–68%), [7, 9] and the sensory defect in the face usually clears more quickly than that on the body/limbs. Although a selective loss of spinothalamic sensation is a rule, vibration sensation is occasionally involved as well in the hypalgic body/limbs, [9] due probably to the fact that some of the vibratory sensations are carried through the lateral column [17].

Crossed (ipsilateral trigeminal-contralateral limb/body) sensory changes have been considered a classical sensory pattern in LMI. However, sensory manifestations are much more diverse in the acute stage [9]. In the largest series [10], the patterns included ipsilateral trigeminal-contralateral limb/body in 26%, contralateral trigeminal-contralateral limb/body in 25%, bilateral trigeminal-contralateral limb/body in 14%, limb/body involvement without trigeminal involvement in 21%, and trigeminal involvement without limb/body involvement in 10%. Although the arm and leg are usually equally involved, in approximately 30% of the patients, there is a discrepancy; some have more severe sensory deficits in the arm while others have more severe deficits in the leg [9]. The latter occasion is more common, and some may have a sensory level on the trunk mimicking a spinal cord syndrome [18].

These diverse sensory manifestations are related to the varied patterns of involvement of the spinothalamic tract, descending trigeminal tract, and ascending secondary trigeminal fibers (Fig. 4.1). Notably, approximately 7% of LMI patients have ipsilateral tingling sensation often associated with lemniscal sensory deficits, more

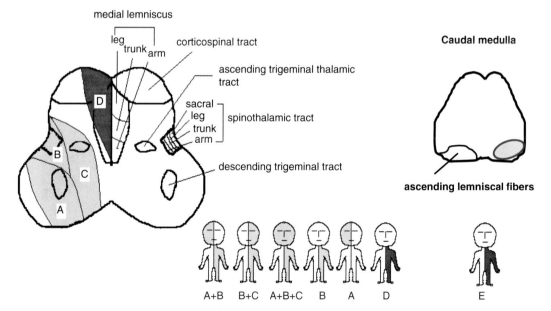

Fig. 4.1 Anatomic structures of the medulla and various patterns of sensory dysfunction caused by medullary infarction (see text for details). Yellow, spinothalamic sensory deficits; red, lemniscal sensory deficits; A + B, ipsilateral trigeminal-contralateral body/limb; B + C, contralateral trigeminal-contralateral body/limb; A + B + C, bilateral trigeminal-contralateral body/limb; B, contralateral body/limb; A, ipsilateral trigeminal; D, contralateral body/limb (lemniscal sensation); E, ipsilateral body/limb (lemniscal sensation). (Modified from Kim et al., Neurology 1997; Brain 2003)

marked in the arm than in the leg. Due to the leminscal sensory impairment, these patients often have feeling of "clumsiness" or "weakness" in the ipsilateral extremities. This sensory pattern is related to involvement of the lowermost medulla and explained by involvement of lemniscal sensory fibers at the upper-most part of the fasciculus cuneatus/gracilis or crossing fibers to the medial lemniscus [19] (Figs. 4.1E and 4.2).

In the descending trigeminal tract, the V3-representing area is located most dorsally and V1 most anteriorly, but in the ascending secondary trigeminal tracts, V3 is located most medially and V1 most laterally. Therefore, trigeminal sensory involvement is often inhomogeneous, more so on the contralateral side than the ipsilateral side. On both sides, the inhomogeneity is either divisional or segmental (onion-skin) pattern [4, 5, 9]. Bilateral perioral paresthesia, often observed in patients with large infarcts extending medially [9], may be caused by the simultaneous involve-

ment of the descending and ascending V3 pathways near its decussation [20, 21].

Patients occasionally complain of facial pain. The pain usually appears at onset, heralding other symptoms and signs [5]. It is described as sharp, stinging, stabbing, or burning, tingling, and numb. The eyeball and the surrounding area are the most commonly affected, but the entire face, including the lips and inside the mouth, may be involved. Although facial pain usually improves, it may last permanently in some patients. Involvement of the sensory nucleus of the descending tract of the fifth cranial nerve may explain the facial pain.

Headache

Headache occurs in about half of the patients [10, 12]. It usually begins at onset or a few days before other symptoms/signs and subsides within several days. It most often occurs in the ipsilateral occipital or upper nuchal area followed by the frontal region and is usually described as dull, aching, or

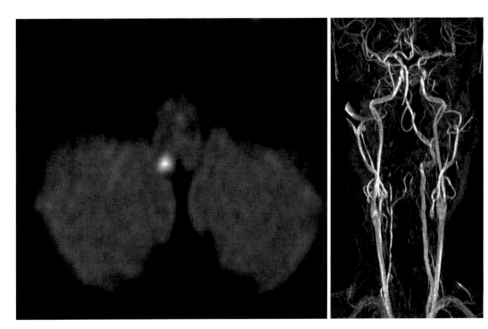

Fig. 4.2 A 69-year-old hypertensive man developed gait instability and numb sensation in the right hand, most markedly in the first-third finger tips. Neurological examination showed slightly decreased position and vibration sensation in the right fingers and impaired tandem gait. Diffusion-weighted MRI (left image) showed dorsally located infarct in the medullary-spinal cord junction. MRA (right image) showed right distal vertebral artery (VA) atherosclerotic occlusion. The ipsilateral sensory symptoms are probably due to involvement of the most rostral part of the ipsilateral lemniscal fibers (nucleus cuneatus) before decussation. The infarct was probably caused by occlusion of perforators (or posterior spinal artery) associated with VA atherosclerotic disease

throbbing. Considering that headache occurs before other symptoms and is not related to any symptoms/signs of LMI, [10] headache seems to be caused by an intracranial VA pathology, possibly related to dilated collateral vessels after VA stenosis/occlusion, [12] rather than the medullary lesion itself. Involvement of the descending spinal tract of the fifth cranial nerve and its nucleus may also be responsible for frontal headache. Prominent and persistent nuchal-occipital pain may be a manifestation of VA dissection.

Facial Palsy

Facial palsy, usually mild and upper neuron type, is present in 1/5 to 1/4 of patients [10]. It is presumably caused by involvement of aberrant corticobulbar fibers that loop caudally before traveling rostrally toward the facial nucleus [22]. In patients with upper-most medullary (or pontomedullary junction) lesion, there occurs relatively severe peripheral-type facial palsy due to direct involvement of facial nerve fascicles [23].

Respiratory Difficulty and Other Autonomic Signs

The medullary reticular formation contains neurons related to the control of respiration, and patients may show respiratory arrest or decreased respiratory drive, especially during sleep (Ondine's curse) [24]. Severe respiratory abnormalities calling for medical attention are uncommon unless patients have bilateral or extensive lesions [12]. In pure LMI, aspiration pneumonia associated with dysphagia is the most common reason for respiratory care, in which case, it is often difficult to assess how much respiratory control abnormality contributes to the patients' condition. Other autonomic disturbances such as tachycardia, bradycardia, sweating, orthostatic hypotension, gastric motility dysfunction, and urinary retention are sporadically observed.

Ipsilateral Hemiparesis

Ipsilateral hemiparesis may be associated with other typical symptoms of LMI [25].

The pathogenic mechanism of this so-called Opalski syndrome remains debatable. Recent imaging techniques such as diffusion-weighted MRI (DWI) and diffusion tensor imaging (DTI) showed that infarcts occurring at the lower-most medullary area or the medulla–spinal cord junction involve the ipsilateral corticospinal tract after the pyramidal decussation [26, 27]. This observation corroborates with Opalski's original patients who showed hyperreflexia and Babinski signs.

In addition, patients with ipsilateral ataxia or lemniscal sensory dysfunction (see above) may complain of "clumsiness" or "weakness" in their limbs [19]. In view of transient motor deficits and absent reflex abnormalities in the majority of these patients, most of the patients with ipsilateral "weakness" may have a pseudoparesis unrelated to pyramidal damage [19]. Thus, true Opalski syndrome is a rare entity.

Clinical–Topographical Correlation

The symptoms/signs of LMI differ according to the topography of lesions [5]. Kim et al. [10, 11] analyzed the MRI-identified lesions in a three-dimensional manner and made clinical–topographical correlation (Fig. 4.3).

Generally, rostral lesions tend to involve ventral (Fig. 4.3A), deep areas, while caudal lesions involve lateral-superficial region [10, 11] (Fig. 4.3C). This is probably related to the anatomical course of the VA; the intracranial VAs are located adjacent to the lateral surface at a caudal medulla level, which ascend ventrorostrally to fuse into the BA at the pontomedullary junction. The rostral-ventral lesions tend to produce ipsilateral trigeminal sensory symptoms (Fig. 4.1B+C), whereas caudal-lateral-superficial lesions tend to produce sensory symptoms limited to the extremities (occasionally with a gradient worse in the leg) sparing the face (Fig. 4.1B). A large, wide lesion is associated with a bilateral trigeminal sensory pattern (Fig. 4.1A+B+C), [10] which is quite uncommon in patients with caudal lesions.

The more important rostrocaudal difference is dysphagia, which is distinctly more prevalent and severe in patients with rostral than in caudal lesions [10, 11]. This may be explained by the following: (1) caudal medullary lesions are usually thin (Fig. 4.3C) and do not extend deeply as to involve the nucleus ambiguus and (2) the lower part of the nucleus ambiguus is not directly

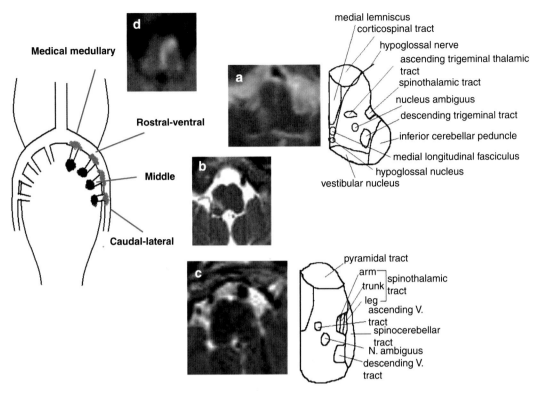

Fig. 4.3 Schematic drawing of stroke mechanism of various types of medullary infarction. Rostral type (**A**), middle type (**B**), and caudal-lateral type (**C**) lesions are categorized as "lateral medullary infarction" and determined according to the rostrocaudal location of the responsible perforating arteries. Medial medullary infarction (MMI) (**D**) seems to be produced by the most rostral vertebral artery disease. Patient A had severe dysphagia due to involvement of upper part of the nucleus ambiguus and contralateral trigeminal type sensory symptoms, whereas patient C had severe gait ataxia and sensory symptoms limited in the lower extremities. Patient B had ipsilateral trigeminal symptoms. Patient D had symptoms of MMI such as contralateral hemiparesis and hemihypesthesia (lemniscal sensation)

related to pharyngeal muscle motility [28]. Facial palsy is also more common in rostral lesions [10]. In patients with most rostral lesions, often at the pontomedullary junction, dysphagia is slight or absent because the nucleus ambiguus is spared at this level [29]. These patients often show severe, ipsilateral, peripheral-type facial palsy.

The caudal lesions are closely associated with severe lateropulsion and gait ataxia, probably due to frequent involvement of the laterodorsally located spinocerebellar tract and vestibular nuclei (Fig. 4.3C). Dissection and headache are also more common, while dysphagia is absent or minimal in this group. The middle medulla shows intermediate characteristics and classical ipsilateral trigeminal-contralateral body/limb pattern sensory deficits (Figs. 4.1B+C, 4.3B).

Stroke Mechanisms

Although Wallenberg initially considered PICA disease as a cause of LMI [1], Fisher et al. [6] found sole involvement of the PICA in only two of their 17 cases of LMI and 14 patients showed VA steno-occlusion. Thus, the most common cause of LMI is occlusion of penetrating branches associated with intracranial VA steno-occlusive disease [6] (Fig. 4.4). In a large series that investigated 123 LMI patients [10], ipsilateral VA steno-occlusive disease was present in 83 (67%) (33 intracranial VA disease, 34 whole VA disease, and 5 extracranial VA disease) and PICA disease in 12 (10%) patients. Atherothrombosis is a dominant pathology, while dissection of the VA or PICA is the cause of steno-occlusive lesions in approximately 14–33% of cases [7, 8, 10] (for

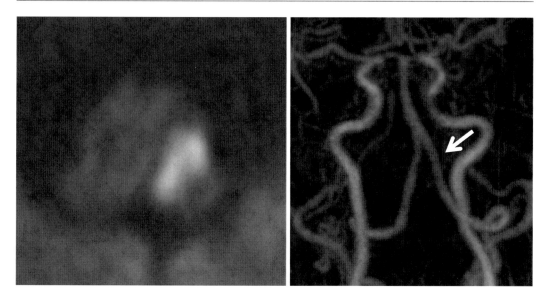

Fig. 4.4 Diffusion-weighted MRI showed an infarction in the left rostral medulla. MRA showed focal, atherosclerotic narrowing (arrow) that probably occluded a perforator

dissection, see Chap. 14). In patients with normal angiographic findings, perforating artery disease seems to be the mechanism of infarction. Embolic occlusion of the PICA or distal VA from diseased heart or proximal artery atherosclerosis may also produce LMI [30, 31], but concomitant infarcts in other parts (mostly, cerebellum) of the brain are usually present in these patients.

Prognosis

The prognosis of pure LMI is benign, mainly due to the absence of significant motor dysfunction. The hospital mortality ranges from 0.8% to 11.6% [2–4, 10]. Patients with large, rostral lesions tend to have severe dysphagia and aspiration pneumonia, requiring ICU care. Sudden respiratory (Ondine's curse) or other autonomic failures may produce respiratory-cardiac arrest, and physicians may have to keep this possibility in mind. Nevertheless, recent studies have shown very low hospital mortality, which is probably related to improved care for respiration, infection, and dysphagia [10]. Old age, having dysphagia [32], and rostral LMI lesions [33] were found to be factors related with unfavorable prognosis.

Despite the relatively benign outcome, the majority of survivors have at least one remaining sequelae. The most important one is sensory symptoms/signs, followed by dizziness and dysphagia [34]. Usually, the persistent and disturbing sequela correlates with the most severe initial symptom. Approximately 1/4 of the patients develop uncomfortable painful paresthesia (central post-stroke pain, CPSP) [35], which are described as numb, burning, or cold [34]. The symptoms usually occur in the body parts where the initial sensory perception deficit was most severe.

Patients with severe and extensive VA diseases more often develop recurrent cerebral infarction or coronary disease than those without [2]. The presence of posterior fossa hypoperfusion may predict poor prognosis [36]. In patients with concomitant infarcts in other areas, the prognosis is influenced by the location and extent of the extramedullar lesions. In patients with large PICA territory cerebellar infarction, massive edema and consequent herniation may yield a poor prognosis. However, a recent study showed that although the short-term outcome is poorer in LMI patients with extramedullar lesions, long-term residual symptoms such as dizziness, dysphagia, and sensory symptoms are more prevalent in pure LMI patients [33]. This is probably because in the former patients, PICA occlusion is the main pathogenesis and LMI lesions are usually limited to a small, dorsal part of the medulla, an area supplied by the PICA. On the contrary, the lesions associated with distal VA disease in pure LMI patients tend to be larger.

Medial Medullary Infarction

Medial medullary infarction (MMI) was initially described by Spiller in 1908 [37]. Dejerine later proposed a triad of symptoms: contralateral hemiplegia sparing the face, contralateral loss of deep sensation, and ipsilateral hypoglossal paralysis [38]. Pathological findings were first reported by Davison in 1937, who described thrombotic occlusion of the anterior spinal artery (ASA) and the adjacent intracranial VA [39].

With the advent of MRI, the premortem diagnosis of MMI can now be easily made. Kim et al. [40] compared their own series of 17 patients diagnosed by MRI, with 26 previously reported patients. They found that in the former group, bilateral lesions, quadriparesis, lingual paresis, and respiratory difficulty were much rarer, and the prognosis was much better. Subsequent studies using MRI showed that patients usually present with relatively benign, unilateral sensorimotor stroke [40–45]. Clinical symptoms/signs of MMI are summarized in (Table 4.2).

Clinical Manifestations

Limb Weakness

Contralateral hemiparesis sparing the face is the most characteristic sign of MMI occurring in approximately 90% [46]. Quadriparesis occurs in less than 10% of the patients [45]. Although rare, hemiparesis may occur on the ipsilateral side due to the lower-most lesion involving the crossed pyramidal tract [40]. The degree of motor dysfunction is variable; in one study [45], it was severe (Medical Research Council scale ≤3) in 37%, 2/3 of whom had a gradual progression of weakness during several days after onset.

Facial Palsy

Although sparing of the face is one of the characteristics of MMI, mild and transient facial paresis

Table 4.2 Neurologic symptoms and signs published in the largest series (In Kim JS, Han Y, Medial medullary infarction: clinical, imaging, and outcome study in 86 consecutive patients, 2009;40: 3221–5)

Symptoms and signs (n = 86)	
Motor dysfunction	78 (91)
	Hemiparesis 68, quadriparesis 8, monoparesis 2
Facial paresis	21 (24)
Sensory dysfunction	59 (73)
	Paresthesia 55
	Impairment of objective sensory perception
	Vibration 48
	Position 41
	Touch 32
	Pinprick 17
	Cold 22
Lim ataxia	36 (42)
Dysarthria	54 (63)
Dysphagia	25 (29)
Ipsilateral hypoglossal palsy	3 (3)
Contralateral tongue deviation	9 (10)
Vertigo/dizziness	51 (59)
Nausea/vomiting	14 (16)
Nystagmus	38 (44)
Diplopia	7 (8)
Headache	9 (10)

Number in parenthesis indicates percentage

occurs in 1/4 to 1/2 [12, 44, 45], probably related to involvement of yet-uncrossed corticobulbar fibers directed to the contralateral cranial nuclei at the level of the upper medulla [22].

Dysarthria and Dysphagia

Dysarthria and dysphagia were reported to occur in 63% and 29%, respectively [45]. These symptoms are much more severe in patients with bilateral MMI. In unilateral cases, a nasogastric tube is required in less than 10%. A study using videofluoroscopic swallowing tests showed that dysphagia in MMI is associated with delayed timing rather than a reduced range of hyolaryngeal excursion [16] and may be attributed to damage to the corticobulbar tract or adjacent pattern generator regulating the nucleus ambiguous.

Ipsilateral Hypoglossal Nerve Palsy

Ipsilateral hypoglossal nerve palsy, if it presents, is an important localizing sign [38]. Its prevalence is reported extremely variably, from 3% to 82% [11, 40–45]. Recent MRI-based studies found a lower prevalence of ipsilateral hypoglossal palsy than earlier studies; a large series showed that definite ipsilateral hypoglossal paresis occurred in only 3% of patients while clumsy tongue movements with occasional contralateral tongue deviation were more common [45]. Because MMI lesions most often involve the rostral medulla, the hypoglossal nerve nucleus and fasciculus, located in the lower medulla, are frequently spared.

Sensory Dysfunction

Sensory dysfunction is the second most important symptom/sign of MMI. Unlike LMI patients, MMI patients typically complain of tingling sensation from the onset. The involved area is usually hemibody/limbs below the ear or neck (Fig. 4.1D). However, sensory symptoms may extend to the face, probably due to additional involvement of the secondary ascending trigeminal sensory tract. The facial sensory symptoms are usually mild, incomplete, and transient. Occasionally, the sensory abnormality is restricted to a certain body part, such as the lower leg [47]. Dermatomal distribution sensory abnormalities are also reported [48]. Although lemniscal sensory deficits are characteristic, mild and transient impairment of pain/temperature perception is occasionally present due possibly to involvement of the spinoreticulothalamic system that regulates the spinothalamic sensory system [41, 42, 44, 45].

Ataxia

Limb incoordination is occasionally noted [42] and is usually attributed to involvement of pontocerebellar fibers and/or associated proprioceptive sensory dysfunction. Gait instability or body lateropulsion may be related to involvement of the vestibulocerebellar tract, inferior olivary nucleus, or more laterally located spinocerebellar tract [42].

Vertigo/Dizziness, Nystagmus, and Ocular Motor Disturbances

These symptoms/signs are closely related to involvement of the dorsal medulla, [44, 49] where the vestibular nuclei, medial longitudinal fasciculus (MLF), and the nucleus prepositus hypoglossi (NPH) are located. In contrast to LMI, nystagmus is mostly ipsilesional, and ocular lateropulsion is to the contralateral side (contrapulsion) [50]. Upbeat nystagmus is observed in 1/10 to 1/5 of patients, [44, 45, 49] which may be explained by involvement of the VOR pathways from both anterior semicircular canals [51]. Unilateral lesion may also produce upbeat nystagmus [45] (see Chap. 7 for detailed mechanisms).

Emotional Disturbances

Previous reports have described patients presenting with pathological crying and laughing, depression, and psychotic behaviors [52, 53]. A recent study showed that emotional incontinence in MMI patients is as common as in those with pontine base infarction [54].

Clinical–Topographical Correlation

The majority of MMI lesions involve the rostral part of the medulla, and lesions limited to the caudal medulla are rare [45]. Ventro-dorsally, ventral lesions are closely related to motor dysfunction, middle lesions to sensory symptoms, and dorsal lesions are associated with vertigo, ataxia, and ocular motor dysfunction (Fig. 4.5). The symptom correlation according to ventrodorsal distribution is similar to that of pontine base infarction (see below, pontine infarction). Unlike pontine infarction, the face is mostly spared because the lesions are below the level of the facial nerve nucleus/fascicles. Sensory abnormalities are mostly lemniscal because lemniscal and spinothalamic tracts are separated in the medulla (Fig. 4.1D). In a large series, the lesion patterns include ventral in 20%, ventral+middle in 33%, and ventral+middle+dorsal in 41% [45].

Bilateral MMI

Bilateral MMI is uncommon. In one study, bilateral lesions occurred in 14%. Because the lesion

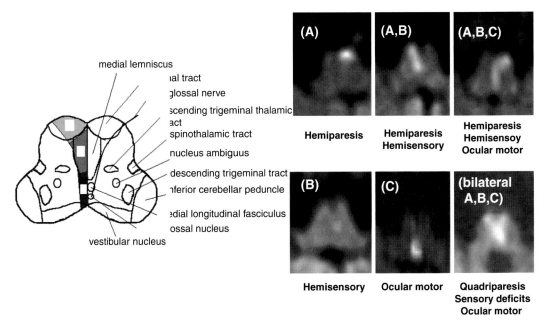

medial lemniscus
ıal tract
ɟlossal nerve
scending trigeminal thalamic
ɔct
spinothalamic tract
nucleus ambiguus
descending trigeminal tract
ɔferior cerebellar peduncle
ɔdial longitudinal fasciculus
ossal nucleus
vestibular nucleus

(A) **(A,B)** **(A,B,C)**

Hemiparesis **Hemiparesis Hemisensory** **Hemiparesis Hemisensoy Ocular motor**

(B) **(C)** **(bilateral A,B,C)**

Hemisensory **Ocular motor** **Quadriparesis Sensory deficits Ocular motor**

Fig. 4.5 Illustrative patients and schematic drawings of patterns of medial medullary infarction. Patterns of involvement of A (pure motor stroke), A + B (sensorimotor stroke), or A + B + C (sensorimotor stroke + ocular dysfunction) are common, while others are uncommon. Selective involvement of B and C produces pure hemisensory stroke and pure ocular motor dysfunction, respectively. Bilateral involvement of A + B + C accounts for less than 10% of medial medullary infarction and leads to quadriparesis, bilateral sensory loss, and ocular motor dysfunction

on the one side is occasionally small and asymptomatic, quadriparesis was observed in 9% [45]. In patients with quadriparesis, MRI lesions are usually symmetrical and heart shaped (Fig. 4.5, bilateral A,B,C). Patients have severe bulbar palsy and sensory symptoms, mimicking pontine locked-in syndrome (see below, pontine infarction). Unless the dorsal pons is concomitantly involved, gaze is generally preserved.

Stroke Mechanism

Although ASA occlusion has traditionally been emphasized, [37–39] recent studies showed that MMI is more often caused by intracranial VA or VA–BA junction atherothrombotic diseases that obliterate perforating branches [55] (Figs. 4.3 and 4.6 upper panel). In one series, relevant intracranial VA atherosclerotic disease was present in 62% of patients while perforator occlusion without VA disease (small artery disease) occurred in 28% of patients [45]. Infarcts associated with intracranial VA atherothrombotic disease tend to extend deeper (Fig. 4.6 upper panel) than those with small vessel disease (Fig. 4.6, lower panel), perhaps associated with either multiple perforator occlusion or more extensive hypoperfusion in the medulla. VA dissection may cause MMI but is less common than in LMI.

ASA occlusion, although uncommon, may produce caudal MMI infarction. Rarely, embolic occlusion of ASA branches by talc [56], fibrocartilaginous material, [57] or syphilitic arteritis [58, 59] can cause MMI. Embolism from the diseased heart or proximal VA disease is an uncommon cause of pure MMI. Bilateral MMI may be caused by occlusion of one ASA supplying both parts of the medulla. However, a large study [45] showed that bilateral MMIs are generally located rostrally in the territory of the distal intracranial VA or proximal BA. It seems that bilateral MMIs are usually caused by intracranial VA–BA atherothrombotic disease that obliterates multiple perforators bilaterally.

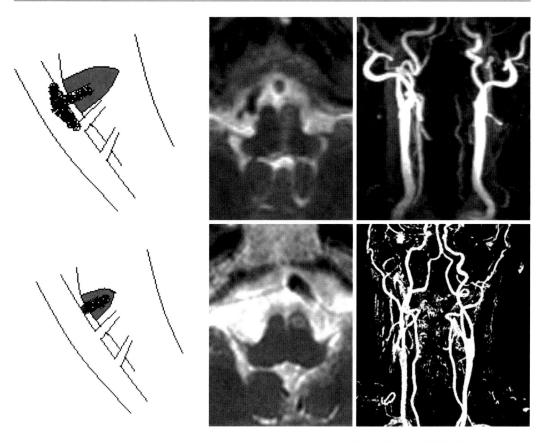

Fig. 4.6 Examples of a patient with large, dorsally extended medial medullary infarction (MMI) that is associated with distal vertebral artery disease (upper panel) and a patient with small, ventral MMI that is associated with small artery disease (lower panel)

Prognosis

Unlike LMI, aspiration pneumonia is uncommon in MMI except for those with bilateral lesions. The prognosis of MMI is better than that reported in the pre-MRI era; in a series of 86 patients, only 3 died during admission [45]. Due to the presence of significant motor dysfunction, functional outcome is generally worse in MMI than in LMI [34]. Severe initial motor dysfunction is a main predictor for poor functional outcome [45]. In the chronic stage, sensory dysfunction is equally prevalent and troublesome, which consists of both joint pain associated with motor dysfunction/spasticity and CPSP. In one study, CPSP defined by visual analog scale ≥4 was present in 36% [45]. The CPSP is most frequently expressed as numb followed by aching, and unlike LMI patients, "burning" sensation is rarely described [34]. Dizziness is reported in approximately 1/3 of the patients [45].

Combined LMI and MMI

LMI and MMI may occur simultaneously or consequently. This hemimedullary syndrome was first described in 1894 by Reinhold [60] and by Babinski and Nageotte [61] 8 years later. Hemimedullary infarction is usually associated with concomitant infarcts in the posterior circulation, and its occurrence in isolation is rare. Clinical symptoms/signs are essentially the combination of LMI and MMI. The usual etiologies are intracranial VA atherosclerosis or dissection that extends to block both lateral and medial medullary perforating branches.

Table 4.3 Clinical manifestations of pontine infarction

Author	Macdonell et al.	Kase et al.	Tohgi et al.
Country	Australia	USA	Japan
Published year	1987	1993	1993
Diagnosis	CT based	CT/MRI based	CT/MRI based
Number of patients	30	66	293
Symptoms			
Dizziness/vertigo	80	50 (vertigo)	70
Nausea/vomiting	63	52	56
Gait difficulty (or truncal ataxia)	77	71	40
Headache	40	53	32
Dysarthria	60		20
Signs			
Limb ataxia	70	61	59
Truncal ataxia	67	62	45
Nystagmus	53	64	38
Decreased consciousness	36		34
Ocular movement disorder	27		
Hemi(mono) paresis	7		20
Facial palsy	13		8

Pontine Infarcts

Pontine infarction may occur in isolation or in association with other posterior circulation infarction. Hospital registry studies showed that patients with isolated pontine infarcts account for 2.6–3% of ischemic stroke and 12–15% of patients with posterior circulation infarcts [62–64]. One study from Asia showed a higher prevalence: 7.6 % of cerebral infarcts and 28% of vertebrobasilar artery territory infarcts [65] (Table 4.3).

Clinical Features

Motor Dysfunction (Including Dysarthria and Ataxia)

The pontine base contains fibers regulating motor function, including descending corticospinal, corticopontocerebellar, and corticobulbar tracts

(Fig. 4.7A). Accordingly, pontine base infarction easily produces motor system dysfunction. Although limb weakness is the most common symptom, the clinical features depend upon the degree of involvement of each fiber tract. Fisher and his colleagues described pure motor stroke [55], ataxic hemiparesis [66], and dysarthria-clumsy hand syndromes [67] as "lacunar" syndromes. However, other combinations are observed such as dysarthria-hemiataxia or dysarthria-facial paresis [68]. The categorization is not strict as patients with ataxic hemiparesis may evolve into pure motor stroke as the limb weakness progresses over time, or vice versa. Patients with ataxic hemiparesis may have additional ataxia on the side ipsilateral to the lesion [68–70] due probably to involvement of the crossing corticopontocerebellar tracts [70].

Severe hemiparesis is usually associated with large lesions affecting the ventral surface of the caudal or middle pons whereas similar sized lesions tend to produce milder limb weakness but relatively prominent dysarthria (producing dysarthria-clumsy hand) when they are located in the rostral pons; here, pyramidal tract fibers are sparsely arranged and located relatively laterally and are therefore not extensively damaged by paramedian lesions [68].

Sensory Dysfunction

Small tegmental pontine infarcts or hemorrhages that selectively involve sensory tracts (medial lemniscus and spinothalamic tract) produce a pure or predominant hemisensory deficit without significant other neurological dysfunctions [71, 72] (Fig. 4.7C). Occasionally, patients have hemi-paresthesias without objectively detectable sensory deficits.

In the pontine medial lemniscal tract, the sensory projections from the arm, trunk, and leg are arranged from a medial to lateral direction. Therefore, a medially located lesion preferentially affects the face and arm, causing a cheiro-oral syndrome, whereas laterally located lesions produce leg-dominant sensory symptoms [71]. The most medially located lesions sometimes produce bilateral facial or perioral sensory symptoms due probably to involvement of trigemino-thalamic fibers bilaterally [71]. Cheiro-oral-pedal

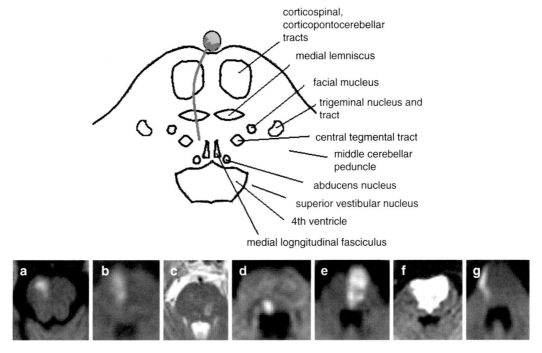

corticospinal,
corticopontocerebellar
tracts

medial lemniscus

facial mucleus

trigeminal nucleus and
tract

central tegmental tract

middle cerebellar
peduncle

abducens nucleus

superior vestibular nucleus

4th ventricle

medial logngitudinal fasciculus

Fig. 4.7 Illustrative patients and schematic drawing showing patterns of infarcts in the pons that is associated with branch occlusion. See the text for details. Patients had left hemiparesis (**A**), left sensorimotor stroke (**B**), right pure sensory stroke (**C**), right internuclear ophthal- moplegia (**D**), left one-and-a-half syndrome and right sen- sorimotor stroke (**E**), quadriparesis, sensory loss, and horizontal gaze palsy (**F**), and left ataxia and sensory change (**G**)

[73] and oro-crural [74] sensory distribution patterns are also reported.

Trigeminal sensory deficits are often noticed in patients with infarcts affecting the lateral pons, usually accompanied by other symptoms of AICA territory infarction. Isolated trigeminal sensory symptoms without other neurological deficits may occur in patients with small strokes affecting the trigeminal fascicles or nucleus in the lateral pons [75]. Trigeminal sensory symptoms restricted to the intraoral area, and isolated involvement of taste sensation [76] were also reported.

Ocular Motor Dysfunction

Structures related to ocular motor function such as abducens nucleus and fascicles, paramedian pontine reticular formation (PPRF), and medial longitudinal fasciculus (MLF) are located in the paramedian, dorsal pontine tegmentum (Fig. 4.7D). Infarcts affecting this region cause various types of ocular motor dysfunctions. For a detailed description and mechanism, see Chap. 7.

6th Nerve Palsy

The abducens nucleus is located in the parame- dian, dorsal, lower pons. Although rare, isolated 6th nerve palsy can result from a small pontine infarct that damages the abducens fascicles [77– 79]. Because the abducens nucleus is surrounded by facial nerve fascicles, dorsal lesions involving the lower pons may produce both 6th and 7th nerve palsies in isolation (Fig. 4.8B), or more fre- quently, in association with contralateral hemipa- resis (Millard–Gubler syndrome).

Internuclear Ophthalmoplegia

Internuclear ophthalmoplegia (INO) due to involvement of the MLF is much more common in patients with pontine infarction than 6th nerve palsy, probably because the MLF is a vertically long structure located in the paramedian area (Fig. 4.7D), easily involved by deep, paramedian pontine infarcts. In the largest series that included 30 patients with INO with minimal neurologic deficits, authors found that they account for

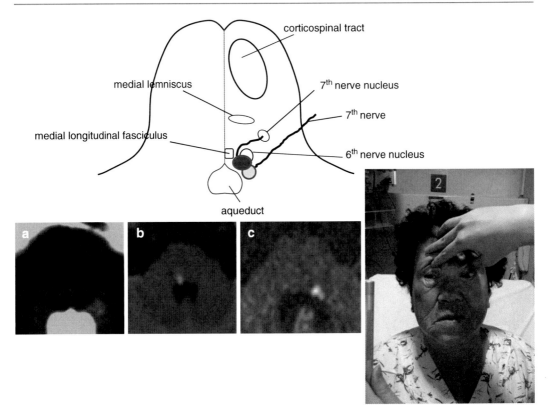

Fig. 4.8 Illustrative patients and schematic drawing of dorsal pontine structures. (**A**) An infarct that produced isolated left facial palsy indistinguishable from peripheral Bell's palsy, due to selective involvement of the genu portion of the seventh nerve (yellow circle). (**B**) An infarct producing right sixth and seventh nerve palsies due to involvement of the sixth nerve nuclei and the genu portion of the seventh nerve (red circle). (**C**) An infarct producing right internuclear ophthalmoplegia and facial palsy (71/2 syndrome) due to involvement of the medial longitudinal fasciculus and seventh nerve fascicle (not indicated in the diagram). Right image: Photography of patient B. She showed lateral gaze limitation of the right eye and decreased nasolabial fold in the right face. Consent was obtained from the patient for this presentation

0.47% of all ischemic stroke patients [80]. If the adjacent medial lemniscus or pontocerebellar fibers are involved, sensory symptoms, ataxia, and dysarthria are added. Lesions that extend laterally may result in additional facial paresis (71/2 syndrome) (Fig. 4.8C).

The symptoms of INO are characterized by (1) paralysis of adduction (or slowed adductive saccade when symptoms are mild) of the ipsilateral eye for all conjugate eye movements and (2) nystagmus in the contralateral eye when this eye is in abduction. Convergence is more often preserved than impaired. Occasionally, the contralateral eye is exotropic on neutral gaze, which is called "paralytic pontine exotropia." The exotropic gaze deviation is attributed to the unop-posed tonic activity of the spared PPRF on the side opposite to a unilateral lesion. Although less common, some patients with bilateral INO show bilateral exotropia, a phenomenon referred to as "wall-eyed bilateral internuclear ophthalmoplegia (WEBINO) [81]." The INO is frequently associated with contraversive ocular tilt reaction (OTR) (subjective visual vertical, ocular torsion, or skew deviation).

Conjugate Horizontal Gaze Palsy

Involvement of the paramedian pontine reticular formation (PPRF) near the 6th nerve nucleus leads to the absence of voluntary lateral gaze to the side of the lesion, including the quick phase of nystagmus. Patients' eyes remain at the midline in attempted ipsilateral saccade, or when they begin in a position contralateral to the lesion, return to the midline slowly [82]. The vestibular ocular reflex (VOR) and ipsilateral smooth pursuit usually remain intact. Bilateral lesions involving the abducens nucleus and PPRF produce paralysis of all horizontal eye movements. Although vertical gaze is mediated at a more rostral level, patients with bilateral horizontal gaze palsies may show slow vertical gaze saccades. This is probably related to the fact that the omnipause neurons that modulate saccadic triggering are also involved in vertical saccades via sending signals to the riMLF [83].

One-and-a-Half Syndrome
One-and-a-half syndrome refers to "a paralysis of eye movements in which one eye lies centrally and fails completely to move horizontally while the other eye lies in an abducted position and cannot be adducted past the midline [84]." A unilateral pontine lesion involving both the PPRF and MLF produces an ipsilateral conjugate gaze palsy, and paralysis of adduction of the ipsilateral eye on conjugate gaze to the opposite side [85].

Ocular Bobbing and Other Related Signs
Fisher [86] introduced the term ocular bobbing: "The eyeballs intermittently dip briskly downward through an arc of a few millimeters and then return to the primary position in a kind of bobbing action." Ocular bobbing is an ominous sign, usually associated with extensive, bilateral pontine infarcts or hemorrhages [86, 87]. Quadriparesis and decreased consciousness are usually present. Bobbing is usually bilateral and symmetric but can be predominantly unilateral or asymmetric [84, 88]. Asymmetric bobbing is common in patients in whom there is an asymmetric paralysis of conjugate gaze. When bobbing is asymmetric, usually the eye ipsilateral to the side of limited gaze bobs when gaze is directed to that side [84, 86]. In patients with extensive pontine lesions, horizontal gaze is lost, but vertical gaze is preserved; the vertical vector of gaze may be accentuated so that the eyes "bob" down. In patients with bilateral pontine

infarcts, ptosis of the upper eyelids is also frequent [89], usually attributed to involvement of descending sympathetic fibers in the lateral pontine tegmentum. The pupils become small (pinpoint pupil) [84], but pupillary response to light is usually preserved if examined by magnifying glass.

Involuntary Movements

Palatal Myoclonus
Palatal myoclonus is a rhythmic involuntary jerking movement of the soft palate and pharyngopalatine arch, often involving the diaphragm and laryngeal muscles as well [90].

Palatal myoclonus does not appear in the acute stage of stroke but develops several months later. Occasionally, rhythmic, jerky movements are also observed in the face, eyeballs, tongue, jaw, vocal cord, or extremities (mostly hands); they may or may not be synchronous with palatal movements. The movements of the palate vary in rate between 40 and 200 beats per minute. The movements may involve the eustachian tube and make a click that the patient can hear.

The posited anatomical lesion involves the "Guillain–Mollaret triangle," which includes the dentate nucleus of the cerebellum, the red nucleus in the midbrain, and the inferior olivary nucleus in the medulla and their interconnections [91]. The pathologic lesion most often seen in these patients is hypertrophic degeneration of the inferior olive. Enlarged neurons and diffuse gliosis are observed usually, though not always, bilaterally. In patients with pontine strokes, damage to the central tegmental tract and consequent hypertrophic degeneration of the inferior olive is considered to be a responsible mechanism. For unclear reason, the palatal myoclonus is more often observed in pontine hemorrhages than infarcts (Fig. 4.9).

Periodic Limb Movements and Restless Leg
Periodic limb movements [92] and restless leglike symptoms [93] may occur after unilateral pontine base infarction. The presumed mechanisms are disinhibited propriospinal/segmental spinal reflexes or dopaminergic fibers involvements due

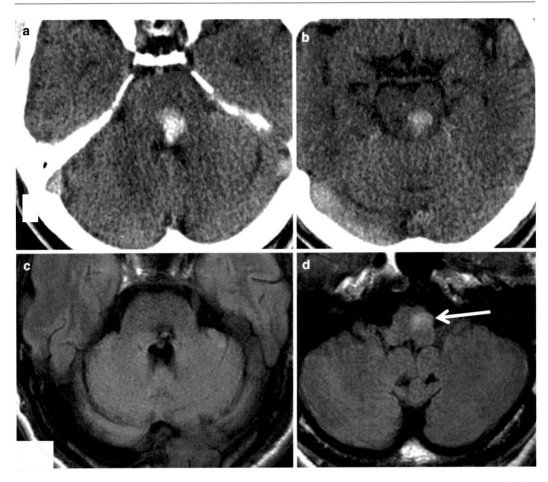

Fig. 4.9 A 68-year-old hypertensive man became drowsy. Neurological examination showed that he had bilateral horizontal gaze paresis, severe dysarthria, quadriparesis, bilateral ataxia, and sensory dysfunction. CT showed paramedian dorsal ponto-mesencephalic hemorrhage (**A**, **B**). He gradually improved but continued to have dizzi-ness, diplopia, and gait ataxia. One year later, examination showed newly developed pendular nystagmus, palatal tremor, and auditory hallucination. MRI showed old, shrunken hemorrhages (**C**) and a high signal intensity in the swollen left medullary olive (arrow, **D**), consistent with inferior olivary hypertrophic degeneration

to lesions involving pontine reticular formation [92, 94].

Other Cranial Nerve Dysfunction

The 5th, 7th, and 8th nuclei or fascicles are involved when lesions are laterally situated. This issue will be discussed in the AICA syndrome (see Chap. 6). A very small infarct selectively damaging the genu portion of the 7th nerve may produce isolated 7th nerve palsy, indistinguish-able from peripheral facial nerve palsy (Fig. 4.8A).

Auditory Symptoms

After entering into the cochlear nucleus, some auditory fibers ascend directly, while others tra-verse through the trapezoid body to the contralat-eral lateral lemniscus. Due to the bilateral, complex auditory pathways, hearing loss is rare in patients with pontine infarction unless the 8th nerve nucleus/fascicles are directly involved in AICA territory infarction.

However, extensive and destructive lesions involving the tegmental area may produce audi-tory symptoms. Bilateral total deafness has been rarely observed [95]. More often, tinnitus and auditory hallucination, usually associated with a certain degree of hearing impairment, are found in patients with pontine strokes [96–98] (Fig. 4.9). The auditory hallucinations are considered a cen-tral "release phenomenon" in the setting of peripheral input deficiency. The hallucination often disappears as the hearing loss improves [98]. For unclear reason, hallucinations are often musical, i.e., songs, drum sound, etc. Contralateral hyperacousis has also been observed in a patient with unilateral pontine tegmental stroke [99], possibly attributed to hypersensitization phenomenon after damage on the sensory tract.

Consciousness Disturbances or Coma

Patients with bilateral, extensive pontine infarcts caused by sudden BA occlusion often present with decreased consciousness or even coma, probably related to involvement of brainstem reticular activating structures responsible for the regulation of alertness.

Abnormalities of Respiration

Abnormalities of respiration are also common, but their mechanism is difficult to determine, partly because of the extensiveness of the infarction and partly because of the usual presence of general medical problems (e.g., aspiration, fever, and hypoventilation) in these patients. Apneustic breathing with a hang-up of the inspiratory phase and grossly irregular breathing (ataxic respirations) occasionally occur in patients with BA occlusion and indicate an ominous prognosis [100].

Emotional Disturbances

Pathological laughing or crying occasionally occurs in patients with pontine infarction [65, 68, 69, 101]. Patients with bilateral pontine lesions have more frequent and severe symptoms. Recent studies [54, 102] focusing on this issue showed that excessive or inappropriate laughing/crying occurs in 33–50% of the patients with pontine base infarction (Fig. 4.10). Depression was less common, occurring in 16% [54]. Patients with tegmental lesions rarely showed emotional disturbances.

The emotional disturbances in patients with pontine base infarction may be attributed to involvement of profuse serotonergic fibers from the brainstem raphe nuclei projecting to the basal ganglia or the cerebellum [54, 103, 104]. Another closely related emotional symptom, excessive or inappropriate anger, is equally

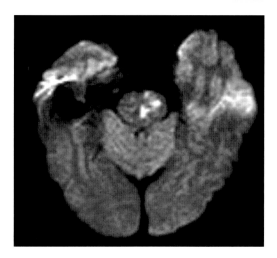

Fig. 4.10 A 58-year-old hypertensive man developed dysarthria and mild right hemiparesis due to left pontine base infarction. The symptoms gradually improved, but he complained of repeated episodes of excessive and inappropriate crying. This was the most distressing symptom of the patient. The symptom, emotional incontinence, improved greatly after escitalopram (10 mg/d) administration

common in patients with pontine base infarction [102]. Mania [105] and psychotic behaviors [106, 107] are also observed but are distinctly uncommon.

Clinical–Topographical Correlation

In the era of MRI, unilateral pontine infarct is much more common than bilateral one, occupying approximately 90% of isolated pontine infarction [62, 63].

Unilateral Infarcts

In one study examining 49 patients with unilateral paramedian infarcts, 27 patients had basal infarcts, 15 basal-tegmental infarcts, and 7 had infarcts limited to the tegmental area [65].

Unilateral Paramedian Basal Infarcts

Paramedian infarction involving mainly the pontine base is the most common pattern occurring in 54–58% of isolated pontine infarction [62, 64, 65]. Motor dysfunction is the main symptom (Fig. 4.7A). Lesions extending dorsally to involve the tegmentum produce sensory symptoms as well (Fig. 4.7B). According to a study that evaluated 37 patients with acute, unilateral infarcts that mainly involved the pontine base [68], the clinical presentations included pure motor hemiparesis in 17, sensorimotor stroke in 3, ataxic hemiparesis in 4, and dysarthria-clumsy hand syndrome in 6 patients. One patient had dysarthria-hemiataxia, two with quadrataxic hemiparesis, and four had dysarthria-facial paresis.

Acute or subacute neurologic progression occurs up to 1/4 of patients with pontine base infarction, along with subacute lesion volume increase [108]. It seems that infarcts in the lower pons are more often associated with progressive worsening and poorer functional outcome than those in the upper pons [65].

Unilateral Paramedian Tegmental Infarction

Unilateral tegmental infarction is the second most common pattern of pure pontine infarction, occurring in 12-31% of patients [62, 63, 65]. Unilateral tegmental infarcts frequently produce hemisensory syndromes [71] (Fig. 4.7C), while more dorsally located lesions produce ocular motor dysfunction, most often INO [80] (Fig. 4.7D). One-and-a-half syndrome and horizontal gaze palsy also occur [65]. Involvement of adjacent structures such as facial nerve/fascicules may produce INO plus peripheral-type facial palsy (Fig. 4.8C). Relatively large lesions result in both hemisensory syndromes and ocular motor dysfunction.

Combined Basal-Tegmental Infarction

Paramedian pontine base infarction may extend dorsally to involve the tegmental portion (Fig. 4.7E). The clinical features are essentially a combination of basal and tegmental syndromes.

Unilateral Circumferential Artery Territory (Ventrolateral) Infarcts

Ventrolateral territory infarcts were reported to occur in 17-25% of patients with isolated pontine infarction [62, 63]. However, it is often difficult to clearly differentiate the ventrolateral from the ventromedial group, and some studies did not separate them [64, 65]. Clinical features are similar to those of paramedian infarcts. However, hemiparesis is relatively mild, probably because pyramidal motor fibers located in the paramedian area are less severely involved (Fig. 4.7G). Accordingly, patients more often present with ataxic hemiparesis, dysarthria-clumsy hand syndrome, or predominant hemisensory symptoms.

Unilateral Dorsolateral Infarcts

The dorsolateral areas are supplied by AICA in the lower pons and SCA in the upper pons.

Infarction of this area is accompanied by concomitant cerebellar infarcts and rarely involved in isolation. Trigeminal sensorimotor dysfunction, 6th nerve palsy, 7th nerve palsy, auditory disturbances, and contralateral sensory dysfunction are usually observed. Contralateral hemiparesis is rare or mild when present.

Bilateral Infarcts

Bilateral infarcts are usually, though not always, associated with BA occlusion and result in grave neurological symptoms. As the bilateral lesions almost always involve the ventral part, involving the corticospinal tracts, quadriparesis is usual [106, 109, 110]. The quadriparesis may start from the beginning; more often, the initial motor dysfunction is lateralized to one side and then progresses [111]. Hemiparetic patients with BA occlusion often show some motor or reflex abnormalities on the nonparetic side such as clumsiness, ataxia, hyperreflexia, and extensor plantar reflex. Occasionally, there are abnormal movements such as shivering, twitching, shaking, or jerking of the relatively spared side, which may be precipitated by painful stimuli [112]. Unless a therapy (e.g., recanalization) is quickly performed, asymmetrical motor disturbances often progress to severe quadriplegia. The progression usually occurs within 24 h [113] but may be delayed up to several days (Fig. 4.7F).

Ataxia or incoordination is another common finding, observed in the limbs that are not severely paretic. The ataxia is invariably bilateral but is frequently asymmetric. Dysarthria and dysphagia due to bilateral bulbar muscle paresis are also common, associated with bilateral facial weakness, tongue weakness, and limited jaw movements. Some patients become totally unable to speak, open their mouth, or protrude their tongue. The jaw, face, and pharyngeal reflexes may be hyperactive and even clonic. Secretions pool in the pharynx and are an important cause of aspiration pneumonia. Somatosensory abnormalities should also be common, but they are usually overshadowed by motor dysfunction and cannot be precisely assessed in patients with severe condition. Occasionally, patients complain of uncomfortable paresthesias or CPSP.

Because large bilateral pontine infarcts frequently involve the dorsal tegmental area, ocular motor dysfunction is also common, which include INO, horizontal gaze palsy, one-and-a-half syndrome, and sixth nerve palsies. Ocular bobbing, ptosis, and pinpoint pupils strongly suggest extensive, bilateral tegmental lesions (see above). Symptoms such as tinnitus, hearing loss, and auditory hallucination are related to involvement of the central auditory tracts or the eighth nerves/fascicles. Some may develop delayed-onset palatal myoclonus.

Altered consciousness is an important sign in patients with sudden BA occlusion and is related to bilateral medial tegmental pontine ischemia. Usually, the level of consciousness improves overtime even if other neurological deficits persist. Patients may show pathological crying and laughing spells that are triggered by minimal social-emotional stimuli. When all voluntary movements are lost, the deficit is referred to as the "locked-in" syndrome. Vertical eye movements are usually spared and are used for simple communications.

Stroke Mechanisms

Unilateral infarcts involving the ventral pons are caused either by large artery disease or penetrating artery disease. Studies primarily using MRA revealed that BA atherosclerotic stenosis was associated with 23% of pontine infarction [62] and 39–50% of pontine base infarction [63, 65, 108]. Therefore, branch occlusion associated with BA stenosis is an important stroke mechanism of pontine base infarction (Figs. 3.4A and 3.5 in Chap. 3). Even in patients without MRA-identified BA stenosis, small plaques that obstruct

the orifice of perforating branches are occasionally seen if high-resolution vessel wall MRI is used [114] (lower panel of Fig. 3.5 in Chap. 3). Pontine infarcts limited to the tegmental area are mostly caused by penetrating artery disease (lipohyalinosis) (Fig. 3.4B in Chap. 3), unassociated with BA disease [62, 65, 71]. Although uncommon, however, the most dorsally located infarcts may be associated with significant, bilateral intracranial VA or BA steno-occlusive disease. Restoration of BA flow through collaterals (e.g., the posterior communicating artery) explains the sparing of the other parts of the pons [80].

In patients with bilateral pontine infarction, significant BA steno-occlusive disease is usually present [106]. Pathologically, the vast majority is atherothrombosis, and dissection is uncommon as compared to medullary infarction. Occasional patients with bilateral pontine infarcts have sequential infarcts caused by occlusion of BA branches on both sides. In these patients, a hemiparesis is followed days, weeks, or months later by another event that leads to paresis on the other side of the body. Embolism is a less common cause of isolated pontine infarction.

Prognosis

Unless accompanied by infarcts in other areas, the prognosis of unilateral pontine infarction is relatively favorable. Most patients survive the acute stage. Their functional deficits depend upon residual neurologic severity. Patients with initially severe hemiparesis, progressive worsening, bilateral ataxia, and lower pontine lesion have relatively unfavorable functional outcomes [62, 65, 68]. The prognosis of patients with tegmental lesions is even better. However, patients with severe sensory deficits may have difficulty in performing fine movements due to sensory deficits. More problematic is the development of CPSP, which usually remains persistent once it develops. When patients have INO as an isolated symptom, INO mostly improves [80]. However, in patients with more extensive ocular dysfunction associated with other major neurologic sequelae, residual ocular motor dysfunction frequently remains, and patients suffer from prolonged diplopia and dizziness. The prognosis of bilateral pontine infarcts presenting with quadriparesis is ominous. Unless promptly and appropriately treated in the early stage, most patients die or remain bed-ridden with quadriparesis. There may be persistent sensory disturbances, diplopia, dizziness, or palatal myoclonus.

Midbrain Infarction

The midbrain is supplied by branches arising from the PCA, upper BA, SCA, and the anterior choroidal artery. It is often affected in patients with embolic stroke occurring in the posterior circulation, usually with the concomitant involvement of other structures such as the thalamus, cerebellum, and occipital lobe [115]. According to the New England Medical Center Registry, midbrain infarction is ten-fold more likely to be accompanied by ischemia of neighboring structures than it is to occur in isolation [116]. Isolated midbrain infarcts account for 0.2–2.3% of admitted ischemic strokes [117–119]. While one study showed that pure midbrain infarct occupied 0.7% of posterior circulation ischemic stroke [116], another reported that it represented 8% of posterior circulation infarcts [118].

Clinical Features

The third nerve palsy has been considered the most important clinical feature indicating midbrain stroke. However, with the advent of MRI, it has been recognized that nonlocalizing "lacunar" syndromes are actually more common. In the largest series that used MRI [117], clinical manifestations included gait ataxia (68%), dysarthria (55%), limb ataxia (50%), sensory symptoms (43%), third nerve palsy (35%), limb weakness (≤IV/V) (23%), and INO (13%).

Ocular Motor Dysfunction

Third Nerve Palsy
Third nerve palsy occurs in 33–50% [117, 118, 120] of patients with pure midbrain infarction due to involvement of either the third nerve fascicles or the nucleus. Lesions that affect the third nerve nucleus often cause bilateral ptosis and upgaze deficits; this is attributed to involvement of the caudal subnucleus supplying both levator palpebrae, and the crossing fibers from the contralateral subnucleus of the superior rectus, respectively, within the third nucleus complex [121].

The third nerve palsy is frequently incomplete, and certain ocular muscles may be selectively involved. For example, divisional oculomotor paresis was reported to be caused by midbrain lesions involving the fascicle suggesting the functional separation of superior (subserving levator palpebrae, superior rectus) and inferior (subserving inferior and medial rectus and inferior oblique) divisions within the brainstem in the fascicular portion of the nerve [122]. Patients with a tiny lesion within the third nucleus may even produce weakness of a single extraocular muscle such as the inferior rectus [79] or medial rectus [123]. A very small infarct was reported to produce isolated inferior rectus palsy due to selective involvement of the relevant fascicle [124].

Internuclear Ophthalmoplegia
The lesions producing an INO are located in the paramedian, dorsal lower midbrain, involving the MLF. A detailed description of INO was included with the topic of pontine infarction. Patients frequently have ocular tilt reaction [125].

Vertical Gaze Disturbances
Involvement of the most rostral part of the midbrain produces vertical gaze paresis (see the section "Top of the Basilar Artery Syndrome").

Fourth Nerve Palsy
The trochlear nucleus lies in the lower midbrain caudal to the oculomotor nuclear complex. Unlike third nerve fascicles that travel in the paramedian area, the fourth nerve fascicles run dorsally around the aqueduct to decussate in the anterior medullary velum just caudal to the inferior colliculus. Because this dorsolateral part of the lower midbrain is mainly supplied by the SCA, fourth nerve palsy is almost always accompanied by concomitant SCA infarction [79, 126] (Fig. 4.11D). Because the lesions mostly dam-

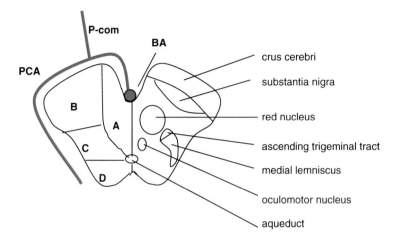

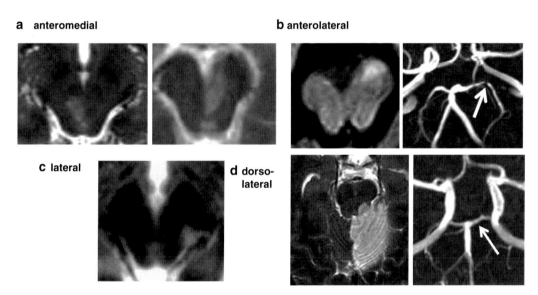

a   anteromedial   **b anterolateral**

c lateral   **d dorso-**
                                     lateral

Fig. 4.11 Illustrative patients and schematic drawing of midbrain indicating important structures, supplying vessels and four topographic subgroups. (**A**) Anteromedial, (**B**) anterolateral, (**C**) lateral, and (**D**) dorsolateral (posterior). (**A**) Both patients had ipsilateral oculomotor disturbances and mild contralateral ataxia. (**B**) The patient had dysarthria and clumsy hand on the right side. MRA showed stenosis in the P2 portion of the left posterior cerebral artery (arrow).

(**C**) The patient presented with pure sensory stroke. (**D**) The patient had concomitant cerebellar infarction. MRA showed occlusion of the superior cerebellar artery (arrow) due to cardiac embolism. He had left limb ataxia, decreased sensory perception on the right side, and right superior oblique palsy. (Modified from Kim JS, Kim J. Pure midbrain infarction: Clinical, radiologic, and pathophysiologic findings. Neurology 2005;64;1227–1232)

age the trochlear nucleus or the fascicle before decussation, superior oblique palsy usually develops in the eye contralateral to the midbrain stroke.

Hemiparesis and Other Motor Dysfunction

Although limb weakness is found in more than half of patients, a significant hemiparesis is pres-

ent in only approximately 1/4 of patients when the pyramidal tract at the crus cerebri was heavily and densely involved [117] (Fig. 4.11). The uncommon occurrence of severe hemiparesis may at least in part be due to sparsely arranged pyramidal fibers in the crus cerebri as compared to the lower brainstem [68]. Dysarthria is invariably present, and hemiataxia may be observed in patients without severe hemiparesis.

Sensory Symptoms/Signs

Unlike the pons, where the sensory tracts are located in the paramedian area, the sensory tracts are located at the dorsolateral portion of the midbrain (Fig. 4.11). In one study, sensory disturbances were observed in 43% of pure midbrain infarction [117]. However, because infarcts preferentially involve the paramedian area, sensory symptoms are often minor and restricted to certain body parts. Cheiro-oral distribution is relatively common [117], probably because face and finger representation areas are located medially in the sensory tract, being vulnerable from paramedian infarction. Mesencephalic pure hemisensory syndrome is rare and is caused by small infarcts or hemorrhages affecting the dorsolateral area [71, 117] (Fig. 4.11C).

Ataxia

Ataxia is one of the most frequently observed symptoms/signs in midbrain infarction [117], probably related to the presence of abundant neuronal fibers connecting with the cerebellum in the midbrain: the descending corticopontocerebellar fibers at the crus cerebri and ascending cerebello-rubro-thalamic tracts in the paramedian area near the red nucleus (Fig. 4.11).

In the cerebral peduncle, descending cerebellar fibers areas are rarely involved in isolation, and concomitant involvement of the pyramidal tracts or corticobulbar tracts lead to syndromes such as ataxic hemiparesis or dysarthria with ataxia. Paramedian lesions affecting ascending cerebello-rubro-thalamic tracts at or near the red nucleus may produce ataxia without significant other motor dysfunction. Because paramedian lesions usually involve the oculomotor nucleus or fascicles, ipsilateral third nerve palsy is often combined with contralateral ataxia (Claude syndrome).

Patients with unilateral lower midbrain lesion may have bilateral ataxia usually worse on the contralateral side [117, 118]. This is attributed to bilateral involvement of crossing efferent dentato-rubral fibers at the lower midbrain level by lesions located in the paramedian area. Bilateral ataxia

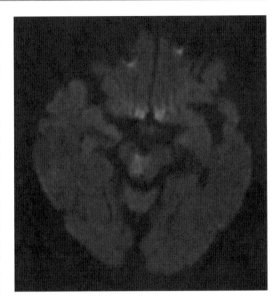

Fig. 4.12 An 81-year-old woman had dizziness, severe dysarthria, bilateral ataxia, and gait difficulty. Diffusion-weighted MRI showed left paramedian infarction in the midbrain. Despite rehabilitation therapy, the symptoms persist, and she was not able to walk alone after 5 years of follow-up

caused by a single lesion is a localizing sign for paramedian lower midbrain infarction. The outcome of such patients is unfavorable; they have marked dysarthria and long-lasting gait instability (Fig. 4.12).

Involuntary Movements

Holmes Tremor

Patients with midbrain strokes occasionally develop a tremor, referred to as "rubral tremor" or "Holmes tremor." The characteristics of the tremor are as follows [127]:

(a) Intention and resting tremor, but some may show postural tremor as well.

　　The tremor may not be as regular as other tremors and occasionally shows jerky components.

(b) Tremor is of low frequency, mostly below 4.5 Hz.

(c) There is a variable delay (mostly 2 weeks to 2 years) between the onset of the lesion and the appearance of tremors.

The tremor is predominantly unilateral and mainly affects the hands and the proximal arm.

The responsible lesions are usually situated at the superior and external part of the red nucleus affecting the rubro-thalamic pathways. Lesions affecting the thalamus, the central tegmental tract in the pons, or deep nuclei of the cerebellum may cause similar movement disorders.

Dopaminergic PET imaging studies showed striatal dopaminergic dysfunction in these patients, probably due to the involvement of the nigrostriatal system [128, 129]. Some suggested that combined damage of the cerebellothalamic and nigrostriatal system may be required to generate Holmes tremor [130, 131]. Ipsilateral third nerve palsy accompanied by contralateral ataxia and tremor is referred to as Benedict syndrome.

Parkinsonism

Midbrain strokes may produce hemi-parkinsonism due to involvement of the substantia nigra [132–134]. The prevalence is very low, probably because parkinsonian symptoms are masked by other major deficits such as hemiparesis or ataxia. However, if carefully tested, subtle symptoms such as micrographia [135] or hypokinetic dysarthria and palilalia [136] are observed. Dopaminergic system dysfunction is documented by PET imaging in these patients.

Dystonia

Unilateral dystonia may be observed in patients with extensive ponto-mesencephalic tegmental lesions [137], usually associated with sensorimotor dysfunction and other involuntary movements such as rubral tremor or excessive twitching.

Asterixis

Paramedian midbrain infarcts may produce asterixis in the contralateral limbs [138], probably related to the involvement of the rubrospinal or cerebellar-rubral tracts that are involved in the regulation of postural/tonic control of extremities.

Neuropsychiatric and Emotional Disturbances

Symptoms such as emotional incontinence [54], agitation, and impulsive behavior [139] have been reported in patients with midbrain infarction. These features may be related to serotonergic or limbic dopaminergic system involvement.

Clinical–Topographical Correlation

According to MRI findings, the lesions are categorized as the following groups (Fig. 4.11).

Anteromedial (or Paramedian) Lesion

Approximately 50–60% of pure midbrain infarctions belong to this group [117, 120] (Fig. 4.11A). The lesions usually involve the third nerve fascicles or nucleus (at the upper midbrain), the MLF (at the lower midbrain), the red nucleus, and the medial part of the cerebral peduncle. The clinical features are characterized by ocular motor disturbances (third nerve palsy or INO), contralateral mild hemiparesis, and ataxia. Ataxia may be bilateral when the paramedian lesion is located in the lower midbrain (Fig. 4.12). Sensory deficits, when present, are usually mild and often present in restricted body parts such as the perioral or perioral-hand areas.

Anterolateral Lesion

Approximately 1/4 of patients belong to this group [117, 120] (Fig. 4.11B). Because the crus cerebri is primarily involved, patients' main symptom is hemiparesis. Although severe motor dysfunction in uncommon (see above), some patients may have progressively worsening hemiparesis. In patients who do not have severe hemiparesis, ataxic hemiparesis, dysarthria-clumsy hand syndrome, pure dysarthria, and dysarthria-ataxia may develop. If adjacent sensory tracts are involved, sensory deficits may be added.

Combined Lesions

Some patients have lesions in both anteromedial and anterolateral areas. Clinical features are the combination of the two: ocular motor disturbances, ataxia, and various motor syndromes.

Lateral Lesion

Although quite uncommon, lesions may be confined to the lateral part of the midbrain (Fig. 4.11C). The clinical features are characterized by hemisensory deficits caused by involvement of the laterally located sensory lemniscus. The clinical features are not distinguishable from a thalamic pure sensory stroke.

Dorsolateral Lesion

This area is supplied by the SCA, and infarcts occurring in this area are almost always accompanied by concomitant cerebellar infarction. Fourth nerve palsy, INO, ataxia, and contralateral sensory disturbances may be present (Fig. 4.11D).

Bilateral Lesions

Bilateral midbrain infarctions are almost always accompanied by extensive infarcts in the other parts of posterior circulation [117, 120]. Patients develop altered consciousness, quadriparesis, severe dysarthria, dysphagia, and, ultimately, a locked-in state. Patients may have bilateral oculomotor palsy [120], but ocular movements may remain intact if dorsal areas are spared [140, 141].

Stroke Mechanism

Approximately 2/3 of pure midbrain infarction is caused by large artery atherosclerotic disease. Anteromedial, anterolateral, and combined type lesions are usually caused by branch occlusion associated with PCA or rostral BA atherothrombosis [117] (Fig. 3.4A in Chap. 3, Fig. 4.11B). Small penetrating artery disease explains stroke in approximately 1/4 of the patients who have deep-seated lesions (Fig. 3.4B in Chap. 3). Cardiac embolism is rare in patients with isolated midbrain infarction [117, 120]. The stroke mechanism of the lateral group is uncertain, but artery-to-artery embolization from tightly stenosed BA was reported [117]. Dorsolateral infarcts are almost always caused by SCA occlusion, which is most often caused by cardiac embolism (Fig. 4.11D).

Prognosis

In patients with pure midbrain infarction, the lesions are mostly unilateral, and the prognosis is relatively good. Initial severe motor dysfunction may predict a worse prognosis. However, in one study, 36 out of 40 patients were functionally independent after 2 years of follow-up [117]. The functional outcome of patients with bilateral ataxia (Fig. 4.12) is unfavorable because they usually have persistent gait difficulty and dysarthria. As in patients with medullary or pontine infarction, underlying vascular diseases (BA or PCA) probably affect the future outcome of these patients. Patients with bilateral infarction have a grave prognosis; they often die due to aspiration pneumonia and frequently remain locked-in.

Top of the Basilar Artery Syndrome

Infarction of rostral brainstem and cerebral hemispheral regions fed by the distal BA causes a clinically recognizable syndrome characterized by visual, ocular motor, and behavioral abnormalities, often without significant motor dysfunction. Caplan [115] described this as "top of the basilar artery syndrome." Typically, there are bilateral, multiple infarcts in the paramedian midbrain, medial thalamus, medial temporal areas, and occipital lobes (Fig. 4.13). The clinical features vary greatly and depend on the topography of the damaged brain. Occasionally, bilateral SCA infarctions are the only manifestation of basilar tip occlusion when bilateral fetal type PCAs are present without anastomosis between the anterior and posterior circulations [142].

Clinical Features

Ocular Motor Dysfunction

See Chap. 7 for details.

Vertical Gaze Palsy

Vertical gaze pathways from the cerebral cortex converge on the periaqueductal region beneath the collicular plate, near the interstitial nucleus of Cajal and the posterior commissure. In this region, there is a cluster of neurons regulating vertical gaze, referred to as rostral interstitial

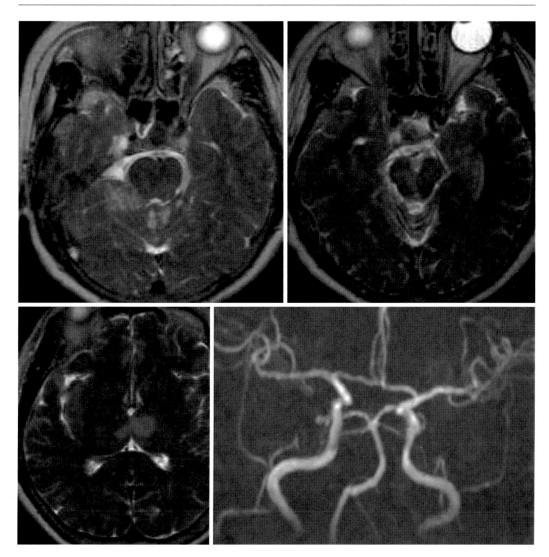

Fig. 4.13 A 75-year-old woman with atrial fibrillation became drowy and confused. Examination showed confused mentality, somnolence, anterograde memory impairment, vertical gaze failure, and gait ataxia. MRI showed multiple infarcts in the cerebellum, midbrain, and bilateral paramedian thalamus. MRA showed normal basilar artery, suggesting that occluded basilar tip was already recanalized

MLF (riMLF) [143, 144]. Extensive lesions occurring in the rostral midbrain result in both upgaze and downgaze failure. Vertical VOR is usually preserved. A unilateral lesion affecting the posterior commissure can cause upward saccadic failure due probably to the fact that fibers involved in upward saccades decussate through the posterior commissure, which connects the riMLF on both sides [145, 146]. Bilateral damage to the riMLF is usually required to produce down gaze paresis; therefore, isolated upgaze palsy is more common than down gaze paresis [147, 148]. If the connections from the riMLF to the third nuclei are selectively damaged just above the nucleus on one side, monocular upgaze palsy may occur [149–151]. A vertical one-and-a-half syndrome (upward gaze paresis with monocular downward gaze paresis or downward gaze paresis with monocular upward gaze paresis) is also observed [152, 153].

Convergence, Eyelid, and Pupillary Abnormalities

Ocular convergence is probably controlled in the medial midbrain tegmentum. Convergence vectors are frequently evident on an attempted upward gaze. Rhythmic convergence nystagmus may be elicited if patients are told to follow a downgoing opticokinetic target with their eyes. Convergence vectors may modify lateral gaze, and patients may show pseudo-sixth nerve palsy [115]. Lid abnormalities are also a sign of rostral brainstem infarction. Unilateral infarction of the third cranial nerve nucleus can lead to complete bilateral ptosis [89]. Retraction of the upper lid (Collier's sign) may be observed in patients with tectal lesions [154]. When ischemia affects the Edinger–Westphal nucleus, the pupils may be fixed and dilated, whereas if the lesion involves sympathetic fibers, the pupil size becomes smaller [155].

Somnolence and Loss of Attention

The medial mesencephalon and diencephalon contain the most rostral portions of the reticular activating system. Infarcts in these regions frequently produce excessive sleep and lack of attention. Because the reticular gray matter is adjacent to the third nerve nuclei, riMLF, and the posterior commissure, somnolence is frequently associated with relevant ocular motor disturbances.

Hallucinations

Patients with rostral brainstem infarction often have hallucinations (peduncular hallucinosis) [156]. The hallucinations tend to occur at twilight or during the night, and such patients usually have sleep disorders (nocturnal insomnia or daytime hypersomnolence) [115]. The hallucinations are usually vivid and mostly visual and contain multiple colors, objects, and scenes. Occasionally, auditory or tactile hallucinations are associated. Bilateral infarcts confined to the medial substantia nigra pars reticulata are reported to cause peduncular hallucinosis [157]. However, similar hallucinations are observed in patients with infarcts that involve the pons or the posterior thalamus [158]. Neuropsychological testing in patients

with hallucination show impairments of episodic memory, confabulation, attention deficits, confusion, delusion, and misidentification for persons and places. It seems that brainstem hallucinosis may be related with the dysfunctional ascending reticular system and thalamocortical circuits [159].

Confabulations

Confabulations are often reported in patients with rostral brainstem infarcts [115]. The features are similar to what were described as Wernicke-Korsakoff psychosis.

Hemiballism and Abnormal Movements

Hemichorea or ballism may occur from infarcts affecting the subthalamic nucleus (corpus Luysii) [160]. Other movement disorders related to midbrain involvement are described above (see the section "**Midbrain Infarction**").

Other Symptoms and Signs

Occipital and thalamic infarcts are common, and relevant symptoms and signs are described in Chap. 5. Embolism may produce infarcts in the other parts of the brainstem, and the relevant symptoms and signs are described in the early part of this chapter.

Stroke Mechanisms and Prognosis

Occlusions of the BA tip are generally embolic [115], more often from the heart than proximal artery atherothrombosis. Although uncommon, atherothrombosis occurring in the distal BA can also result in this syndrome [161]. In patients with embolic occlusion, the embolic fragments may also occlude other vessels such as the PICA, SCA, or pontine branches before they reach to the top of BA. PCA territory infarcts are also commonly found. In patients with cardiac embolism, an embolus is frequently evanescent, and it may already be gone at the time of the angiographic study (Fig. 4.13). In this case, the patient's prognosis is generally good, although they may have residual deficits depending on already damaged structures. However, persistent BA occlusion may lead to downward extension of thrombi to result in catastrophic bilateral brainstem infarction. The recent advent of endovascular thrombectomy is of great help in the early and successful recanalization of the occluded BA (see Chap. 11). Aside from the successful recanalization, adequate collateral system (e.g., the presence of textbook-type posterior communication artery) appears to be associated with better functional outcome in these patients [162].

References

1. Wallenberg A. Acute bulbar affection (Embolie der art. cerebellar post. inf. sinistra ?). Arch f Psychiat Nervenkr. 1895;27:504–40.
2. Norrving B, Cronqvist S. Lateral medullary infarction: prognosis in an unselected series. Neurology. 1991;41((2(Pt 1))):244–8.
3. Lewis GLN, Littman A, Foley EF. The syndrome of thrombosis of the posterior inferior cerebellar artery: a report of 28 cases. Ann Intern Med. 1952;36(2:2):592–602.
4. Peterman AF, Sieker TR. The lateral medullary (Wallenberg) syndrome: clinical features and prognosis. Med Clin North Am. 1960;44:887–96.
5. Currier RD, Giles CL, DeJong RN. Some comments on Wallenberg's lateral medullary syndrome. Neurology. 1961;1:778–92.
6. Fisher CM, Karnes WE, Kubik CS. Lateral medullary infarction-the pattern of vascular occlusion. J Neuropathol Exp Neurol. 1961;20:323–79.
7. Sacco RL, Freddo L, Bello JA, Odel JG, Onesti ST, Mohr JP. Wallenberg's lateral medullary syndrome. Clinical-magnetic resonance imaging correlations. Arch Neurol. 1993;50(6):609–14.
8. Vuilleumier P, Bogousslavsky J, Regli F. Infarction of the lower brainstem. Clinical, aetiological and MRI-topographical correlations. Brain. 1995;118(Pt 4):1013–25.
9. Kim JS, Lee JH, Lee MC. Patterns of sensory dysfunction in lateral medullary infarction. Clinical-MRI correlation. Neurology. 1997;49(6):1557–63.
10. Kim JS. Pure lateral medullary infarction: clinical-radiological correlation of 130 acute, consecutive patients. Brain. 2003;126(Pt 8):1864–72.
11. Kim JS, Lee JH, Suh DC, Lee MC. Spectrum of lateral medullary syndrome. Correlation between clinical findings and magnetic resonance imaging in 33 subjects. Stroke. 1994;25(7):1405–10.
12. Caplan LR. Posterior circulation disease: clinical findings, diagnosis, and management. Boston: Blackwell Science; 1996. p. 262–323.
13. Dieterich M, Brandt T. Wallenberg's syndrome: lateropulsion, cyclorotation, and subjective visual vertical in thirty-six patients. Ann Neurol. 1992;31(4):399–408.
14. Marx JJ, Iannetti GD, Thomke F, Fitzek S, Galeotti F, Truini A, et al. Topodiagnostic implications of hemiataxia: an MRI-based brainstem mapping analysis. NeuroImage. 2008;39(4):1625–32.
15. Meyer KT, Baloh RW, Krohel GB, Hepler RS. Ocular lateropulsion. A sign of lateral medullary disease. Arch Ophthalmol. 1980;98(9):1614–6.
16. Kwon M, Lee JH, Kim JS. Dysphagia in unilateral medullary infarction: lateral vs medial lesions. Neurology. 2005;65(5):714–8.
17. Calne DB, Pallis CA. Vibratory sense: a critical review. Brain. 1966;89(4):723–46.
18. Matsumoto S, Okuda B, Imai T, Kameyama M. A sensory level on the trunk in lower lateral brainstem lesions. Neurology. 1988;38(10):1515–9.
19. Kim JS. Sensory symptoms in ipsilateral limbs/body due to lateral medullary infarction. Neurology. 2001;57(7):1230–4.
20. Caplan L, Gorelick P. "Salt and pepper on the face" pain in acute brainstem ischemia. Ann Neurol. 1983;13(3):344–5.
21. Reutens DC. Burning oral and mid-facial pain in ventral pontine infarction. Aust NZ J Med. 1990;20(3):249–50.
22. Kuypers HG. Corticobular connexions to the pons and lower brain-stem in man: an anatomical study. Brain. 1958;81(3):364–88.
23. Fisher CM, Tapia J. Lateral medullary infarction extending to the lower pons. J Neurol Neurosurg Psychiatry. 1987;50(5):620–4.
24. Bogousslavsky J, Khurana R, Deruaz JP, Hornung JP, Regli F, Janzer R, et al. Respiratory failure and unilateral caudal brainstem infarction. Ann Neurol. 1990;28(5):668–73.
25. Opalski A. Un nouveau syndrome sous-bulbaire: syndrome partiel de l'artère vertébro-spinale postérieur. Paris Med. 1946;1:214–20.
26. Hermann DM, Jung HH, Bassetti CL. Lateral medullary infarct with alternating and dissociated sensorimotor deficits: Opalski's syndrome revisited. Eur J Neurol. 2009;16(4):e72–4.
27. Nakamura S, Kitami M, Furukawa Y. Opalski syndrome: ipsilateral hemiplegia due to a lateral-medullary infarction. Neurology. 2010;75(18):1658.
28. Carpenter MBSJ. Human neuroanatomy. 8th ed. Baltimore: Williams & Wilkins; 1983. p. 315–57.
29. Vuillier F, Tatu L, Dietsch E, Medeiros E, Moulin T. Pontomedullary sulcus infarct: a variant of lateral medullary syndrome. J Neurol Neurosurg Psychiatry. 2006;77(11):1276–8.
30. Castaigne P, Lhermitte F, Gautier JC, Escourolle R, Derouesne C, Der Agopian P, et al. Arterial occlusions in the vertebro-basilar system. A study of 44 patients with post-mortem data. Brain. 1973;96(1):133–54.
31. Caplan LR. Occlusion of the vertebral or basilar artery. Follow up analysis of some patients with benign outcome. Stroke. 1979;10(3):277–82.

32. Kim TJ, Nam H, Hong JH, Yeo MJ, Chang JY, Jeong JH, et al. Dysphagia may be an independent marker of poor outcome in acute lateral medullary infarction. J Clin Neurol. 2015;11(4):349–57.

33. Kang HG, Kim BJ, Lee SH, Kang DW, Kwon SU, Kim JS. Lateral medullary infarction with or without extra-lateral medullary lesions: what is the difference? Cerebrovasc Dis. 2018;45(3–4):132–40.

34. Kim JS, Choi-Kwon S. Sensory sequelae of medullary infarction: differences between lateral and medial medullary syndrome. Stroke. 1999;30(12):2697–703.

35. MacGowan DJ, Janal MN, Clark WC, Wharton RN, Lazar RM, Sacco RL, et al. Central poststroke pain and Wallenberg's lateral medullary infarction: frequency, character, and determinants in 63 patients. Neurology. 1997;49(1):120–5.

36. Kim SJ, Ryoo S, Bang OY, Chung CS, Lee KH, Kim GM. Perfusion-weighted MRI as a predictor of clinical outcomes following medullary infarctions. Cerebrovasc Dis. 2010;29(4):382–8.

37. Spiller WG. The symptom-complex of a lesion of the upper most portion of the anterior spinal and adjoining portion of the vertebral arteries. J Nerv Mednt Dis. 1908;35:775–8.

38. Dejerine J. Semiologie des affections du système nerveux. Paris: Masson; 1914. p. 226–30.

39. Davison C. Syndrome of the anterior spinal artery of the medulla oblongata. Arch Neurol Psychiatr. 1937;37:91–107.

40. Kim JS, Kim HG, Chung CS. Medial medullary syndrome. Report of 18 new patients and a review of the literature. Stroke. 1995;26(9):1548–52.

41. Toyoda K, Imamura T, Saku Y, Oita J, Ibayashi S, Minematsu K, et al. Medial medullary infarction: analyses of eleven patients. Neurology. 1996;47(5):1141–7.

42. Bassetti C, Bogousslavsky J, Mattle H, Bernasconi A. Medial medullary stroke: report of seven patients and review of the literature. Neurology. 1997;48(4):882–90.

43. Kumral E, Afsar N, Kirbas D, Balkir K, Ozdemirkiran T. Spectrum of medial medullary infarction: clinical and magnetic resonance imaging findings. J Neurol. 2002;249(1):85–93.

44. Park JY, Chun MH, Kang SH, Lee JA, Kim BR, Shin MJ. Functional outcome in poststroke patients with or without fatigue. Am J Phys Med Rehabil. 2009;88(7):554–8.

45. Kim JS, Han YS. Medial medullary infarction: clinical, imaging, and outcome study in 86 consecutive patients. Stroke. 2009;40(10):3221–5.

46. Ropper AH, Fisher CM, Kleinman GM. Pyramidal infarction in the medulla: a cause of pure motor hemiplegia sparing the face. Neurology. 1979;29(1):91–5.

47. Kim JS, Koh JY, Lee JH. Medial medullary infarction with restricted sensory symptom. Eur Neurol. 1998;39(3):174–7.

48. Lee SH, Kim DE, Song EC, Roh JK. Sensory dermatomal representation in the medial lemniscus. Arch Neurol. 2001;58(4):649–51.

49. Kim JS, Choi KD, Oh SY, Park SH, Han MK, Yoon BW, et al. Medial medullary infarction: abnormal ocular motor findings. Neurology. 2005;65(8):1294–8.

50. Kim JS, Moon SY, Kim KY, Kim HC, Park SH, Yoon BW, et al. Ocular contrapulsion in rostral medial medullary infarction. Neurology. 2004;63(7):1325–7.

51. Choi KD, Jung DS, Park KP, Jo JW, Kim JS. Bowtie and upbeat nystagmus evolving into hemiseesaw nystagmus in medial medullary infarction: possible anatomic mechanisms. Neurology. 2004;62(4):663–5.

52. Brown WJ, Fang HC. Spastic hemiplegia in man associated with unilateral infarct of the cortico spinal tract at the pontomedullary juncture. Trans Am Neurol Assoc. 1956;(81st Meeting):22–6.

53. Paulson GW, Yates AJ, Paltan-Ortiz JD. Does infarction of the medullary pyramid lead to spasticity? Arch Neurol. 1986;43(1):93–5.

54. Kim JS, Choi-Kwon S. Poststroke depression and emotional incontinence: correlation with lesion location. Neurology. 2000;54(9):1805–10.

55. Fisher CM, Curry HB. Pure motor hemiplegia of vascular origin. Arch Neurol. 1965;13:30–44.

56. Mizutani T, Lewis RA, Gonatas NK. Medial medullary syndrome in a drug abuser. Arch Neurol. 1980;37(7):425–8.

57. Kase CS, Varakis JN, Stafford JR, Mohr JP. Medial medullary infarction from fibrocartilaginous embolism to the anterior spinal artery. Stroke. 1983;14(3):413–8.

58. Tyler KL, Sandberg E, Baum KF. Medical medullary syndrome and meningovascular syphilis: a case report in an HIV-infected man and a review of the literature. Neurology. 1994;44(12):2231–5.

59. Meyer JS, Herndon RM. Bilateral infarction of the pyramidal tracts in man. Neurology. 1962;12:637–42.

60. Reinhold H. Beitrage zur Pathologie der akuten Erweichungen des Pons und der Oblongata. Zugleich ein Beitrag zur Lehre von der "Bulbaeren Ataxie.". Dtsch Zeit Nervenheilk. 1894;5:351–74.

61. Babinski J, Nageotte J. Hdmiasynergie, lateropulsion et myosis bulbaires avec hemianesthesie et hemiplegie croisees. Rev Neurol (Paris). 1902;10:358–65.

62. Bassetti C, Bogousslavsky J, Barth A, Regli F. Isolated infarcts of the pons. Neurology. 1996;46(1):165–75.

63. Kumral E, Bayulkem G, Evyapan D. Clinical spectrum of pontine infarction. Clinical-MRI correlations. J Neurol. 2002;249(12):1659–70.

64. Erro ME, Gallego J, Herrera M, Bermejo B. Isolated pontine infarcts: etiopathogenic mechanisms. Eur J Neurol. 2005;12(12):984–8.

65. Kataoka S, Hori A, Shirakawa T, Hirose G. Paramedian pontine infarction. Neurological/topographical correlation. Stroke. 1997;28(4):809–15.

66. Fisher CM. Ataxic hemiparesis. A pathologic study. Arch Neurol. 1978;35(3):126–8.

67. Fisher CM. A lacunar stroke. The dysarthria-clumsy hand syndrome. Neurology. 1967;17(6):614–7.

68. Kim JS, Lee JH, Im JH, Lee MC. Syndromes of pontine base infarction. A clinical-radiological correlation study. Stroke. 1995;26(6):950–5.

69. Helgason CM, Wilbur AC. Basilar branch pontine infarction with prominent sensory signs. Stroke. 1991;22(9):1129–36.

70. Caplan LR, Goodwin JA. Lateral tegmental brainstem hemorrhages. Neurology. 1982;32(3):252–60.

71. Kim JS, Bae YH. Pure or predominant sensory stroke due to brain stem lesion. Stroke. 1997;28(9):1761–4.

72. Shintani S, Tsuruoka S, Shiigai T. Pure sensory stroke caused by a pontine infarct. Clinical, radiological, and physiological features in four patients. Stroke. 1994;25(7):1512–5.

73. Kim JS. Restricted acral sensory syndrome following minor stroke. Further observation with special reference to differential severity of symptoms among individual digits. Stroke. 1994;25(12):2497–502.

74. Combarros O, Berciano J, Oterino A. Pure sensory deficit with crossed orocrural topography after pontine haemorrhage. J Neurol Neurosurg Psychiatry. 1996;61(5):534–5.

75. Holtzman RN, Zablozki V, Yang WC, Leeds NE. Lateral pontine tegmental hemorrhage presenting as isolated trigeminal sensory neuropathy. Neurology. 1987;37(4):704–6.

76. Sunada I, Akano Y, Yamamoto S, Tashiro T. Pontine haemorrhage causing disturbance of taste. Neuroradiology. 1995;37(8):659.

77. Donaldson D, Rosenberg NL. Infarction of abducens nerve fascicle as cause of isolated sixth nerve palsy related to hypertension. Neurology. 1988;38(10):1654.

78. Fukutake T, Hirayama K. Isolated abducens nerve palsy from pontine infarction in a diabetic patient. Neurology. 1992;42(11):2226.

79. Kim JS, Kang JK, Lee SA, Lee MC. Isolated or predominant ocular motor nerve palsy as a manifestation of brain stem stroke. Stroke. 1993;24(4):581–6.

80. Kim JS. Internuclear ophthalmoplegia as an isolated or predominant symptom of brainstem infarction. Neurology. 2004;62(9):1491–6.

81. Daroff R, Hoyt W. Supranuclear disorders of ocular control systems in man. In: Bach Y, Rita P, Collins C, editors. The control of eye movements. Orlando, FL: Academic Press; 1977. p. 175.

82. Pierrot-Deseilligny C, Chain F, Lhermitte F. The pontine reticular formation syndrome. Physiopathologic data on voluntary eye movement abnormalities. Rev Neurol (Paris). 1982;138(6–7):517–32.

83. Miura K, Optican LM. Membrane channel properties of premotor excitatory burst neurons may underlie saccade slowing after lesions of omnipause neurons. J Comput Neurosci. 2006;20(1):25–41.

84. Fisher CM. Some neuro-ophthalmological observations. J Neurol Neurosurg Psychiatry. 1967;30(5):383–92.

85. Pierrot-Deseilligny C, Chain F, Serdaru M, Gray F, Lhermitte F. The 'one-and-a-half' syndrome. Electro-oculographic analyses of five cases with deductions about the physiological mechanisms of lateral gaze. Brain. 1981;104(Pt 4):665–99.

86. Fisher CM. Ocular Bobbing. Arch Neurol. 1964;11:543–6.

87. Nelson JR, Johnston CH. Ocular bobbing. Arch Neurol. 1970;22(4):348–56.

88. Newman N, Gay AJ, Heilbrun MP. Disjugate ocular bobbing: its relation to midbrain, pontine, and medullary function in a surviving patient. Neurology. 1971;21(6):633–7.

89. Caplan LR. Ptosis. J Neurol Neurosurg Psychiatry. 1974;37(1):1–7.

90. Tahmoush AJ, Brooks JE, Keltner JL. Palatal myoclonus associated with abnormal ocular and extremity movements. A polygraphic study. Arch Neurol. 1972;27(5):431–40.

91. Lapresle J, Hamida MB. The dentato-olivary pathway. Somatotopic relationship between the dentate nucleus and the contralateral inferior olive. Arch Neurol. 1970;22(2):135–43.

92. Kim JS, Lee SB, Park SK, Han SR, Kim YI, Lee KS. Periodic limb movement during sleep developed after pontine lesion. Mov Disord. 2003;18(11):1403–5.

93. Han SH, Park KY, Youn YC, Shin HW. Restless legs syndrome and akathisia as manifestations of acute pontine infarction. J Clin Neurosci. 2014;21(2):354–5.

94. Lee SJ, Kim JS, Song IU, An JY, Kim YI, Lee KS. Poststroke restless legs syndrome and lesion location: anatomical considerations. Mov Disord. 2009;24(1):77–84.

95. Egan CA, Davies L, Halmagyi GM. Bilateral total deafness due to pontine haematoma. J Neurol Neurosurg Psychiatry. 1996;61(6):628–31.

96. Cascino GD, Adams RD. Brainstem auditory hallucinosis. Neurology. 1986;36(8):1042–7.

97. Lanska DJ, Lanska MJ, Mendez MF. Brainstem auditory hallucinosis. Neurology. 1987;37(10):1685.

98. Murata S, Naritomi H, Sawada T. Musical auditory hallucinations caused by a brainstem lesion. Neurology. 1994;44(1):156–8.

99. Lee E, Sohn HY, Kwon M, Kim JS. Contralateral hyperacusis in unilateral pontine hemorrhage. Neurology. 2008;70(24 Pt 2):2413–5.

100. Fisher CM. The neurological examination of the comatose patient. Acta Neurol Scand. 1969;45(Suppl 36):1–56.

101. Kim JS. Pathologic laughter after unilateral stroke. J Neurol Sci. 1997;148(1):121–5.

102. Kim JS, Choi S, Kwon SU, Seo YS. Inability to control anger or aggression after stroke. Neurology. 2002;58(7):1106–8.

103. Andersen G, Ingeman-Nielsen M, Vestergaard K, Riis JO. Pathoanatomic correlation between poststroke pathological crying and damage to brain areas involved in serotonergic neurotransmission. Stroke. 1994;25(5):1050–2.

104. Choi-Kwon S, Han SW, Kwon SU, Kang DW, Choi JM, Kim JS. Fluoxetine treatment in poststroke

depression, emotional incontinence, and anger proneness: a double-blind, placebo-controlled study. Stroke. 2006;37(1):156–61.

105. Drake ME Jr, Pakalnis A, Phillips B. Secondary mania after ventral pontine infarction. J Neuropsychiatry Clin Neurosci. 1990;2(3):322–5.

106. Ferbert A, Bruckmann H, Drummen R. Clinical features of proven basilar artery occlusion. Stroke. 1990;21(8):1135–42.

107. Kim JS, Lee JH, Lee MC, Lee SD. Transient abnormal behavior after pontine infarction. Stroke. 1994;25(11):2295–6.

108. Kim JS, Cho KH, Kang DW, Kwon SU, Suh DC. Basilar artery atherosclerotic disease is related to subacute lesion volume increase in pontine base infarction. Acta Neurol Scand. 2009;120(2):88–93.

109. Kubik CS, Adams RD. Occlusion of the basilar artery; a clinical and pathological study. Brain. 1946;69(2):73–121.

110. Voetsch B, DeWitt LD, Pessin MS, Caplan LR. Basilar artery occlusive disease in the New England Medical Center Posterior Circulation Registry. Arch Neurol. 2004;61(4):496–504.

111. Fisher CM. The 'herald hemiparesis' of basilar artery occlusion. Arch Neurol. 1988;45(12):1301–3.

112. Ropper AH. 'Convulsions' in basilar artery occlusion. Neurology. 1988;38(9):1500–1.

113. Biemond A. Thrombosis of the basilar artery and the vascularization of the brain stem. Brain. 1951;74(3):300–17.

114. Klein IF, Lavallee PC, Schouman-Claeys E, Amarenco P. High-resolution MRI identifies basilar artery plaques in paramedian pontine infarct. Neurology. 2005;64(3):551–2.

115. Caplan LR. "top of the basilar" syndrome. Neurology. 1980;30(1):72–9.

116. Martin PJ, Chang HM, Wityk R, Caplan LR. Midbrain infarction: associations and aetiologies in the New England Medical Center Posterior Circulation Registry. J Neurol Neurosurg Psychiatry. 1998;64(3):392–5.

117. Kim JS, Kim J. Pure midbrain infarction: clinical, radiologic, and pathophysiologic findings. Neurology. 2005;64(7):1227–32.

118. Bogousslavsky J, Maeder P, Regli F, Meuli R. Pure midbrain infarction: clinical syndromes, MRI, and etiologic patterns. Neurology. 1994;44(11):2032–40.

119. Kumral E, Bayulkem G, Akyol A, Yunten N, Sirin H, Sagduyu A. Mesencephalic and associated posterior circulation infarcts. Stroke. 2002;33(9):2224–31.

120. Ogawa K, Suzuki Y, Oishi M, Kamei S. Clinical study of twenty-one patients with pure midbrain infarction. Eur Neurol. 2012;67(2):81–9.

121. Leigh RJ, Zee DS. The neurology of eye movements. 3rd ed. New York: Oxford University Press; 1999. p. 321–404.

122. Ksiazek SM, Repka MX, Maguire A, Harbour RC, Savino PJ, Miller NR, et al. Divisional oculomotor nerve paresis caused by intrinsic brainstem disease. Ann Neurol. 1989;26(6):714–8.

123. Rabadi MH, Beltmann MA. Midbrain infarction presenting isolated medial rectus nuclear palsy. Am J Med. 2005;118(8):836–7.

124. Lee DK, Kim JS. Isolated inferior rectus palsy due to midbrain infarction detected by diffusion-weighted MRI. Neurology. 2006;66(12):1956–7.

125. Halmagyi GM, Brandt T, Dieterich M, Curthoys IS, Stark RJ, Hoyt WF. Tonic contraversive ocular tilt reaction due to unilateral meso-diencephalic lesion. Neurology. 1990;40(10):1503–9.

126. Lee SH, Park SW, Kim BC, Kim MK, Cho KH, Kim JS. Isolated trochlear palsy due to midbrain stroke. Clin Neurol Neurosurg. 2010;112(1):68–71.

127. Deuschl G, Bain P, Brin M. Consensus statement of the Movement Disorder Society on tremor. Ad Hoc Scientific Committee. Mov Disord. 1998;13(Suppl 3):2–23.

128. Remy P, de Recondo A, Defer G, Loc'h C, Amarenco P, Plante-Bordeneuve V, et al. Peduncular 'rubral' tremor and dopaminergic denervation: a PET study. Neurology. 1995;45(3 Pt 1):472–7.

129. Paviour DC, Jager HR, Wilkinson L, Jahanshahi M, Lees AJ. Holmes tremor: application of modern neuroimaging techniques. Mov Disord. 2006;21(12):2260–2.

130. Deuschl G, Wilms H, Krack P, Wurker M, Heiss WD. Function of the cerebellum in Parkinsonian rest tremor and Holmes' tremor. Ann Neurol. 1999;46(1):126–8.

131. Kim DG, Koo YH, Kim OJ, Oh SH. Development of Holmes' tremor in a patient with Parkinson's disease following acute cerebellar infarction. Mov Disord. 2009;24(3):463–4.

132. Morgan JC, Sethi KD. Midbrain infarct with parkinsonism. Neurology. 2003;60(12):E10.

133. Akyol A, Akyildiz UO, Tataroglu C. Vascular parkinsonism: a case of lacunar infarction localized to mesencephalic substantia nigra. Parkinsonism Relat Disord. 2006;12(7):459–61.

134. Gonzalez-Alegre P. Monomelic parkinsonian tremor caused by contralateral substantia nigra stroke. Parkinsonism Relat Disord. 2007;13(3):182–4.

135. Kim JS, Im JH, Kwon SU, Kang JH, Lee MC. Micrographia after thalamo-mesencephalic infarction: evidence of striatal dopaminergic hypofunction. Neurology. 1998;51(2):625–7.

136. Kwon M, Lee JH, Kim J, Kim JS. Hypokinetic dysarthria and palilalia in midbrain infarction. J Neurol Neurosurg Psychiatry. 2008;79(12):1411–2.

137. Loher TJ, Krauss JK. Dystonia associated with pontomesencephalic lesions. Mov Disord. 2009;24(2):157–67.

138. Kim JS. Asterixis after unilateral stroke: lesion location of 30 patients. Neurology. 2001;56(4):533–6.

139. Park HK, Kim HJ, Kim SJ, Kim JS, Shin HW. From Jekyll to Hyde after limbic subthalamic nucleus infarction. Neurology. 2011;77(1):82–4.

140. Zakaria T, Flaherty ML. Locked-in syndrome resulting from bilateral cerebral peduncle infarctions. Neurology. 2006;67(10):1889.

141. Kobayashi K, Matsubara R, Kurachi M, Sano J, Isaki K, Yamaguchi N, et al. Locked-in syndrome with bilateral midbrain infarcts—report of an autopsy. No To Shinkei. 1983;35(2):115–21.

142. Silverman IE, Geschwind MD, Vornov JJ. Cerebellar top-of-the-basilar syndrome. Clin Neurol Neurosurg. 1998;100(4):296–8.

143. Trojanowski JQ, Wray SH. Vertical gaze ophthalmoplegia: selective paralysis of downgaze. Neurology. 1980;30(6):605–10.

144. Buttner-Ennever JA, Buttner U, Cohen B, Baumgartner G. Vertical glaze paralysis and the rostral interstitial nucleus of the medial longitudinal fasciculus. Brain. 1982;105(Pt 1):125–49.

145. Pierrot-Deseilligny CH, Chain F, Gray F, Serdaru M, Escourolle R, Lhermitte F. Parinaud's syndrome: electro-oculographic and anatomical analyses of six vascular cases with deductions about vertical gaze organization in the premotor structures. Brain. 1982;105(Pt 4):667–96.

146. Bhidayasiri R, Plant GT, Leigh RJ. A hypothetical scheme for the brainstem control of vertical gaze. Neurology. 2000;54(10):1985–93.

147. Halmagyi GM, Evans WA, Hallinan JM. Failure of downward gaze: the site and nature of the lesion. Arch Neurol. 1978;35(1):22–6.

148. Jacobs L, Anderson PJ, Bender MB. The lesions producing paralysis of downward but not upward gaze. Arch Neurol. 1973;28(5):319–23.

149. Jampel RS, Fells P. Monocular elevation paresis caused by a central nervous system lesion. Arch Ophthalmol. 1968;80(1):45–57.

150. Lessell S. Supranuclear paralysis of monocular elevation. Neurology. 1975;25(12):1134–43.

151. Thomke F, Hopf HC. Acquired monocular elevation paresis. An asymmetric upgaze palsy. Brain. 1992;115(Pt 6):1901–10.

152. Bogousslavsky J, Regli F. Upgaze palsy and monocular paresis of downward gaze from ipsilateral thalamo-mesencephalic infarction: a vertical "one-and-a-half" syndrome. J Neurol. 1984;231(1):43–5.

153. Deleu D, Buisseret T, Ebinger G. Vertical one-and-a-half syndrome. Supranuclear downgaze paralysis with monocular elevation palsy. Arch Neurol. 1989;46(12):1361–3.

154. Collier J. Nuclear ophthalmoplegia with special reference to retraction of the lids and ptosis and to lesions of the posterior commissure. Brain. 1927;50:488.

155. Seybold ME, Yoss RE, Hollenhorst RW, Moyer NJ. Pupillary abnormalities associated with tumors of the pineal region. Neurology. 1971;21(3):232–7.

156. van Bogaert L. L'hallucinose pdonculaire. Rev Neurol (Paris). 1927;43:608–17.

157. McKee AC, Levine DN, Kowall NW, Richardson EP Jr. Peduncular hallucinosis associated with isolated infarction of the substantia nigra pars reticulata. Ann Neurol. 1990;27(5):500–4.

158. Serra Catafau J, Rubio F, Peres SJ. Peduncular hallucinosis associated with posterior thalamic infarction. J Neurol. 1992;239(2):89–90.

159. Benke T. Peduncular hallucinosis: a syndrome of impaired reality monitoring. J Neurol. 2006;253(12):1561–71.

160. Martin JP. Hemichorea resulting from a local lesion of the brain (the syndrome of the body of Luys). Brain. 1927;50:637–42.

161. Mehler MF. The rostral basilar artery syndrome: diagnosis, etiology, prognosis. Neurology. 1989;39(1):9–16.

162. Ahn SH, Kim BJ, Kim YJ, Kang DW, Kwon SU, Kim JS. Patterns and outcomes of the top of the basilar artery syndrome: the role of the posterior communicating artery. Cerebrovasc Dis. 2018;46(3–4):108–17.

Thalamic and Other Posterior Cerebral Artery Stroke Syndromes

5

Stefania Nannoni and Patrik Michel

Introduction

Approximately 20–40% of all ischaemic events in the brain affect posterior circulation [1, 2]. According to registry-based studies, isolated posterior cerebral artery (PCA) territory strokes occur in 5–10% of cerebral infarctions [3, 4], while up to 40% of patients have concomitant infarcts elsewhere in the posterior circulation or in the carotid territory [4, 5]. Among patients with pure PCA territory infarction, the confined involvement of deep structures (i.e. the thalamus and midbrain) varies from 34 to 64% across studies, with the ventrolateral thalamus emerging as the most frequently affected structure [4, 5]. The proportion of pure PCA cortical infarcts ranges from 14% to 51% of the total PCA infarctions, with the occipital lobe being most frequently involved [6, 7].

In the Acute Stroke Registry and Analysis of Lausanne (ASTRAL), from 5120 acute ischaemic stroke patients collected between 2003 and 2018, 184 (3.6%) patients presented with multi-level posterior stroke involving the PCA territory, whereas 336 (6.6%) patients exhibited pure PCA territory infarctions. Of these, 226 (67.3%) cases were authentic thalamic strokes (unpublished results from the ASTRAL registry) [2].

The involvement of supratentorial posterior structures supplied by the posterior cerebral arteries (PCAs) causes typical stroke syndromes. Knowledge of the clinical features allows characterizing the diverse spectrum of symptoms associated with the vascular topography of lesions.

Clinical identification of supratentorial PCA syndromes has several clinical implications: Precise localization to the anterior vs. posterior circulation may allow (a) correlating findings on arterial and cardiac workup with the stroke location; (b) making inferences on stroke mechanism in recurrent events, especially if a parenchymal lesion is not evident on imaging (such as in transient ischaemic attacks, TIA); and (c) deciding on acute recanalization in cases of multiple occlusions in pre- and intracranial arteries.

However, posterior circulation ischaemia can be challenging to recognize, particularly in patients with a TIA, and discriminating between anterior and posterior vascular territory may be difficult on a purely clinical basis. Studies comparing anterior vs. posterior circulation stroke symptoms have shown that vestibulo-cerebellar signs (including nystagmus and oculomotor palsy), visual field abnormalities and crossed sensory-motor deficits are very specific to posterior strokes, while dysarthria, hemiparesis and cognitive symptoms are not [8, 9].

In some situations, clinical distinction between a stroke in the middle cerebral artery (MCA) and PCA is impossible [10–12]. This is typically the case with an acute proximal PCA occlusion,

S. Nannoni · P. Michel (✉)
Stroke Centre, Neurology Service, Lausanne University Hospital, Lausanne, Switzerland
e-mail: Patrik.Michel@chuv.ch

© Springer Nature Singapore Pte Ltd. 2021
J. S. Kim (ed.), *Posterior Circulation Stroke*, https://doi.org/10.1007/978-981-15-6739-1_5

where contralateral hemiparesis results from isch-aemia in the cerebral peduncle and hemispheric symptoms from the large-volume thalamic isch-aemia. It has been shown, however, that clinical distinction between anterior and posterior circula-tion strokes are very reliable in patients with large (proximal) artery occlusions that are eligible for acute endovascular treatment [13].

This chapter will review the major clinical syndromes associated with posterior circulation ischaemia in the thalamus as well as other supra-tentorial structures. The clinical features of mid-brain infarctions are described in Chap. 4.

Anatomy of the Posterior Cerebral Circulation

The posterior cerebral arteries (PCAs) are the ter-minal branches of the basilar artery (BA) and supply blood to the midbrain (rostral part), thala-mus (medial and posterolateral regions), hippo-campus, occipital lobes, temporal lobes (inferior and medial portions) and partially to the parietal lobes (posterior and inferior portions) [14].

Each PCA originates from the bifurcation of the BA at the pontomesencephalic junction and is traditionally divided into four segments: P1, from the termination of the BA up to the posterior communicating artery (PCom); P2, between the PCom and the posterior part of the midbrain; P3, from the pulvinar to the anterior limit of the cal-carine fissure; and P4, the cortical segment within the calcarine fissure becoming the calcarine artery [15].

Classically, the PCAs have two main territo-ries of vascular supply: a proximal or deep PCA territory, including the thalamus, and a distal or superficial PCA territory, including the hemi-spheric occipital and temporoparietal lobes [16, 17].

Blood Supply to the Thalamus

The thalamus receives most of its blood supply from four arterial pedicles that arise from the proximal portions of the PCAs and the P-com. Consequently, the vascular territories of the thal-

amus can be divided into four major regions: (a) the anterior region supplied by the polar or tuber-othalamic artery; (b) the medial region supplied by the paramedian or thalamic–subthalamic arteries; (c) the inferolateral region supplied by the thalamogeniculate arteries; and (d) the poste-rior region supplied by the posterior choroidal arteries [15, 18]. Similar to the lenticulostriate arteries that irrigate the basal ganglia and the internal capsule, the thalamic arteries may show wide interindividual variation, regarding the ori-gin, the number of arteries and the supplied nuclei [15, 18].

Cortical Branches of the PCA

As the PCAs reach the dorsal surface of the mid-brain, they divide into four cortical branches: the anterior temporal, posterior temporal, parieto-occipital and calcarine arteries. The anterior tem-poral arteries arise first from the distal P3 segment; then, the posterior temporal arteries arise and course laterally, travelling along the hippocampal gyrus. The posterior temporal arteries course between the tentorium and the medial temporal lobe, including the fusiform gyrus. The parieto-occipital arteries usually originate from the P4 segment and supply the occipital and medial infe-rior parietal lobes, usually giving off the posterior pericallosal arteries, which circle the splenium of the corpus callosum. Usually, the calcarine arter-ies arise as single branches from the P4 segment, travelling at first lateral to the parieto-occipital arteries and then following a winding course, medially along the calcarine fissure [17, 19].

Important anatomical variants of the poste-rior circulation are frequent but commonly asymptomatic. Although typically discovered incidentally, their clinical significance is impor-tant so as not to mistake them for pathological findings and may be of relevance when determin-ing stroke aetiology.

A carotid or foetal (fPCA) origin of the PCA refers to a PCA arising directly from the intracranial internal carotid artery (ICA) and occurs in 10–29% of the population [20, 21]. In this variant of the circle of Willis, the internal carotid artery contributes to the PCA via a patent

Pcom, while the connection of the PCA to the BA is hypoplastic or even aplastic. fPCA is mainly unilateral and is either partial or complete depending on whether or not a hypoplastic P1 segment is present. Bilateral fPCAs are associated with a small calibre BA, as the BA does not contribute to mesencephalic, temporal or occipital lobe flow.

Even though there is no established association between unilateral or bilateral fPCAs and stroke risk, such a foetal anastomosis may allow thromboemboli from the carotid artery to pass into the PCA [22]. Therefore, the etiologic evaluation of occipital stroke in patients with an ipsilateral fPCA should include an assessment of carotid artery disease. Moreover, in patients with haemodynamically significant carotid occlusive disease, the ipsilateral fPCAs and a nonfunctioning anterior communicating artery may be particularly vulnerable to ischaemia and infarction due to haemodynamic failure.

Another form of foetal anastomosis with a prevalence of 0.1–0.6% is the persistent trigeminal artery that connects the carotid to the basilar artery [23]. This artery originates from the internal carotid artery after its exit from the carotid canal and anastomoses with the mid-basilar artery. The part of the basilar artery caudal to the anastomosis is usually hypoplastic. In such patients, atherosclerotic carotid stenosis may lead to bilateral occipital infarction [24].

The artery of Percheron refers to an anatomical variant of thalamus supply, characterized by a single thalamic perforating artery arising from the proximal PCA (P1 segment) and suppling the rostral mesencephalon and both paramedian thalami [15]. Hypoplastic or absent P1 segments are more likely to be seen with this variant. The occlusion of this artery leads to bilateral infarction of the paramedian thalami, with or without rostral midbrain involvement [25].

Thalamic Stroke Syndromes

Ischaemic strokes involving the thalamus can give rise to a large variety of syndromes due to the complex anatomy and vascularization of this structure.

Isolated thalamic infarctions are traditionally classified into four territories (i.e. anterior, paramedian, inferolateral and posterior infarctions), which correspond, respectively, to the vascular territory of the polar, paramedian, thalamogeniculate and posterior choroidal arteries. This classification was initially based on neuroanatomical and neuropathological data [15] and later confirmed by imaging techniques (CT and MRI) [18, 26]. Some variant topographic patterns of thalamic infarction with distinct clinical manifestations, including the anteromedian, central and posterolateral infarct types, were also described [15, 27]. These result from variations in the thalamic arterial supply or reflect border-zone ischaemia.

The main types of thalamic infarctions, with their vascular supply and typical clinical presentation, are described below and summarized in Table 5.1. Examples of thalamic strokes are depicted in Fig. 5.1.

Table 5.1 Thalamic infarcts, vascular supply and corresponding clinical syndromes, including the four classical thalamic stroke syndromes (a-d), less frequent variants (e-g) and the syndrome from occlusion of the artery of Percheron (h)

Thalamic infarct type	Frequency	Main aetiology	Vascular supply	Clinical stroke syndrome
(a) Anterior	11–13% [26, 27]	SVD 60% [26]	Polar arteries	– Personality changes, apathy, aboulia – Executive failure, perseverations – Superimposition of temporally unrelated information (*palipsychism*) – Anterograde amnesia – Aphasia if left; hemispatial neglect if right-sided – Emotional facial paresis, acalculia, apraxia

(continued)

Table 5.1 (continued)

Thalamic infarct type	Frequency	Main aetiology	Vascular supply	Clinical stroke syndrome
(b) Paramedian	23–27% [26, 27]	CE 33%, SVD 33% [26]	Paramedian arteries	– Decreased or fluctuating arousal – Impaired learning and memory, confabulation, temporal disorientation – Altered social skills and personality, including apathy, aggression, agitation – Vertical gaze paresis – Aphasia if left-sided, spatial deficits if right-sided
(c) Inferolateral	27–45% [26, 27]	SVD 33%, LAA 33% [26]	Thalamogeniculate arteries	– Sensory loss (variable extent, all modalities) – Hemiataxia – Hemiparesis – Post-lesion painful syndrome (Dejerine–Roussy)
(d) Posterior	6% [26]	SVD 33% [26]	Posterior choroidal arteries	– Visual field loss (hemianopia, quadrantanopia, sectoranopia) – Variable sensory loss, weakness, aphasia, memory impairment, dystonia, hand tremor
(e) Anteromedian	13% [27]	CE 56% [27]	Variant anteriomedian arteries	– Cognitive and memory impairment – Decreased consciousness – Vertical eye paresis – Aphasia (left-sided lesion)
(f) Central	6% [27]	SVD 50% [27]	Border-zone vascular territory	– Hypoaesthesia – Memory impairment
(g) Posterolateral	11% [27]	SVD 38%, LAA 38% [27]	Variant posterolateral arteries	– Hypoaesthesia – Ataxia – Hemiparesis – Aphasia and executive dysfunction (left-sided)
(h) Bilateral paramedian	12% [26]	40% CE [26]	Artery of Percheron	– Disorders of vigilance – Anterograde and retrograde memory deficit – Behavioural changes (with a mixture or irritability and apathy) – Vertical gaze palsy

Legend: *SVD* small vessel disease, *CE* cardioembolic, *LAA* large artery disease

Anterior Thalamic Infarct

Anterior thalamic infarct is caused by the occlusion of the polar artery (also known as the tuberothalamic artery) [28]. This artery originates from the middle-third of the PCom artery but is absent in about one-third of cases (in these cases, the anterior territory is supplied by the paramedian arteries from the same side). It irrigates the reticular nucleus, ventral anterior nucleus, rostral part of the ventrolateral nucleus, ventral pole of the medial dorsal nucleus, mamillothalamic tract, ventral amygdalofugal pathway, ventral part of the internal medullary lamina and anterior thalamic nuclei. The anterior thalamic nuclei receive projections from the mamillothalamic tract and are connected to the anterior limbic system.

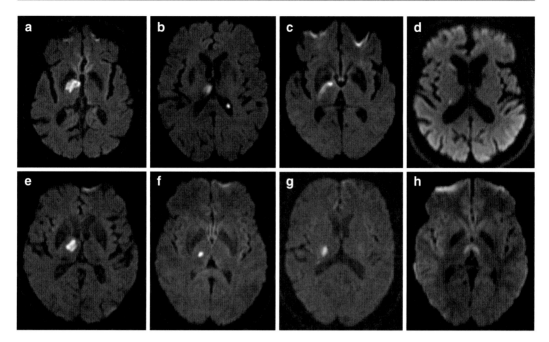

Fig. 5.1 Diffusion-weighted MRI showing a right thalamic infarction in anterior (**a**), paramedian (**b**), inferolateral (**c**) and posterior (**d**) infarctions. Localization in the anteriomedian (**e**), central (**f**), posterolateral (**g**) and bilateral paramedian (**h**) territories are also shown. (From Department of Radiology, Lausanne University Hospital)

Anterior thalamic infarcts account for about 13% of all thalamic infarcts but are rarely isolated, being most often part of anteromedian infarctions [26]. The most frequent aetiology is small vessel disease.

The clinical syndrome of anterior thalamic strokes is dominated by severe and various neuropsychological deficits [28, 29]. For this reason, such strokes are often underdiagnosed or missed initially. Patients can exhibit changing levels of consciousness in the early stages, while persistent personality changes are seen in the later course. They typically appear apathetic and aboulic, with a lack of spontaneity and emotional concern [28]. Disorientation in time and place, executive failure and perseverations can be present. Moreover, patients may show increased sensitivity to interference and have improper superimposition of temporally unrelated information (the latter called "palipsychism") [29, 30].

Another common finding in anterior thalamic infarct is the impairment of anterograde memory, likely from involvement of the mamillothalamic tract, with inability to make new memories. Left-sided lesions tend to affect more often the verbal and right-sided, the visual memory function [29, 31, 32].

Language disturbances, named transcortical motor aphasia, have been described in anterior thalamic lesions affecting the dominant hemisphere, i.e. typically left-sided lesions. They are characterized by impaired verbal fluency, anomia, semantic and phonemic paraphasia, with impaired comprehension but well-preserved repetition.

Right-sided lesions may be associated with hemispatial neglect.

"Emotional central facial paralysis," characterized by impaired activation of face muscles with emotion but normal voluntary activation, is also described [18].

Paramedian Thalamic Infarct

Paramedian thalamic infarct is due to the occlusion of the thalamic–subthalamic arteries (also called the paramedian or thalamoperforating arteries), which arise from the proximal P1 segment of the PCA, mainly as a pair from each P1. In about one-third of cases, these small arteries both originate from one side (asymmetric variant) or from a common pedicle of one P1 (artery of Percheron). They supply the paramedian parts of the upper midbrain and the posteromedial thalamus, including the posteroinferior portion of the dorsomedial nucleus and the intralaminar nuclei. When the polar artery is absent, the paramedian artery supplies this territory as well, and thus, infarction in this vascular territory is clinically severe.

Paramedian infarctions are the second most frequent after lateral infarcts and may occur unilaterally or bilaterally, accounting overall for about 35% of all thalamic infarcts [26]. The main aetiology is embolism.

Patients with unilateral infarcts of the paramedian arteries are described by a classic triad of symptoms: an acute decrease of consciousness, neuropsychological disturbances and abnormalities of vertical gaze [28, 33]. Impairment of arousal, with patients being lethargic, hypersomnolent or even comatose, is a dominant feature during the early stages. It is probably related to involvement of the intralaminar nuclei and the rostral portion of the midbrain reticular activating system [30]. As the impairment of consciousness diminishes and patients become more alert, memory and behavioural disturbances may be more evident. Amnesia is predominant, with patients being unable to learn and make new memories. Confusion, agitation, aggression and apathy are common personality disturbances and may persist in the long term [33, 34]. It has been suggested that memory loss and behavioural syndromes are related to the interruption of the mamilothalamic tract or ventral amygdalofugal pathway [31].

Vertical gaze palsy is characteristically present, with up-gaze palsy or combined up- and down-gaze palsy, depending on the volume of the lesion, its bilaterality and the degree of rostral midbrain involvement. Skew deviation is also common, with the eye elevated on the side of the lesion. Also, speech and language impairments are described in left-sided infarction. They are characterized by hypophonia and dysprosody, with frequent perseveration and mark-

edly reduced verbal fluency, but normal repetition and preserved syntactic structure. This was named the adynamic aphasia of Guberman and Stuss [25]. Temporary and spatial neglect may be observed in patients with right-sided infarction.

An alternate syndrome characterized by central Horner syndrome (i.e. ptosis, myosis, pseudoenophthalmos and hypohidrosis of the ipsilateral hemibody) and contralateral mild ataxic hemiparesis has been described in ischaemic stroke patients due to paramedian (and anterior) thalamic lesions [35]. In these patients, infarction extended to the hypothalamic or rostral paramedian mesencephalic region, also irrigated by branches arising from the P1 segment. This syndrome likely results from impairment of the sympathoexcitatory and motor pathways in the thalamic–hypothalamic–rostral mesencephalic region [35, 36].

Inferolateral Thalamic Infarct

This type of thalamic stroke is caused by occlusion of the inferolateral arteries (also known as thalamogeniculate arteries), a group of 6–10 arteries that arise from the P2 segment of the PCA after the level of the PCom. They supply the ventrolateral thalamus, including the ventrolateral and ventroposterior nuclear groups, the lateral part of the centromedian nucleus and the rostrolateral portion of the pulvinar [15].

Infarcts in the inferolateral territory are the most common type of ischaemic stroke in the thalamus, accounting for about 45% of all thalamic infarcts [26]. Their major aetiology is small vessel disease.

The clinical features of inferolateral artery infarction were initially described as "thalamic syndrome" by French neurologists Dejerine and Roussy, with intense central post-stroke pain as the most characteristic symptom [37]. Patients may present a pure sensory stroke, a sensorimotor stroke or, in cases of extensive involvement of lateral thalamus, a sensorimotor stroke with abnormal movement patterns.

A pure sensory stroke is due to the selective involvement of the ventrolateral nucleus. It usually starts with paraesthesia or numbness on the contralateral side, followed by an isolated hemisensory deficit. Sensory loss may involve all modalities of sensation, though a dissociated loss, with sparing of pain and temperature, may be observed. A typical distribution in face-arm-leg is suggestive of a lateral thalamic infarction, even if a predominant acral distribution may occur [38, 39]. Some patients may develop an intense and delayed pain in the affected area, usually unrelieved by analgesics. This post-stroke painful syndrome has an apparent preference for right thalamic infarcts [40].

In sensorimotor stroke, the above-mentioned sensory disturbances are associated with hemiparesis on the same side, due to the extension of the infarcted area to the posterior limb of the internal capsule.

Abnormal movement patterns, such as ataxic hemiataxia or hemydystonia, result from the interruption of cerebellar or extrapyramidal tracts that synapse in the lateral thalamus. In some patients, an inability to stand and walk is predominant, and Masdeu and Gorelick called this "thalamic astasia" [41]. Another motor abnormality was described by Foix and Hillemand as flexed and pronated hand, with the thumb tucked under the other fingers, called the "thalamic hand" [42].

Cognitive and behavioural performances are usually preserved in inferolateral thalamic infarcts, although mild transcortical motor aphasia with reduced fluency is occasionally reported in dominant hemisphere lesions [30].

Posterior Thalamic Infarct

Posterior thalamic infarct is caused by the occlusion of the posterior choroidal arteries, also arising from the P2 segment of the PCA, just after the inferolateral arteries. They consist of a group of small vessels, with 1–2 branches (medial) arising adjacent to the origin of the Pcom artery and 1–6 branches (lateral) originating from the distal P2 segment of the PCA. They supply the pulvinar and lateral dorsal and posterior nucleus, the geniculate bodies and partially the anterior nucleus. Infarction limited to the dorsal part of

the thalamus is rare [26], and the most characteristic clinical findings are visual field defects (due to involvement of the lateral geniculate body) [43].

Medial posterior choroidal artery infarction causes visual field cuts including upper or lower quadrantanopia, whereas involvement of the lateral posterior choroidal artery causes horizontal wedge-shaped or tubular sectoranopias [44].

Involvement of the pulvinar and posterior nuclei can produce numerous less-specific symptoms, including impairment of ipsilateral pursuit, contralateral saccades, mild hemiparesis or hemisensory abnormalities, abnormal dystonic movement and neuropsychological disturbances (such as aphasia, amnesia, aboulia and visual hallucinosis) [30].

A delayed complex hyperkinetic motor syndrome that includes myoclonus, ataxia, chorea, pseudorubral tremor, dystonic posture of the fingers and worsened by voluntary activities, termed the "jerky dystonic unsteady hand," was also observed in a small subset of patients with infarcts restricted to the pulvinar according to CT or MRI assessment, raising the question of additional nuclei involved [18, 45].

Variant: Anteromedian Thalamic Infarct

This stroke involves the posterior part of the anterior territory and the anterior part of the paramedian territory [27]. It is likely related to the occlusion of variant anteromedian arteries, originating from the proximal segment of the PCA [15]. Similar to paramedian thalamic strokes, cardioembolism is the most frequent aetiology [27].

The dominant feature is a wide range and severe neuropsychological disturbance [27]. Severe anterograde amnesia is a common feature, particularly prominent when involving the anterior part of the dorsomedian nucleus and intralaminar nuclei. Loss of initiative and executive dysfunction is frequently found. Contrary to infarcts restricted to the anterior territory, patients with anteromedian territory infarcts do not exhibit issues with perseverance. Instead, the main behavioural change in anteromedian infarct is a severe loss of self-activation, requiring constant external stimulation. Aphasic troubles with word-finding difficulties, reduced fluency and denomination are also described. Decreased consciousness is uncommon in unilateral anteromedian territory infarcts, but a frequent finding in bilateral lesions. Vertical gaze palsy has been reported and postulated to be due to involvement of fronto-cortical fibres that may be decussating in the medial thalamus [46].

Variant: Central Thalamic Infarct

Infarct of the central territory is characterized by the involvement of parts of all four adjacent classic territories. It may be expression of a borderzone infarction between adjacent territories [27].

In the four patients observed by Carrera et al., hypoesthesia was a common feature, likely due to involvement of the medial portion of the ventroposterolateral nucleus. Anterograde amnesia and short-term memory impairment are also dominant and more severe than in anteromedian territory infarcts [27]. Ataxia, vertical gaze paresis and neuropsychological signs are also described in patients with bilateral lesions.

Variant: Posterolateral Thalamic Infarct

The posterolateral territory is formed by combining the posterior portion of the inferolateral territory and the anterior portion of the posterior territory. This is likely supplied by variant posterolateral arteries. Microangiopathy is the predominant stroke aetiology, as well as for inferolateral infarcts [27].

The clinical picture is characterized by contralateral hypaesthesia and ataxia, with transient hemiparesis. Compared to patients with inferolateral infarcts, an unusual finding in posterolateral territory infarct is the impaired cognition from a left-sided lesion. Aphasia with impaired repetition that resembles cortical motor aphasia is described; this differs from transcortical aphasia due to anteromedian infarcts. Executive dys-

function may also be seen because of the disruption of thalamocortical fibres arising from the posterolateral nuclei of the thalamus [27, 47].

Variant: Bilateral Paramedian Thalamic Infarct

Occlusion of the artery of Percheron leads to bilateral infarction of the paramedian thalami, with or without rostral midbrain involvement, and causes severe stroke [15, 33]. Asymmetric thalamic involvement is seen in two-thirds of cases, and midbrain infarction is present in over half [48]. Artery-to-artery embolism or cardioembolism are thought to be the most common aetiology of stroke in patients carrying this anatomic variant [49].

The most typical clinical features of bilateral paramedian thalamic infarction are altered sensorium such as stupor or coma, prominent memory impairment, behavioural changes and vertical gaze palsy. Overall, the neuropsychological disturbances are more severe than in those with unilateral infarcts and can be persistent [25, 34, 50].

Patients are usually apathetic and aboulic, with reduced spontaneity and increased inertia. Disorientation, confusion and akinetic mutism (i.e. awake unresponsiveness) can be observed. Patients may show perseveration and a marked tendency to confabulate. A compulsive use of objects out of a behavioural context, as observed in patients with frontal-lobe lesions, is also described [48, 51].

The amnestic syndrome resulting from paramedian territory infarction is similar to thiamine-deficient Korsakoff's syndrome, destroying the medial dorsal thalamic nuclei and the mammillary bodies. The addition of the other behavioural features produces a constellation of symptoms that led to the term "thalamic dementia" [18, 52].

Non-thalamic PCA Stroke Syndromes

The syndromes of infarction in the PCA territory are conventionally associated with homonymous visual field defects. However, patients with PCA territory infarcts often present clinically with multiple symptoms and signs, including sensory and motor abnormalities and cognitive and neuropsychological deficits [5, 7, 16, 19]. These strokes can simulate strokes in the middle cerebral artery (MCA) territory, especially in the presence of significant motor deficits [10–12].

In this section, we first describe typical signs and symptoms found in infarcts affecting the PCA territory and not related to thalamic involvement, followed by a description of the main clinical syndromes associated with proximal and distal PCA occlusion.

Clinical Features in PCA Strokes without Thalamic Involvement

Hemispheric infarctions in the PCA territory potentially involve the occipital, posterior temporal and parietal lobes, with variable clinical manifestations. The most frequent symptom is visual field abnormality, which is reported in more than 90% of patients with cortical PCA infarctions [4, 6, 7]. Among cognitive deficits, memory impairment and aphasia are reported in 18 and 15% of patients, respectively [6]. Cognitive deficits associated with visual function, such as visual neglect or visual agnosia, seem less common in clinical practice, being reported in less than 10% of patients with cortical PCA infarctions [6].

Visual Field Defects

Homonymous hemianopia is the most frequent visual field defect after unilateral PCA infarctions, involving either the two right or two left-halves of the visual fields of each eye [16, 53]. It is caused by contralateral lesions of the optic radiations (also called geniculocalcarine tracts) in the occipital lobe and/or by contralateral lesions in the cerebral visual (occipital) cortex (Brodmann area 17). Hemianopia from PCA infarctions is traditionally described as sparing the macula, i.e. the central or medial part of the visual field is preserved [4, 6, 7].

Homonymous hemianopia is often disabling, causing difficulties with reading and visual scanning. Patients usually fail to notice relevant objects or avoid obstacles on the affected side,

causing collisions with approaching people or cars. The visual defect is often described as a void, blackness, or a limitation of vision to one side, and patients recognize after some training that they must focus extra attention on the hemianopic field.

Hemianopia is in most cases complete, but upper or lower quadrantanopsia can also be found. A *superior quadrant field defect* (*"pie in the sky"*) is seen if the infarct is limited to the lower-bank of the calcarine fissure (the lingual gyrus), or if it affects the inferior (temporal) radiations of the optic tract. An *inferior quadrantanopia* results if the lesion affects the cuneus on the upper-bank of the calcarine fissure, or the upper (parietal) optic radiations [6].

Cortical bilateral visual field defects including complete "cortical" blindness are found as a result of bilateral PCA territory strokes, usually after "top of the basilar" embolism [54, 55]. Interestingly, such patients may exhibit *visual anosognosia* for their blindness, despite the sparing of parietal and thalamic structures. This so-called "Anton's syndrome" is characterized by the patients' affirmation of seeing normally despite objective evidence of blindness [56]. If patients do not admit that they cannot see, they may use confabulation or increased verbosity to try to compensate for the lack of visual input.

Neuropsychological Features in Dominant PCA Strokes

Language-related disorders such as dysphasia, dyslexia (without dysgraphia), dyscalculia and colour anomia may occur when the dominant PCA territory is infarcted (usually the left side) [16, 57].

Aphasia can be due to an infarction large enough to cover the left parietal lobe or temporal lobe [58]. "Transcortical sensory aphasia," similar to Wernicke's sensory aphasia but with preserved repetition, is caused by infarctions into the parietal–occipital region on the left side. The patient may alternatively show "amnestic (or anomic) aphasia" (inability to name but repetition and comprehension intact) due to infarction to the left temporal lobe of the PCA territory.

Alexia refers to difficulty in reading, with patients being unable to read single letters or numbers, while writing, speaking and other language functions are preserved. In less-severe deficit, patients may need more time to read, depending on sequential identification of letters. Alexia without agraphia (pure alexia) is caused by a lesion of the dominant occipital lobe and splenium of the corpus callosum and is often accompanied by right homonymous hemianopia. The pathophysiological basis is a disconnection between the visual information and the language-processing area [59]. In patients with extensive infarction that damages the left angular gyrus, *alexia with agraphia* will develop, but oral-language functions are still preserved [60].

Elements of "Gerstmann's syndrome" (i.e. dyscalculia, dysgraphia, finger agnosia and right–left disorientation) may be found in patients with inferior parietal lobe lesions (especially involving the angular gyrus and adjacent structures) [61].

Bilateral or unilateral dominant PCA infarction may produce significant *memory impairment* by damaging the hippocampus, parahippocampus and connecting fibres [19, 57, 62]. Patients demonstrate the impaired acquisition of new memories (anterograde amnesia), while the retrieval of memories encoded prior to the onset of the infarction (retrograde amnesia) is usually less affected.

Amnesia in patients with unilateral lesions is generally transient on bedside examination, lasting a few days, but may not be detected at all. Sometimes, patients appear frankly confused. They cannot recall what has happened recently, and when given new information, do not recall it moments later. They often repeat statements and questions spoken only minutes before.

Clinically isolated amnesia from stroke may be difficult to distinguish from transient global amnesia (TGA). The latter often shows a small punctate DWI lesion ("pixel") in the hippocampus at 12–48 h after symptom onset. Still, TGA is not considered an ischaemic stroke and its pathophysiology remains uncertain [63]. As described by our group, a typical TGA presentation is very rare due to ischaemic stroke [64]. Red flags that may indicate stroke include associated focal neurological symptoms and signs, such as visual field deficits or

transient hemisyndromes. Also, a very long or very short duration of amnesia and the presence of major stroke sources increase the likelihood of an ischaemic origin of amnesia, which are located in or close to the Papez circuit [64].

Radiologically, DWI lesions from TGA are located in the CA1 region of the hippocampus and are usually unique. In 10–15%, a second similar lesion in the same or contralateral hippocampus may occur [65]. On the contrary, patients with ischaemic hippocampal lesions often have other acute lesions in the same or other territories, with lesions of a larger size that are visible more quickly (i.e. within 12 h) and that tend to enhance with gadolinium if repeat MRI is performed beyond 5–7 days [66].

After the acute phase, amnestic signs in PCA territory strokes may persist up to 6 months on a detailed neuropsychological exam. However, in bilateral medial temporal lobe lesions, amnesia may be permanent and severe.

Neuropsychological Features in Non-dominant PCA Strokes

Disorders of visual cognitive functions with visual agnosia including prosopagnosia, spatial disorientation, dyschromatopsia and palinopsia may be found in patients with non-dominant hemisphere (usually right-sided) infarcts [16, 19].

Visual agnosia is the inability to recognize visually presented objects despite the preservation of elementary visual function. This is usually found in patients where the PCA supplies adjacent parietal structures and PCA branch occlusions cause a disconnection between language and visual systems [67, 68]. Patients have difficulty in understanding the nature and use of objects presented visually, but they can name objects when they touch them or when the objects are described to them. Two forms of visual agnosia are described: "apperceptive" agnosia involves poor perception and ability to understand, while "associative" agnosia involves poor ability to match and use. Close to associative agnosia, patients may present *optic aphasia,* i.e. a naming deficit confined to the visual modality [69]. Patients typically present with extensive left

PCA territory infarction with right homonymous hemianopia.

Prosopagnosia is a form of visual agnosia characterized by difficulty in recognizing previously familiar faces. It is due to lesions in the inferior occipital areas, the lingual and fusiform gyri and the anterior temporal cortex. In the literature, this deficit is described as associated with the right PCA territory [70].

Achromatopsia refers to difficulty perceiving colours [71]. It is due to infarctions in the ventral occipital cortex and/or infracalcarine. The patient may present with hemiachromatopsia if the infarction is unilateral.

Visual hallucinations are uncommon but may develop from PCA strokes on any side of the brain, often during the recovery phase [6]. They can be either simple or complex and usually criticized by the patient.

Palinopsia refers to images persisting even after the image has been removed from the visual fields. Infarctions can be in the lingual and fusiform gyri [72].

Spatial and geographic disorientation and an inability to recall routes or to read or visualize the location of places on maps are also common. This is named *topographagnosia* and may comprise heterogeneous manifestations, including difficulty identifying familiar environmental landmarks such as buildings and street corners. This deficit is associated with the right posterior parahippocampal gyrus and the anterior part of the lingual and fusiform gyri [73].

Moreover, unusual aggressive behaviour can be caused by PCA strokes as well, especially with the involvement of the right occipital lobe. These patients may become anxious, aggressive and frustrated when they are stimulated by the environment [74].

PCA Stroke Syndromes According to Occlusion Site

Patients with PCA occlusion present with clinical stroke syndromes that vary according to the site of occlusion and to the corresponding location and extent of infarction. As described above, cognitive symptoms are often side-related [7, 16, 75, 76].

Depending on the location of the vascular occlusion, we identify three groups of unilateral PCA infarctions and a heterogeneous syndrome associated with bilateral infarction, which are listed below and summarized in Table 5.2.

Table 5.2 Infarct topography and clinical findings of the main PCA stroke syndromes

PCA infarction	Vascular site of occlusion	Infarct location	Clinical stroke syndrome
Unilateral			
Proximal	(a) Proximal P1 segment (near its origin from the basilar artery)	*Deep and superficial infarct*, involving: medial midbrain, posterolateral thalamus, and hemispheric occipito-parieto-temporal PCA territory	– Decrease in consciousness – Lethargy, aboulia – Oculomotor abnormalities (partial or complete ipsilateral third nerve palsy, bilateral ptosis and vertical gaze palsy) – Contralateral hypoaesthesia and hemiplegia – Visual agnosia, colour anomia, visual hallucinations
	(b) P2 segment (before the branching of the thalamogeniculate arteries)	*Deep and superficial infarct*, involving: lateral thalamus and hemispheric PCA territory	– Severe contralateral sensory loss – Hypotonia, clumsiness and abnormal movements (but not hemiplegia) – Short-term memory impairment – Variable language and visual cognitive dysfunctions

(continued)

Table 5.2 (continued)

PCA infarction	Vascular site of occlusion	Infarct location	Clinical stroke syndrome
Distal	(c) Single or multiple PCA branch(es)	*Superficial infarct*, involving the calcarine, parieto-occipital and posterior temporal artery territories	– Homonymous hemianopia – Language disorders including dysphasia, dyslexia, dyscalculia, colour dysnomia (dominant hemisphere) – Visual cognitive dysfunctions including visual agnosia, dyschromatopsia and spatial disorientation (non-dominant hemisphere)
Bilateral	(d) Bilateral PCA occlusion from embolus or fragmentation of a thrombus in the basilar artery	*Deep and superficial infarct*: variable extended bilateral hemispheric infarction with thalamic involvement	– Cortical blindness – Possible visual anosognosia and confabulation (Anton's syndrome) – Amnesia and cognitive dysfunctions – Emotional and behavioural disturbances (agitated delirium) – Visual field defects with visual cognitive abnormalities (for bilateral inferior-bank infarct) – Optic ataxia, oculomotor apraxia, simultagnosia (Balint's syndrome) (for bilateral superior-bank infarct)

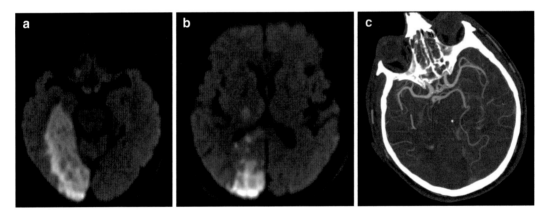

Fig. 5.2 Diffusion-weighted MRI showing a large right PCA infarction involving the temporal lobe (**a**), the occipital lobe and the median and lateral thalamus (**b**). CT-angiography shows a right-side P1 occlusion (**c**, red arrow). (From Department of Radiology, Lausanne University Hospital. Right P1 occlusion on CTA)

(a) *Occlusion of the very proximal PCA (P1-segment occlusion)*: Occlusion near its origin from the BA causes a total PCA territory infarction, which includes the cerebral peduncle of the midbrain, lateral thalamus and the hemispheric territory (Fig. 5.2).

The midbrain infarction can also be bilateral, even when only one PCA is occluded, if penetrating arteries to the bilateral paramedian rostral brainstem structures

arise from one PCA. In this case, patients often exhibit prolonged stupor or coma, or, later, hypersomnolence and vertical gaze palsies [17].

Occlusions of the proximal PCA origins are usually embolic (from the heart, aorta or proximal vertebrobasilar arteries) [4].

Sensory and motor abnormalities are described in approximately 70% of patients, with sensory deficits being more common. In patients with PCA territory ischaemia, lateral thalamic infarction is likely the major reason for sensory symptoms and signs. A severe hemiparesis or hemiplegia is mainly due to infarction in the lateral midbrain as a result of involvement of the corticospinal and/or corticobulbar tracts in the cerebral peduncles.

Partial or complete ipsilateral third-nerve palsy, bilateral ptosis, loss of vertical gaze, lethargy and aboulia are also variable features associated with proximal PCA occlusion. Other signs of posterior hemispheric cortical involvement, such as visual agnosia, colour anomia, visual hallucinations or illusions can also be present.

Such proximal P1 occlusion can also produce the historical syndromes of Weber [77] or Parinoud [78].

(b) *Occlusion of the P2 segment of the proximal PCA*, beyond the origin of the posterior communicating artery but before the branching of the thalamogeniculate arteries, will lead to a combined deep and superficial infarction mainly involving the inferolateral thalamus and the hemispheric PCA territory [16, 17]. The pulvinar (posterior choroidal artery) may also be affected.

The combination of infarctions of the lateral thalamus and cortical PCA branches (with or without involvement of the pulvinar) will lead to a variable combination of contralateral sensory hemisyndromes (sometimes with ataxia and minor corticospinal signs). Abnormal spontaneous contralateral limb movements may occur, and pain may develop weeks or months after the stroke, as described above. Dejerine–Roussy syndrome may occur after the acute phase. Consciousness disturbances are more frequent than in patients with pure cortical PCA infarctions [7]. Ischaemia in superficial PCA branches will lead to variable combinations of homonymous visual field defects and cognitive signs, as described above. Visual inattention and prosopagnosia are seen in patients with right temporal and parieto-occipital branch involvement, while patients with left-side lesions show mostly transcortical sensorial aphasia [7].

Clinically, it is sometimes impossible to distinguish whether signs stem from the thalamic or superficial lesions; similarly, strokes from P2 occlusion may imitate occlusions of parietal and temporal (posterior) branches of the MCA.

(c) *Occlusions of cortical PCA branches* (from the P3 segment of the PCA) mainly affect the calcarine arteries, leading to homonymous visual field defects [5, 17]. Parieto-occipital branch occlusions will lead to visual associative agnosia and visual neglect with right-sided lesions. Anterior temporal branch occlusions will affect mainly memory function specific to the side of the lesion, with language disturbance if localized in the dominant hemisphere, as described above. Occlusions of the posterior temporal branch lead to spatial/geographic disorientation and prosopagnosia, mainly if located on the right. Simple and complex visual hallucinations may occur with an occlusion of any of these branches, typically beginning hours to days after the stroke, and usually disappear spontaneously [4, 7].

Occlusion of multiple cortical PCA branches leads to variable combinations of signs described in this chapter.

(d) *Bilateral PCA territory infarction* occurs in about 6–13% of all PCA strokes [6, 7, 76]. We already described bilateral thalamic stroke from a single occlusion of the paramedian thalamic artery (artery of Percheron) [15]. Moreover, in "top of the basilar" syndrome, thalamic and/or superficial PCA territory lesions are frequently bilateral and occur simultaneously [54] (Fig. 5.3).

In such extensive lesions, patients usually have decreased levels of consciousness. In cases of bilateral occipital involvement, they present "cortical" blindness, with or without Anton's syndrome, i.e. anosognosia of blindness. Confabulations are commonly used to compensate blindness. Less-severe visual field defects, like bilateral hemianopia or bilateral scotoma, may be observed in cases of compensatory blood supply, including from the middle cerebral artery.

Cognitive dysfunction from bilateral thalamic involvement may dominate the clinical

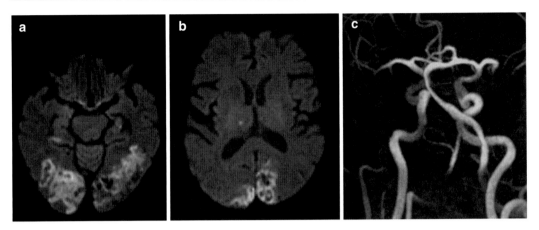

Fig. 5.3 Diffusion-weighted MRI showing a bilateral PCA infarction involving the occipital lobe (**a**) and the central thalamus (**b**). MR-angiography shows a focal ste-nosis in the mid-basilar artery (**c**, red arrow). (From Department of Radiology, Lausanne University Hospital)

picture in the long term ("thalamic dementia") [52]. Amnesia may also be a permanent sequela of bilateral infarction of the medial temporal lobes.

The most frequent structures involved in bilateral PCA strokes are those located below the calcarine fissure, including both occipital and temporal lobes [17]. These produce upper quadrantopsia, achromatopsia, apperceptive visual agnosia and prosopagnosia. Patients may present hyperactive and restless behaviour, with motor agitation and aggressive reactions, especially when stimulated. This agitated delirium seems to be attributed to the limbic system involvement in patients with bilateral inferior temporal lobe infarction [19, 74].

The infarction of the bilateral occipitoparietal border may result in features of Balint's syndrome. This presents with optic ataxia (inability to reach targets under visual guidance), oculomotor apraxia (inability to intentionally move eyes towards an object) and simultagnosia (inability to synthesize objects within a visual field) [79].

Moreover, patients with bilateral upperbank lesions may have difficulties in recognizing where objects, people or places are topographically [80].

Prognosis of PCA Stroke

After thalamic infarction, prognosis is generally regarded as more favourable compared with lesions of the cerebral cortex or other subcortical structures [26, 81]. This generally reflects the low incidence of mortality and the good recovery from motor deficit. However, patients with tuberothalamic or paramedian artery stroke could be affected by the persistence of cognitive and psychiatric manifestations, even if systematic longitudinal analyses have not been performed [18].

Similarly, the functional outcome of patients with superficial PCA territory infarction is usually good [16]. Compared with MCA infarctions, they showed higher frequency of symptom-free at discharge and lower in-hospital mortality rate [3, 4]. Early mortality in PCA infarction is low, ranging from 0% to 7% in different series [1, 3, 4, 6, 75]. Recurrent vertebrobasilar ischaemia, myocardial infarction, sudden unexplained death and pneumonia are the main reported causes of death [3, 7].

Unlike MCA territory infarction, malignant infarctions of the PCA with cerebral edema, mass effect and transtentorial herniation are rarely reported, given the more limited vascular territory that is involved. Gogela et al. described three cases of unilateral occipital infarction, which resulted in massive edema and herniation [82], while Pfefferkorn et al. reported one case of extensive bilateral PCA infarction, which produced fatal herniation [83].

Long-term prognosis after PCA strokes seemed heavily associated with the localization of the infarct: patients with extensive involvement of deep structures, especially the midbrain, showed worse prognosis than those with infarction limited to the superficial territory [84]. Similarly, PCA-plus patients (i.e. patients with coincident infarct outside the PCA territory) had increased disability at 6 months and long-term mortality compared to pure PCA strokes [85]. In a retrospective cohort study of PCA strokes from our institution, we observed a trend for a lower cognitive, visual and functional disability at 3 months in patients treated with intravenous thrombolysis and/or mechanical thrombectomy compared to conservative treatment [86].

Stroke recurrence is an important cause of morbidity and mortality after posterior ischaemic stroke. Patients with PCA infarcts of atherothrombotic aetiology showed a higher risk of recurrence compared to other etiologies [16]. Moreover, patients with PCA stroke and proximal large artery disease (i.e. BA and intracranial vertebral artery disease) demonstrated a higher risk of a second ischaemic event than patients with intrinsic PCA atherosclerosis [7].

Similarly to anterior circulation stroke, functional outcome after PCA stroke mainly depends on recovery from motor dysfunction (due to the involvement of the midbrain or internal capsule). Also, the size of infarction of the dominant hemisphere is crucial for the persistence and severity of neuropsychological deficits [16]. Moreover, patients with PCA stroke might be specifically affected by long-term sequelae concerning visual field defects, sensory deficits and involuntary movements.

Visual field defects after PCA stroke can result in significant disability and reduction in quality of life [87]. The impact of visual impairment on daily activities can be wide ranging, including a general reduction in mobility, reduced ability to judge distance, higher risk of falls, reading impairment and inability to drive [88]. Spontaneous visual field improvement can occur

post-stroke in varying degrees, mostly depending on the severity of the initial severity of symptoms and lesion extension. This has been reported in up to 50% of patients, usually within the first 3–6 months, mostly due to the resolution of cerebral edema and the recovery of neurotransmission [89]. After this period, spontaneous recovery is possible, but usually at a much slower rate and likely related to improvement in the patient's functional ability despite persistent defects [89].

Sequelae related to sensory dysfunction are relatively common after thalamic infarction. Central post-stroke pain syndrome (CPSP) is a debilitating sequelae that can follow laterothalamic sensory stroke. It has been originally described as part of the "thalamic syndrome of Dejerine and Roussy" [37], even if it is now recognized that strokes occurring anywhere along the spinothalamic or trigemino-thalamic pathways (including lateral medullary stroke and parietal cortical stroke) can produce similar symptoms [90]. Frequency of CPSP appears to depend upon lesion location: in inferior lateral thalamic infarctions, 17% to 18% of cases were described to develop CPSP, while this percentage was higher in the lateral medullary infarction, and much lower in parietal cortex infarction [90]. At the nuclear level, CPSP following thalamic stroke seemed to be critically related to the damage of the ventral posterolateral nucleus [91], although the exact pathogenesis of this delayed sensory syndrome remains unclear. Symptoms usually develop weeks or months after the onset of stroke and affect the areas where the sensory deficits were the most severe in the acute phase. Patients may describe sharp, stabbing or burning pain and experience hyperpathia and especially allodynia [92, 93]. Pharmacological therapy, magnetic stimulation and invasive electrical stimulation are therapeutical options [94].

Patients with thalamic stroke may also develop post-stroke involuntary movements, such as asterixis, dystonia, chorea/athetosis, tremors, and myoclonus [95]. These represent a rare complication of posterior or infcrolateral thalamic strokes, usually appearing several months after the event and following full recovery of initially severe motor deficits. Affected patients often show a complex combination of hyperkinetic movements, also described as "jerky dystonic unsteady hand" syndrome [45]. Dystonia and choreoathetosic patterns have been associated with severe positional sensory deficits, whereas tremor/myoclonus patterns were related to severe cerebellar ataxia. Therefore, it has been proposed that these involuntary movements result from failure of the proprioceptive sensory and cerebellar inputs in addition to successful, but unbalanced, recovery of the motor dysfunction [96].

References

1. Caplan LR, Wityk RJ, Glass TA, Tapia J, Pazdera L, Chang HM, et al. New England Medical Center posterior circulation registry. Ann Neurol. 2004;56(3):389–98.
2. Michel P, Odier C, Rutgers M, Reichhart M, Maeder P, Meuli R, et al. The Acute STroke Registry and Analysis of Lausanne (ASTRAL): design and baseline analysis of an ischemic stroke registry including acute multimodal imaging. Stroke. 2010;41(11):2491–8.
3. Arboix A, Arbe G, Garcia-Eroles L, Oliveres M, Parra O, Massons J. Infarctions in the vascular territory of the posterior cerebral artery: clinical features in 232 patients. BMC Res Notes. 2011;4:329.
4. Yamamoto Y, Georgiadis AL, Chang HM, Caplan LR. Posterior cerebral artery territory infarcts in the New England Medical Center Posterior Circulation Registry. Arch Neurol. 1999;56(7):824–32.
5. Lee E, Kang DW, Kwon SU, Kim JS. Posterior cerebral artery infarction: diffusion-weighted MRI analysis of 205 patients. Cerebrovasc Dis. 2009;28(3):298–305.
6. Cals N, Devuyst G, Afsar N, Karapanayiotides T, Bogousslavsky J. Pure superficial posterior cerebral artery territory infarction in The Lausanne Stroke Registry. J Neurol. 2002;249(7):855–61.
7. Kumral E, Bayulkem G, Atac C, Alper Y. Spectrum of superficial posterior cerebral artery territory infarcts. Eur J Neurol. 2004;11(4):237–46.
8. Tao WD, Liu M, Fisher M, Wang DR, Li J, Furie KL, et al. Posterior versus anterior circulation infarction: how different are the neurological deficits? Stroke. 2012;43(8):2060–5.
9. Zurcher E, Richoz B, Faouzi M, Michel P. Differences in ischemic anterior and posterior circulation strokes: a clinico-radiological and outcome analysis. J Stroke Cerebrovasc Dis. 2019;28(3):710–8.
10. Chambers BR, Brooder RJ, Donnan GA. Proximal posterior cerebral artery occlusion simulating middle cerebral artery occlusion. Neurology. 1991;41(3):385–90.
11. North K, Kan A, de Silva M, Ouvrier R. Hemiplegia due to posterior cerebral artery occlusion. Stroke. 1993;24(11):1757–60.
12. Maulaz AB, Bezerra DC, Bogousslavsky J. Posterior cerebral artery infarction from middle cerebral artery infarction. Arch Neurol. 2005;62(6):938–41.
13. Vanacker P, Faouzi M, Eskandari A, Maeder P, Meuli R, Michel P. Large arterial occlusive strokes as a medical emergency: need to accurately predict clot location. Eur J Emerg Med. 2017;24(5):353–8.
14. Tatu L, Moulin T, Bogousslavsky J, Duvernoy H. Arterial territories of the human brain: cerebral hemispheres. Neurology. 1998;50(6):1699–708.
15. Percheron G. The anatomy of the arterial supply of the human thalamus and its use for the interpretation of the thalamic vascular pathology. Z Neurol. 1973;205(1):1–13.
16. Brandt T, Steinke W, Thie A, Pessin MS, Caplan LR. Posterior cerebral artery territory infarcts: clinical features, infarct topography, causes and outcome. Multicenter results and a review of the literature. Cerebrovasc Dis. 2000;10(3):170–82.
17. Chaves CJ, Caplan LR. Posterior cerebral artery. In: Caplan LR, editor. Stroke syndromes. Cambridge: Cambridge University Press; 2012. p. 405–18.
18. Schmahmann JD. Vascular syndromes of the thalamus. Stroke. 2003;34(9):2264–78.
19. Fisher CM. The posterior cerebral artery syndrome. Can J Neurol Sci. 1986;13(3):232–9.
20. Jongen JC, Franke CL, Soeterboek AA, Versteege CW, Ramos LM, van Gijn J. Blood supply of the posterior cerebral artery by the carotid system on angiograms. J Neurol. 2002;249(4):455–60.
21. Nouh A, Remke J, Ruland S. Ischemic posterior circulation stroke: a review of anatomy, clinical presentations, diagnosis, and current management. Front Neurol. 2014;5:30.
22. de Monye C, Dippel DW, Siepman TA, Dijkshoorn ML, Tanghe HL, van der Lugt A. Is a fetal origin of the posterior cerebral artery a risk factor for TIA or ischemic stroke? A study with 16-multidetector-row CT angiography. J Neurol. 2008;255(2):239–45.
23. Okahara M, Kiyosue H, Mori H, Tanoue S, Sainou M, Nagatomi H. Anatomic variations of the cerebral arteries and their embryology: a pictorial review. Eur Radiol. 2002;12(10):2548–61.
24. Gasecki AP, Fox AJ, Lebrun LH, Daneault N. Bilateral occipital infarctions associated with carotid stenosis in a patient with persistent trigeminal artery. The collaborators of the North American Carotid Endarterectomy Trial (NASCET). Stroke. 1994;25(7):1520–3.
25. Guberman A, Stuss D. The syndrome of bilateral paramedian thalamic infarction. Neurology. 1983;33(5):540–6.
26. Bogousslavsky J, Regli F, Uske A. Thalamic infarcts: clinical syndromes, etiology, and prognosis. Neurology. 1988;38(6):837–48.
27. Carrera E, Michel P, Bogousslavsky J. Anteromedian, central, and posterolateral infarcts of the thalamus: three variant types. Stroke. 2004;35(12):2826–31.
28. Bogousslavsky J, Regli F, Assal G. The syndrome of unilateral tuberothalamic artery territory infarction. Stroke. 1986;17(3):434–41.

29. Ghika-Schmid F, Bogousslavsky J. The acute behavioral syndrome of anterior thalamic infarction: a prospective study of 12 cases. Ann Neurol. 2000;48(2):220–7.

30. Carrera E, Bogousslavsky J. The thalamus and behavior: effects of anatomically distinct strokes. Neurology. 2006;66(12):1817–23.

31. von Cramon DY, Hebel N, Schuri U. A contribution to the anatomical basis of thalamic amnesia. Brain. 1985;108(Pt 4):993–1008.

32. Clarke S, Assal G, Bogousslavsky J, Regli F, Townsend DW, Leenders KL, et al. Pure amnesia after unilateral left polar thalamic infarct: topographic and sequential neuropsychological and metabolic (PET) correlations. J Neurol Neurosurg Psychiatry. 1994;57(1):27–34.

33. Castaigne P, Lhermitte F, Buge A, Escourolle R, Hauw JJ, Lyon-Caen O. Paramedian thalamic and midbrain infarct: clinical and neuropathological study. Ann Neurol. 1981;10(2):127–48.

34. Graff-Radford NR, Eslinger PJ, Damasio AR, Yamada T. Nonhemorrhagic infarction of the thalamus: behavioral, anatomic, and physiologic correlates. Neurology. 1984;34(1):14–23.

35. Rossetti AO, Reichhart MD, Bogousslavsky J. Central Horner's syndrome with contralateral ataxic hemiparesis: a diencephalic alternate syndrome. Neurology. 2003;61(3):334–8.

36. Amonoo-Kuofi HS. Horner's syndrome revisited: with an update of the central pathway. Clin Anat. 1999;12(5):345–61.

37. Dejerine J, Roussy J. Le syndrome thalamique. Rev Neurol. 1906;14:521–32.

38. Fisher CM. Thalamic pure sensory stroke: a pathologic study. Neurology. 1978;28(11):1141–4.

39. Kim JS. Pure sensory stroke. Clinical-radiological correlates of 21 cases. Stroke. 1992;23(7):983–7.

40. Déjerine J, Roussy G. Le syndrome thalamique. Rev Neurol (Paris). 1906;14:521.

41. Masdeu JC, Gorelick PB. Thalamic astasia: inability to stand after unilateral thalamic lesions. Ann Neurol. 1988;23(6):596–603.

42. Foix CH, P. Les syndromes de la région thalamique. Presse Med. 1925;1:113–7.

43. Neau JP, Bogousslavsky J. The syndrome of posterior choroidal artery territory infarction. Ann Neurol. 1996;39(6):779–88.

44. Frisen L, Holmegaard L, Rosencrantz M. Sectorial optic atrophy and homonymous, horizontal sectoranopia: a lateral choroidal artery syndrome? J Neurol Neurosurg Psychiatry. 1978;41(4):374–80.

45. Ghika J, Bogousslavsky J, Henderson J, Maeder P, Regli F. The "jerky dystonic unsteady hand": a delayed motor syndrome in posterior thalamic infarctions. J Neurol. 1994;241(9):537–42.

46. Clark JM, Albers GW. Vertical gaze palsies from medial thalamic infarctions without midbrain involvement. Stroke. 1995;26(8):1467–70.

47. Annoni JM, Khateb A, Gramigna S, Staub F, Carota A, Maeder P, et al. Chronic cognitive impairment following laterothalamic infarcts: a study of 9 cases. Arch Neurol. 2003;60(10):1439–43.

48. Lazzaro NA, Wright B, Castillo M, Fischbein NJ, Glastonbury CM, Hildenbrand PG, et al. Artery of percheron infarction: imaging patterns and clinical spectrum. AJNR Am J Neuroradiol. 2010;31(7):1283–9.

49. de la Cruz-Cosme C, Marquez-Martinez M, Aguilar-Cuevas R, Romero-Acebal M, Valdivielso-Felices P. Percheron artery syndrome: variability in presentation and differential diagnosis. Rev Neurol. 2011;53(4):193–200.

50. Reilly M, Connolly S, Stack J, Martin EA, Hutchinson M. Bilateral paramedian thalamic infarction: a distinct but poorly recognized stroke syndrome. Q J Med. 1992;82(297):63–70.

51. Arauz A, Patino-Rodriguez HM, Vargas-Gonzalez JC, Arguelles-Morales N, Silos H, Ruiz-Franco A, et al. Clinical spectrum of artery of Percheron infarct: clinical-radiological correlations. J Stroke Cerebrovasc Dis. 2014;23(5):1083–8.

52. Segarra JM. Cerebral vascular disease and behavior. I. the syndrome of the mesencephalic artery (basilar artery bifurcation). Arch Neurol. 1970;22(5):408–18.

53. Margolis MT, Newton TH, Hoyt WF. Cortical branches of the posterior cerebral artery.Anatomic-radiologic correlation. Neuroradiology. 1971;2(3):127–35.

54. Caplan LR. "Top of the basilar" syndrome. Neurology. 1980;30(1):72–9.

55. Aldrich MS, Alessi AG, Beck RW, Gilman S. Cortical blindness: etiology, diagnosis, and prognosis. Ann Neurol. 1987;21(2):149–58.

56. Kondziella D, Frahm-Falkenberg S. Anton's syndrome and eugenics. J Clin Neurol. 2011;7(2):96–8.

57. De Renzi E, Zambolin A, Crisi G. The pattern of neuropsychological impairment associated with left posterior cerebral artery infarcts. Brain. 1987;110(Pt 5):1099–116.

58. Servan J, Verstichel P, Catala M, Yakovleff A, Rancurel G. Aphasia and infarction of the posterior cerebral artery territory. J Neurol. 1995;242(2):87–92.

59. Leff AP, Spitsyna G, Plant GT, Wise RJ. Structural anatomy of pure and hemianopic alexia. J Neurol Neurosurg Psychiatry. 2006;77(9):1004–7.

60. Geschwind N. Disconnexion syndromes in animals and man. I. Brain. 1965;88(2):237–94.

61. Benton AL. Gerstmann's syndrome. Arch Neurol. 1992;49(5):445–7.

62. Benson DF, Marsden CD, Meadows JC. The amnesic syndrome of posterior cerebral artery occlusion. Acta Neurol Scand. 1974;50(2):133–45.

63. Bartsch T, Deuschl G. Transient global amnesia: functional anatomy and clinical implications. Lancet Neurol. 2010;9(2):205–14.

64. Michel P, Beaud V, Eskandari A, Maeder P, Demonet JF, Eskioglou E. Ischemic amnesia: causes and outcome. Stroke. 2017;48(8):2270–3.

65. Sedlaczek O, Hirsch JG, Grips E, Peters CN, Gass A, Wohrle J, et al. Detection of delayed focal MR changes in the lateral hippocampus in transient global amnesia. Neurology. 2004;62(12):2165–70.

66. Szabo K, Forster A, Jager T, Kern R, Griebe M, Hennerici MG, et al. Hippocampal lesion patterns in acute posterior cerebral artery stroke: clinical and MRI findings. Stroke. 2009;40(6):2042–5.

67. Larrabee GJ, Levin HS, Huff FJ, Kay MC, Guinto FC Jr. Visual agnosia contrasted with visual-verbal disconnection. Neuropsychologia. 1985;23(1):1–12.

68. Martinaud O, Pouliquen D, Gerardin E, Loubeyre M, Hirsbein D, Hannequin D, et al. Visual agnosia and posterior cerebral artery infarcts: an anatomical-clinical study. PLoS One. 2012;7(1):e30433.

69. Coslett HB, Saffran EM. Preserved object recognition and reading comprehension in optic aphasia. Brain. 1989;112(Pt 4):1091–110.

70. Landis T, Cummings JL, Christen L, Bogen JE, Imhof HG. Are unilateral right posterior cerebral lesions sufficient to cause prosopagnosia? Clinical and radiological findings in six additional patients. Cortex. 1986;22(2):243–52.

71. Zeki S. A century of cerebral achromatopsia. Brain. 1990;113(Pt 6):1721–77.

72. Meadows JC, Munro SS. Palinopsia. J Neurol Neurosurg Psychiatry. 1977;40(1):5–8.

73. Takahashi N, Kawamura M. Pure topographical disorientation--the anatomical basis of landmark agnosia. Cortex. 2002;38(5):717–25.

74. Botez SA, Carrera E, Maeder P, Bogousslavsky J. Aggressive behavior and posterior cerebral artery stroke. Arch Neurol. 2007;64(7):1029–33.

75. Pessin MS, Lathi ES, Cohen MB, Kwan ES, Hedges TR 3rd, Caplan LR. Clinical features and mechanism of occipital infarction. Ann Neurol. 1987;21(3):290–9.

76. Steinke W, Mangold J, Schwartz A, Hennerici M. Mechanisms of infarction in the superficial posterior cerebral artery territory. J Neurol. 1997;244(9):571–8.

77. Weber HD. A contribution to the pathology of the crura cerebri. Med Chir Trans. 1863;46:121–39.

78. Parinaud H. Paralysie des mouvements associés des yeux. Arch Neurol. 1883;5:145–72.

79. Hecaen H, De Ajuriaguerra J. Balint's syndrome (psychic paralysis of visual fixation) and its minor forms. Brain. 1954;77(3):373–400.

80. Levine DN, Warach J, Farah M. Two visual systems in mental imagery: dissociation of "what" and "where" in imagery disorders due to bilateral posterior cerebral lesions. Neurology. 1985;35(7):1010–8.

81. Steinke W, Sacco RL, Mohr JP, Foulkes MA, Tatemichi TK, Wolf PA, et al. Thalamic stroke. Presentation and prognosis of infarcts and hemorrhages. Arch Neurol. 1992;49(7):703–10.

82. Gogela SL, Gozal YM, Rahme R, Zuccarello M, Ringer AJ. Beyond textbook neuroanatomy: the syndrome of malignant PCA infarction. Br J Neurosurg. 2015;29(6):871–5.

83. Pfefferkorn T, Deutschlaender A, Riedel E, Wiesmann M, Dichgans M. Malignant posterior cerebral artery infarction. J Neurol. 2006;253(12):1640–1.

84. Milandre L, Brosset C, Botti G, Khalil R. A study of 82 cerebral infarctions in the area of posterior cerebral arteries. Rev Neurol (Paris). 1994;150(2):133–41.

85. Ntaios G, Spengos K, Vemmou AM, Savvari P, Koroboki E, Stranjalis G, et al. Long-term outcome in posterior cerebral artery stroke. Eur J Neurol. 2011;18(8):1074–80.

86. Strambo D, Bartolini B, Beaud V, Nannoni S, Marto JP, Sirimarco G, et al. Thrombectomy and thrombolysis of isolated posterior cerebral artery occlusion: cognitive, visual and disability outcomes. Eur Stroke J. 2019;4(1_suppl):501–2.

87. Gray CS, French JM, Bates D, Cartlidge NE, Venables GS, James OF. Recovery of visual fields in acute stroke: homonymous hemianopia associated with adverse prognosis. Age Ageing. 1989;18(6):419–21.

88. Romano JG. Progress in rehabilitation of hemianopic visual field defects. Cerebrovasc Dis. 2009;27(Suppl 1):187–90.

89. Zhang X, Kedar S, Lynn MJ, Newman NJ, Biousse V. Natural history of homonymous hemianopia. Neurology. 2006;66(6):901–5.

90. Klit H, Finnerup NB, Jensen TS. Central post-stroke pain: clinical characteristics, pathophysiology, and management. Lancet Neurol. 2009;8(9):857–68.

91. Krause T, Brunecker P, Pittl S, Taskin B, Laubisch D, Winter B, et al. Thalamic sensory strokes with and without pain: differences in lesion patterns in the ventral posterior thalamus. J Neurol Neurosurg Psychiatry. 2012;83(8):776–84.

92. Hansson P. Post-stroke pain case study: clinical characteristics, therapeutic options and long-term follow-up. Eur J Neurol. 2004;11(Suppl 1):22–30.

93. Kim JS. Post-stroke pain. Expert Rev Neurother. 2009;9(5):711–21.

94. Flaster M, Meresh E, Rao M, Biller J. Central post-stroke pain: current diagnosis and treatment. Top Stroke Rehabil. 2013;20(2):116–23.

95. Lehericy S, Grand S, Pollak P, Poupon F, Le Bas JF, Limousin P, et al. Clinical characteristics and topography of lesions in movement disorders due to thalamic lesions. Neurology. 2001;57(6):1055–66.

96. Kim JS. Delayed onset mixed involuntary movements after thalamic stroke: clinical, radiological and pathophysiological findings. Brain. 2001;124(Pt 2):299–309.

Cerebellar Infarction

6

Cristina Hobeanu, Elena Viedma-Guiard,
and Pierre Amarenco

Introduction/Epidemiology

The cerebellum is a structure that is located at the back of the brain, underlying the occipital and temporal lobes of the cerebral cortex. It accounts for approximately 10% of the brain's volume, but it contains more neurons than the rest of the brain. The cerebellum is involved in the maintenance of balance and posture, coordination of voluntary movements, motor learning, and cognitive functions.

Infarcts in the cerebellum are an uncommon localization, with a frequency of 2% [1] but a higher mortality than that of other vascular territories, which makes it important to diagnose in early stages.

As cerebellar infarction frequently manifests by nonspecific symptoms such as nausea, vomiting, dizziness, unsteadiness, and headache, its true frequency may be higher, as suggested by autopsy series [2] and MRI series [3].

Compared to hemorrhagic stroke, infarcts are three to four times more frequent in autopsy series [4] and in CT series [5]. There is a male preponderance of two to three times [4, 6]. The mean age is 65 ± 13 years, with one-half of the cases occurring between the ages of 60 and 80 years [7].

C. Hobeanu · E. Viedma-Guiard · P. Amarenco (✉)
Department of Neurology and Stroke Center, Bichat Hospital, Paris University, Paris, France
e-mail: cristina.hobeanu@aphp.fr; elena.viedma@aphp.fr; pierre.amarenco@aphp.fr

Classification

Classically, cerebral infarcts are classified based on arterial territories (Table 6.1) as a function of the three long circumferential arteries arising from the vertebrobasilar system in a rostrocaudal disposition: the posterior inferior cerebellar artery (PICA), anterior inferior cerebellar artery (AICA), and superior cerebellar artery (SCA) (Fig. 6.1). The PICA and SCA are arterial pairs with medial branches that supply mostly the vermian and paravermian portions of the cerebellum, and lateral branches for the cerebellar hemispheres (Fig. 6.2).

Posterior Inferior Cerebellar Artery Infarcts

Infarcts in the PICA territory were extensively studied and once considered to be the most frequent of cerebellar infarcts, but further autopsy studies showed that SCA infarcts may be as or more frequent [2, 6, 8]. The overestimation was partly due to the erroneous consideration that all lateral medullary infarcts (i.e., Wallenberg's syndrome) were due to PICA occlusion. But as Miller Fisher showed, the lateral region of the medulla is mainly supplied by three or four small direct branches arising from the termination of the vertebral artery between the PICA ostium and origin of the basilar artery, and less frequently by small branches arising from the PICA, and in

Table 6.1 Cerebellar stroke syndromes (Amarenco 1991, with permission)

Location of cerebellar infarct	Associated infarcts	Clinical syndrome
Rostral (SCA)	Mesencephallum, subthalamic area, thalamus, occipitotemporal lobes Laterotegmental area of the upper pons	Rostral basilar artery syndrome or coma from onset+/−tetraplegia Dysmetria and Horner's syndrome (ipsilateral), temperature and pain sensory loss, and IVth nerve palsy (contralateral) Dysarthria, headache, dizziness, vomiting, ataxia, and delayed coma (pseudotumoral form)
Dorsomedia (mSCA)		Dysarthria ataxia
Ventrolateral (lSCA)		Dysmetria, axial lateropulsion (ipsilateral), ataxia, and dysarthria
Medial (AICA)	Lateral area of the lower pons	VII, V, VIII, Horner's syndrome, dysmetria (ipsilateral), temperature and pain sensory loss (contralateral) Pure vestibular syndrome
Caudal (PICA)		Vertigo, headache, vomiting, ataxia, and delayed coma (pseudotumoural form)
Dorsomedial (mPICA)	Dorsolateromedullary area	Wallenberg's syndrome Isolated vertigo or vertigo with dysmetria and axial lateropulsion (ipsilateral) and ataxia
Ventrolateral (lPICA)		Vertigo, ipsilateral limb dysmetria AICA syndrome+/−delayed coma (pseudotumoral form)
Caudal and medial	Lateral area of the lower pons and/or lateromedullary area	Vertigo, vomiting, headache, ataxia, dysarthria, and delayed coma (pseudotumoral form)
Rostrocaudal	Brainstem, thalamus, occipitotemporal lobes	Coma from onset+/−tetraplegia

only up to 22% of individuals, this region is supplied by PICA [9].

The posterior inferior cerebellar artery is usually the largest branch of the vertebral artery, and it arises extracranially from its intradural segment, approximately 1.5 cm from the origin of the basilar artery. PICA may also be the termination of the vertebral artery, which, in this case, is smaller than the contralateral vertebral artery. After its origin, it reaches the caudal part of the cerebellar hemisphere and vermis.

It courses transversely and downward along the medulla, and then it makes a first caudal loop, ascending in the sulcus separating the dorsal medulla from the tonsil of the cerebellum. It then makes a second loop above the cranial part of the tonsil and descends, following the inferior vermis, where it divides into a medial branch (mPICA) and a lateral branch at a variable level between the two first loops [10, 11], On an axial mid-medullary and cerebellar section, the mPICA

supplies a triangular area with a dorsal base and a ventral apex toward the fourth ventricle, first described in 1990 [12]. The medial branch of the PICA supplies the inferior vermis (nodulus, uvula, pyramis, tuber, and sometimes clivus) and the internal parts of the lobulus semilunaris inferior, lobulus gracilis, and tonsil; mPICA exists even when the PICA is hypoplasic. In this case, the lateral branch of the PICA arises from the anterior and inferior cerebellar artery [13] as there is a reciprocal relation between these two arteries. At times, the sole medial branch participates in the blood supply of the medulla [14] in its dorsal region, and sometimes in the lateral retro-olivary area [15]. This latter region is usually supplied by small short circumferential arteries arising from the vertebral artery [9, 16].

Infarcts of the medial branch may be clinically silent [6, 7, 17]. Its anatomo-clinical manifestations have been first described in 1990 [17] and present with three main patterns: (1) Wallenberg's

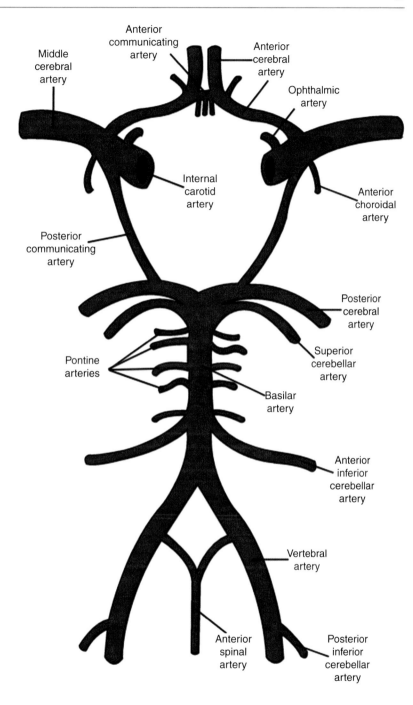

Fig. 6.1 Schematic representation of the basilar and vertebral arteries and their branches Gross anatomy

syndrome when the medulla is also involved, (2) vertigo together with ipsilateral axial lateropulsion of trunk and gaze, and dysmetria or unsteadiness (hence, cerebellar signs can be minimal, and MRI may be required for diagnosis), and (3) isolated vertigo often misdiagnosed as labyrinthitis [6, 7, 17].

1. When PICA includes the dorsal lateral part of the medulla, patients present with Wallenberg's syndrome that can be complete or not, including vertigo, nystagmus, Vth, IXth, and Xth cranial nerve palsies, ipsilateral Horner's syndrome, appendicular ataxia, and contralateral temperature and pain sensory loss (Fig. 6.3).

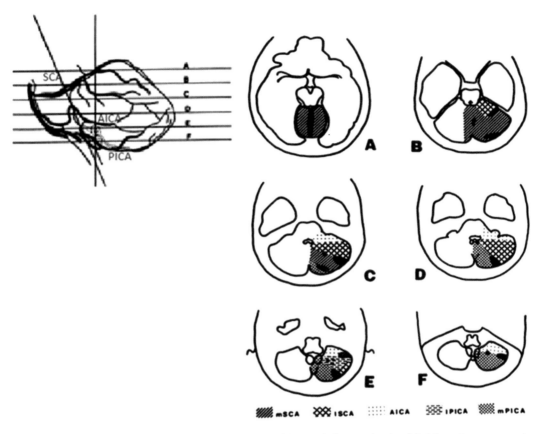

Fig. 6.2 Anatomical drawings of the territory of branches of the cerebellar arteries (modified from Amarenco et al., 1993b, with permission)

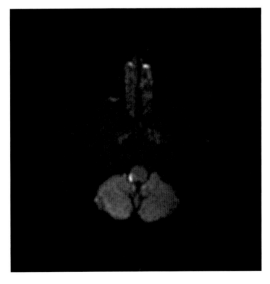

Fig. 6.3 A 70-year-old patient with dorsolateral medullar stroke

2. When PICA territory infarcts spare the medulla (Fig. 6.4), they mainly present with vertigo, headache, gait ataxia, appendicular ataxia, and horizontal nystagmus. Headache is cervical, occipital, or both plus occasional periauricular or hemifacial-ocular radiation. Unilateral headaches are ipsilateral to the cerebellar infarction [18]. Nystagmus is the most frequent sign (75%) either horizontal (ipsilateral in 47% of patients, contralateral in 5%, bilateral in 11%) or vertical (11% of patients) [19]. In addition to vertigo, one of the most striking findings in PICA infarcts is ipsilateral axial lateropulsion [17] as if there was a lateral projection of the central representation of the center of gravity. This sign is totally different from the lateral deviation of the limbs (i.e., past-pointing) and gait veering. Attempts at

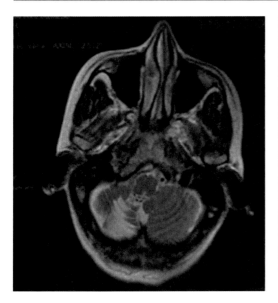

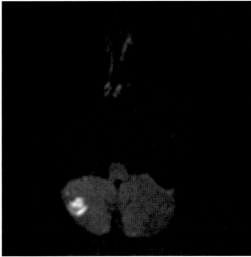

Fig. 6.5 Infarct in the lateral branch of the right PICA

Fig. 6.4 Right medial PICA stroke in a 45-year-old patient

standing or walking led to falling toward the side of the cerebellar infarction [18]. In one-quarter of patients, there may be signs of brainstem compression such as drowsiness and lateral gaze palsy, followed by progressive coma [18].

3. An isolated acute vertigo form, mimicking labyrinthitis [17], may be seen in patients with medial and caudal cerebellar infarct with involvement of the uvulonodular complex of the vermis, which is part of the vestibular portion of the cerebellum. The MRI has shown the high frequency of such infarcts [8], which should be done when there are vascular risk factors or in the circumstances supporting a vascular mechanism. Normal caloric responses and direction-changing nystagmus on gaze to each side, or after changing of head posture, or lying down, are two other signs that can suggest a "pure" vestibular syndrome in a patient with a PICA territory infarct [6, 20].

PICA infarcts may be in association with AICA or SCA infarcts with a more severe clinical presentation.

These multiple cerebellar infarcts, constituting about 20% of all cerebellar infarcts in autopsy series, often present with a pseudotumoral pattern or deep coma with quadraplegia [7].

The lateral branch of the posterior inferior cerebellar artery (lPICA) supplies the anterolateral region of the caudal part of the cerebellar hemisphere. Infarcts of the lateral branch of PICA (Fig. 6.5) are less frequent, initially described as chance autopsy findings with no available clinical information [6]. With time, clinical manifestations were described, mainly rotatory vertigo and isolated ipsilateral dysmetria or nystagmus [8].

The main cause of infarcts in the PICA territory is arterial occlusion, mainly involving the intracranial portion of the vertebral artery facing the PICA ostium and the origin of the PICA. The mechanisms of occlusion are equally divided into cardioembolic and atherosclerotic causes [6, 18], with maybe the predominance of atherosclerosis for infarcts of lPICA [8]. Other mechanisms are vertebral artery dissection [18], ulcerated plaques in the aortic arch [7], PFO (Fig. 6.6), and occlusion of the mPICA by tonsillar herniation due to raised posterior fossa pressure [21].

The evolution of infarcts in PICA territory is usually favorable with good outcome [18].

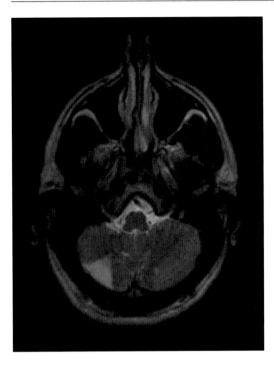

Fig. 6.6 Bilateral PICA infarcts in a 33-year-old patient with PFO

Anterior Inferior Cerebellar Artery Infarcts

The infarction in the territory of the anterior inferior cerebellar artery (AICA) is rare, but it is probably underestimated.

The anterior cerebellar artery is an almost constant artery. It usually arises from the basilar artery, from its lower third in 75% of cases. It can also arise from the vertebral artery or by a common trunk with the posterior inferior cerebellar artery (PICA) from the basilar artery. Infrequently, there are small arteries directly from the basilar artery that replace the AICA [13].

It supplies a small area of the anterior and medial cerebellum, the middle cerebellar peduncle, and the floculus. Proximal branches of the AICA usually supply the lateral portion of the pons, including the facial, trigeminal, and vestibular nuclei, the root of the VIIth and VIIIth cranial nerves, and the spinothalamic tract.

The clinical presentation typically involves several cranial ipsilateral nerves: trigeminal sensory impairment, facial palsy, deafness, vestibular syndrome, or lateral gaze palsy. Frequently, we can find cerebellar signs, and, at times, there is contralateral pain and temperature sensory loss. This last characteristic and the other signs associated (like sometimes Horner's syndrome and the cranial nerve involvement with ataxia) may be confused with Wallenberg's syndrome due to lateral medullar infarction. Considering some signs that are unusual in Wallenberg's syndrome, such as deafness with or without tinnitus or lateral gaze palsy, may help in clinical differential diagnosis [13, 19].

Dysphagia can be due to an extension of the infarction to the superior part of the lateral medulla, and contralateral limb weakness can be observed when the corticospinal tract in the pons or mesencephalon is involved [22].

There may be an isolated vestibular manifestation but is rare. AICA infarcts can also cause isolated cerebellar signs.

The classic syndrome of AICA occlusion was described by Adams from a single neuropathologic case [23]. It involved vertigo, tinnitus, ipsilateral hearing loss, dysarthria, peripheral facial palsy, Horner's syndrome, multimodal facial hypoesthesia, and ipsilateral limb ataxia accompanied by contralateral thermanalgesia of the limbs and trunk [23]. The AICA syndromes were fully described in 1990 in the only large clinico-neuropathological series available [13].

The main cause is atherosclerotic occlusion. Pure AICA infarcts are usually due to basilar branch occlusion. Plaques in the basilar artery extent into AICA, or small atheroma occludes the AICA origin. We can also find arterial occlusion that involves the lower basilar artery and less frequently the end of the vertebral artery above the PICA ostium at postmortem examination [24]. Patients with "AICA plus" infarcts mainly have proximal basilar artery occlusion.

Nevertheless, atrial fibrillation should not be ruled out. Other less frequent etiologies such as vasculitis or dolichoectasia are also described (Fig. 6.7).

These patients usually present with vascular risk factors like high blood pressure or diabetes.

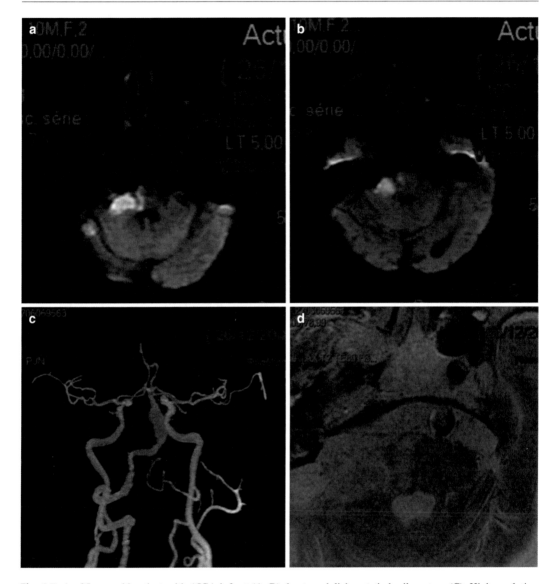

Fig. 6.7 An 85-year-old patient with AICA infarct (A, B) due to a dolichoectatic basilar artery (C). High-resolution MRI (D) showing a thrombus inside the basilar artery

Superior Cerebellar Artery Infarcts

Infarctions in the territory of the superior cerebellar artery (SCA) are among the most common of the cerebellar stroke syndromes.

The SCA supplies the rostral half of the cerebellar hemisphere and vermis as well as the dentate nucleus. This artery also vascularizes a small portion of the brainstem, the laterotegmental portion of the rostral pons, and lower midbrain.

Full clinicopathological description of SCA infarcts has been done in the largest clinical-neuropathological series available [25]. Infarcts in the full territory of the SCA are usually accompanied by other infarcts in the rostral territory of the basilar artery, involving uni- or bilateral occipitotemporal lobes, thalamic and subthalamic areas, and the mesencephalon [25].

The typical clinical features of the infarcts in the SCA territory are dysarthria and ipsilateral limb ataxia. Dysarthria can be useful for differentiating from the PICA stroke [2]. Nystagmus is caused by involvement of the medial longitudinal fasciculus and the cerebellar pathways.

When the dorsal mesencephalic territory is involved, the clinical presentation may include Horner's syndrome, fourth nerve palsy, and contralateral temperature and pain sensory loss. Ipsilateral abnormal limb movements (choreiform or athetotic) can be associated. These features characterize the classic SCA syndrome as described by Guillain, Bertrand, and Péron, but it is rare to find [26].

Isolated occlusion of the lateral branch of the SCA was also described in 1991 [27, 28]. The lateral SCA syndrome includes ipsilateral limb dysmetria, ipsilateral axial lateropulsion, dysarthria, and gait unsteadiness. Similarly, an involvement of the medial branch of SCA can cause a dorsomedial SCA infarction with a clinical manifestation that includes unsteadiness of gait and dysarthria [27].

In the case of infarcts in the occipitotemporal lobes or in the thalamic or subthalamic areas, we can find other clinical signs such as hemianopsia, memory loss or confusion, Balint's syndrome, multimodal sensory loss, transcortical aphasia, and motor weakness.

There is sometimes a deep coma from onset, with or without quadriplegia when there is sudden occlusion of the basilar artery.

SCA infarcts may have a pseudotumoral presentation, especially if the territory of the PICA is also involved, with rapidly progressive cerebellar edema that leads to obstructive hydrocephalus and acute intracranial hypertension [1, 21].

In the SCA territory, more than one-half of infarcts are due to cardioembolism (with atrial fibrillation as the main cause) (Fig. 6.8).

Sometimes, the responsible stroke mechanism is artery-to-artery embolism either atherosclerotic, from vertebral artery occlusion, or ulcerated plaques in the aortic arch. There are also cases described with embolisms from vertebral artery dissection.

Multiple Infarcts

Initially described in autopsy series [2], the occurrence of multiple infarcts in the posterior circulation territory was further documented with the development of imaging techniques, such as CT and MRI. Multiple infarcts can appear in the cerebellum in different arterial territories, PICA and SCA or PICA, AICA, and SCA, or may be associated with ischemic lesions in the brain stem or other regions of the posterior circulation. Basilar occlusion or occlusion of the dominant

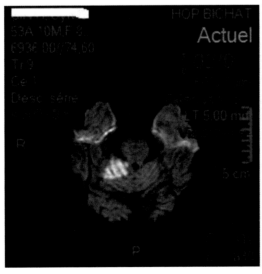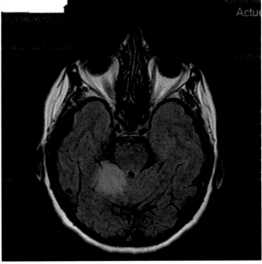

Fig. 6.8 Lateral SCA infarct in a 53-year-old woman with atrial fibrillation

vertebral artery may manifest in the same way with infarcts in multiple cerebellar territories and brainstem that can a have a severe course.

In the New England Medical Center Posterior Circulation Registry [29], the multiple territory infarcts were divided into two groups: proximal and distal intracranial territories (PICA and SCA), and those that included the middle intracranial territory (PICA and AICA, AICA and SCA, and PICA, AICA, and SCA). Embolism was the predominant stroke mechanism in patients with proximal and distal territory cerebellar infarction: emboli from the extracranial vertebral artery or cardiac sources like cardiomyopathy, atrial fibrillation, valvular disease, and PFO. In patients with emboli that arose from the extracranial vertebral artery (ECVA), the emboli presumably first stopped at the intracranial part of the vertebral artery (ICVA) and then it traveled distally, or a part to the SCA-distal basilar artery region.

In contrast to the proximal+distal territory, when the middle territory was involved, the most common cause was large artery intracranial occlusive disease. Embolism was a less common cause occurring in about one-third of patients. Basilar artery lesions are more often due to in situ occlusive disease of the basilar artery itself or to propagation of thrombus from the ICVA. ICVA and basilar artery occlusive disease often coexist.

Small Cerebellar Infarcts

With the MRI gaining its place in diagnosing cerebellar infarcts, very small cerebellar infarcts (<2 cm) are now a frequent finding and were first described in 1993 [30]. These small infarcts, also known as border-zone cerebellar infarcts, have yet unclear mechanism. They are located in boundary zones (or end zones), also called nonterritorial infarcts [8], between the SCA and PICA or between left and right SCAs on the cortex [8, 30], and between SCA and PICA in the deep cerebellar white matter.

The location can be divided into three groups: cortical border-zone infarcts, very small deep infarcts in the deep watershed territory, usually limited to a small hole outside the dentate nucleus, cortical and superficial small infarcts along the boundary zone between cortical superficial branches of the SCA and PICA.

1. Cortical border-zone infarcts in a parallel direction with the penetrator branches, which are perpendicular to the cortex, are most frequent and located at the boundary zones between SCA and PICA territories, corresponding to the AICA-PICA, mPICA-lPICA, mPICA-SCA, and mSCA-lSCA border zones. Other border-zone infarcts involved the medial rostral cerebellum between the right and left SC [30].
2. Very small deep infarcts in the deep watershed territory [30] in a small hole outside the dentate nucleus: The infarcts involve usually the caudal cerebellum and are located at the deep boundary zones of the AICA, lPICA, mPICA, lSCA, and mSCA territories. These arteries supply the dentate nucleus area, and they anastomose with superficial branches penetrating the cortex perpendicularly.
3. Cortical dorsal border-zone infarcts between PICA and SCA: They are strictly cortical and superficially located along the boundary zone between cortical superficial branches of the SCA and PICA.

Small cerebellar infarcts were classified according to border zones in between perfusion territories, but a functional topographic classification according to an anatomical location in the cerebellum was also proposed [31]. Thus, they were classified according to their midline or hemispheric location in either the anterior, posterior, or flocculonodular lobe. Thus, they can be localized in the anterior or posterior vermis, in the nodulus, in the anterior or posterior hemisphere, or in the flocculus. A more precise classification in terms of affected lobule(s) was proposed for research purpose [31].

Border-zone infarcts do not differ clinically from territorial infarcts [8, 30]. Some patients may have transient loss of consciousness, postural trunk or head position-related symptoms for days, weeks, months, or years before or after the infarct, light headedness, pitching sensations, vertigo, and disequilibrium, resulting from a low flow state in the posterior circulation.

The etiology also does not differ from territorial infarct [8, 30]. Small nonterritorial cerebellar infarcts have the same high rate of embolic mechanism (47%) with the same frequency of the cardiac source of embolism (42%) and of large artery occlusive disease (19%). They differ by the presence of more frequent low flow states distal to bilateral vertebral artery occlusion (14% in nonterritorial infarcts vs. 0% in territorial infarcts) and by the presence of more frequent hypercoagulable states resulting in end-artery disease (17% in nonterritorial infarcts vs. 1.25% in territorial infarcts) [8, 32].

Three circumstances can be distinguished.

1. Focal hypoperfusion distal to large artery occlusion is the most frequent mechanism [30]. It often involves the proximal basilar artery+/− AICA and sometimes a distal vertebral artery occlusion ipsilateral to the border-zone cerebellar infarct. The rostral basilar artery can be supplied by retrograde filling from the superior cerebellar arteries or posterior communicating arteries. Other cases are due to bilateral vertebral artery occlusion, either distal, or proximal on one side and distal on the other, and the lack of anastomoses causes the infarct in a border-zone area.
2. Small or end (pial) artery disease associated with primary or secondary hypercoagulable states, which are known to give border-zone infarcts: thrombocythemia, polycythemia, hypereosinophilia, and disseminated intravascular coagulation [8]. Arteritis and cholesterol emboli are occasionally encountered [8]. Other patients have severe intracranial distal atheroma with MRI showing multiple small cortical and deep infarcts of the cerebral hemispheres and angiography demonstrating multiple intracranial arterial stenoses and no extracranial atheroma.
3. Systemic hypotension due to cardiac arrest is seldom the cause of border-zone cerebellar infarcts as the cerebellum seems to be relatively protected from deep systemic hypotension [30].

The more recent SMART-Medea study [3] showed that small cerebellar infarcts predominantly involved the posterior lobes, sparing the subcortical white matter and occurring in characteristic topographic patterns. This could be explained by the distribution of the white matter in shape of a tree with branches of subcortical white matter and stem of deep white matter. These branches with the surrounding cortex form the cerebellar folia. These folia receive arterial supply from arterial branches in two fissures. This dual cortical arterial supply accounts for the subcortical white matter sparing of the observed cortical infarcts [33] in larger infarcts caused by a more proximal occlusion of a cerebellar artery. However, arterial branches may be occluded in both the fissure above and beneath the infarcted folium, leaving no collateral arterial supply [3] (Fig. 6.9).

Four patterns of small cerebellar infarct were described: infarcts occurring in the apex of a large (pattern 1) or a small fissure (pattern 2), infarcts occurring more superficially alongside one (pattern 3) or opposite sides (pattern 4) of a fissure, and infarcts bridging multiple fissures.

Lacunar Infarction

Lipohyalinosis has never been reported in the cerebellum in association with a stroke syndrome. Lacunes of vascular origin have been scarcely described in postmortem studies and rarely seen in radiologic studies [34]. The arterial anatomic disposition with progressively tapered arteries reaching the deep cerebellar white matter does not favor lacunar stroke [34]. Small deep infarcts with CT and MRI appearance of lacunae have been described in the watershed area between the SCA, PICA, and AICA and were associated with large artery occlusive disease, cardiac source of embolism, and end-artery disease, aortic arch atheroma, and intracranial atheroma.

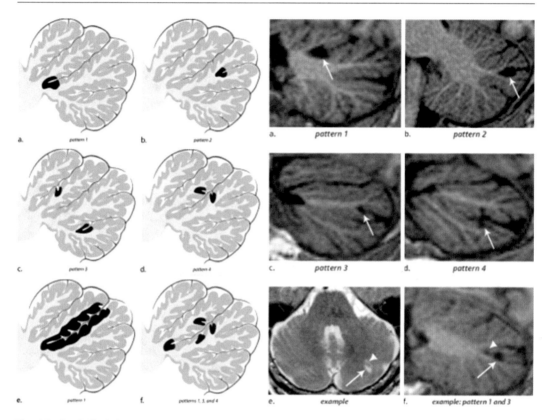

Fig. 6.9 Cerebellar infarct patterns: the SMART-Medea study (with permission)

Etiology of Cerebellar Infarcts

The causes and risk factors of cerebellar infarcts do not differ from other cerebral infarcts [2, 7, 8], and we can find large vessel atherosclerosis, cardioembolism, and arterial dissection as well as less frequent causes like hypercoagulable states or vasculitis [8].

Cardioembolic causes seem to be more frequent, and up to 54% of small nonterritorial infarcts as well as large territorial infarcts [8, 25] may be of cardiac origin. Infarcts in the SCA and PICA territory are more associated with a cardiac source, and up to 80% of SCA infarcts and 50% for PICA [8, 18, 25] come from cardiac causes such as atrial fibrillation, valvular disease, cardiomyopathy, PFO, or angiographic complication. Certain studies have shown that PFO was associated with strokes more often in the vertebrobasilar territory [35].

An atheromatous mechanism is described in 23–32% of infarcts, mainly in the AICA territory [2].

The histologic features do not differ qualitatively from atherosclerosis elsewhere, but ulceration in plaques is less frequent than in the anterior circulation [7, 36]. When ulceration is present, it affects the subclavian artery or the vertebral arteries in their proximal segments [7]. Ulcerated atherosclerotic plaques in the aortic arch can also be a source of arterio-arterial embolism and were first described as a cause of cerebellar infarcts [6, 7, 13, 21] before being described in ischemic stroke overall [37].

Atherosclerotic stenosis is common at the origin of the vertebral arteries and also in the intracranial portion of them (V4). Thrombus formed in V4 frequently extends into the proximal basilar artery [7, 38, 39].

For the basilar artery, stenosis is more frequently found in the proximal 2 cm of the vessel. At its distal end, the origin of the posterior cere-

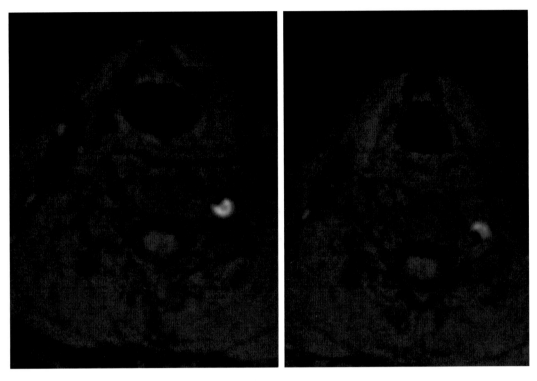

Fig. 6.10 Fat-saturated T1 axial images in MRI: left vertebral artery dissection (intramural hemorrhage seen as hyperintensity)

bral arteries is also a common site of atheromatous lesions [7].

Thrombi within the basilar artery frequently extend to the orifice of the next long circumferential cerebellar artery (the AICA or SCA) [7].

Atherosclerosis may also affect the branches of the vertebral and basilar arteries. AICA occlusions are atherothrombotic and in situ in most cases [6, 7, 13, 21].

Small artery disease can also be the cause of cerebellar infarcts. A process called lipohyalinosis is the responsible mechanism for this type of infarcts, which are generally small, usually less than one/two centimeters of diameter. This process is characterized by fibrinoid vessel wall necrosis and segmental arteriolar disorganization that can obliterate the lumen and leads to ischemia distal to the lesion. This same mechanism can produce hemorrhage due to the weakness of the wall. The small artery disease is usually associated with vascular risk factors such as high blood pressure or diabetes.

In the case of artery dissection, the vessel most commonly affected in the posterior circulation is the extracranial vertebral artery. It is important to evaluate all the arterial axes as we can find bilateral artery dissection or concomitant dissection of the internal carotid. The diagnosis is based on echographic, tomographic, and MRI findings. Fat-saturated T1 axial images in MRI are more sensitive at imaging intramural hemorrhage.

Vertebral artery dissection [8] should be especially considered in young patients with no known predisposing vascular risk factors for atherosclerosis or cerebral embolism, especially if there is neck pain, recent trauma, or neck manipulation, or in patients with Marfan's syndrome, Ehlers–Danlos syndrome (Fig. 6.10), systemic lupus erythematosus, fibromuscular dysplasia, or pseudoxanthoma elasticum.

Dissection of the basilar artery and its major branches is very uncommon but real with possible fatal complications (Fig. 6.11).

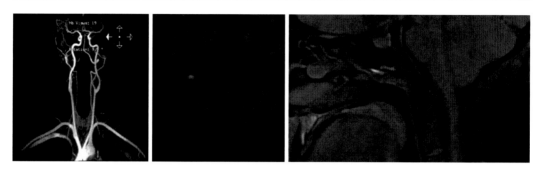

Fig. 6.11 Right vertebral artery dissection extending to the basilar artery in a 38-year-old patient with vertebrobasilar stroke due to Ehlers–Danlos syndrome

Less common causes include hypercoagulable states (like antiphospholipid syndrome) or vasculitis (Wegener more frequently) [30].

In 20–30% of patients, the etiology remains undetermined.

Treatment

The acute management of cerebellar infarction is similar to the management of the rest of strokes.

The fibrinolysis with rTPA iv has proven its efficacy within the 4 or 5 h of symptom onset in selected patients (after evaluating radiological and clinical information, absence of contraindications) [40].

In the case of basilar artery occlusion, mechanical thrombectomy within 6 h of symptom onset in carefully selected patients may be indicated, but its benefits have not been proven yet (there are clinical trials ongoing). Nevertheless, the clinical data are in favor of this procedure [40], also given the high mortality and complications of this condition. There are experts who considered that the therapeutic window could be extended up to 8–12 h after onset (always considering the clinical features and radiological findings).

During the surveillance after a cerebellar infarction, if clinical deterioration occurs (decreasing level of consciousness, new oculomotor signs, etc.), it is indicated to repeat brain imaging to distinguish brainstem ischemia from secondary brainstem compression or hydrocephalus [40].

Suboccipital decompressive craniectomy should be considered in the case of pronounced edema with brainstem compression. The decompressive craniectomy may or may not be combined with resection of the necrotic tissue.

External ventricular drainage should be considered if an obstructive hydrocephalus occurs [40] (Fig. 6.12). Hydrocephalus usually occurs in the first 48–72 h, although it can occur any time within the first week.

The secondary stroke prevention with antiplatelet/anticoagulant agents and control of the risk factors is the same as the treatment for the ischemic stroke in the anterior circulation and depends on the cause and the identified vascular risk factors.

The optimal time to start oral anticoagulation in acute cardioembolic infarction is uncertain. However, it is probably between 4 and 14 days after stroke onset, depending on the balance between the risk of recurrent stroke and the risk of hemorrhagic transformation of the infarcted brain.

Dual antiplatelet therapy might be indicated for 3 months if there is significant aortic arch atheroma (>4 mm) or intracranial stenosis. Dual antiplatelet therapy can also be administrated during the first weeks after the stroke, especially if the cause is atherosclerosis (currently there are ongoing trials). The individual risk of bleeding and the potential benefits before starting should be evaluated.

In the case of artery dissection, anticoagulation has no proven better efficacy than antiplatelet therapy [41], but it can be used within the first

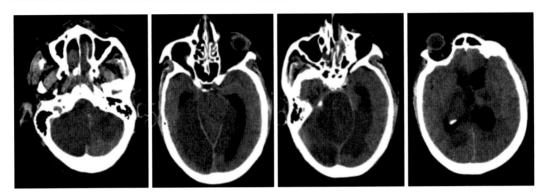

Fig. 6.12 Ventricular drainage was performed in a patient with multiple, bilateral infarcts in the cerebellum and posterior cerebral artery territories associated with ventricular hydrocephalus

6–12 weeks. Some authors recommend antico-agulation if there is an arterial occlusion or severe stenosis. After a few weeks, antiplatelet or anti-coagulant therapy can be stopped if *"restitution ad integrum"* is achieved or the occlusion persists, and it is unclear whether it should be continued if in the follow-up imaging there are aneurysms or remaining stenosis. Intravenous thrombolysis is not contraindicated in this case, only in the case of subarachnoid hemorrhage, which also contraindicates the anticoagulation.

In the case of discovery of a patent foramen ovale with no other stroke etiology found, if it is associated with atrial septal aneurysm or large interatrial shunt, in patients up to 60 years, the closure of the foramen ovale can be proposed [42].

Prognosis

Patients with cerebellar stroke usually have a good prognosis and good recovery, more frequent than that of stroke in the anterior circulation. Excellent recovery with a little or no assistance, as evaluated by the Functional Independence Measure, may be obtained in over 80% of survivors [43]. In most series, more than two-thirds of patients have Rankin scores consistent with independence at 3 months.

Nevertheless, in the early phase, cerebellar infarction has greater fatality rate than any other location of brain infarction, and significant morbidity, due to rapidly progressing cerebellar

edema with acute hydrocephalus, brainstem compression, and death.

The rapid diagnosis and the surveillance in stroke units with an early recognition (using a combination of clinical and radiological findings) of patients eligible for surgical decompression may improve the outcome. About half of the patients who progress to coma and who are treated with decompressive craniectomy have good outcomes (modified Rankin scale score ≤ 2) [44].

We can distinguish different groups of patients according to their clinical course [1]:

– Patients whose conscious state remains unimpaired.
– Some patients suffer a sudden deterioration of consciousness, within the first few hours, usually due to extension of the ischemic process to the brainstem.
– Patients with delayed alteration of consciousness, from a few hours to 10 days, due to compressive edema. Decompressive surgery is needed when deterioration of consciousness appears. Total recovery is obtained in 63% of published cases after ventricular drainage or opening of the dura mater by suboccipital craniectomy, but prognosis depends on whether there is an associated brainstem infarct or not [21].

As regards functional outcome, the modified Rankin Score should be preferred to the NIHSS, which is a score mainly oriented for anterior circulation strokes, since patients with a low NIHSS may have disability. Worse outcome occurs for lesions >20 cc, and there is also an association with the development of hydrocephalus and brainstem compression. The outcome is also worse if there is more than one arterial territory affected.

Regarding the arterial territory, functional disability occurred most frequently in those with SCA infarcts compared with those with lesions in other single artery regions [21, 45].

Several studies have reported that a reduced level of consciousness at the initial presentation is strongly correlated with poor outcome. On the other hand, the presenting syndrome of vertigo/vomiting/ataxia/headache is correlated with a better functional recovery (probably related with an isolated cerebellar involvement) [2].

An activation of contralateral cerebellar and neocortical areas may explain a good recovery of the territorial infarcts [46].

References

1. Macdonell RA, et al. Cerebellar infarction: natural history, prognosis, and pathology. Stroke. 1987;18:849–55.
2. Amarenco P. The spectrum of cerebellar infarctions. Neurology. 1991;41(7):973–9.
3. De Cocker LJL, Geerlings MI, Hartkamp NS, Grool AM, Mali WP, Van der Graaf Y, Kloppenborg RP, Hendrikse J, SMART study group. Cerebellar infarct patterns: the SMART-Medea study. Neuroimage Clin. 2015;8:314–21. https://doi.org/10.1016/j.nicl.2015.02.001.
4. Sypert GW, Alvord EC. Cerebellar infarction: a clinicopathologic study. Arch Neurol. 1975;32:357–63.
5. Shenkin HA, Zavala M. Cerebellar strokes: mortality, surgical indications, and results of ventricular drainage. Lancet. 1982;11:429–31.
6. Amarenco P, Hauw J-J, Hénin D, et al. Les infarctus du territoire de l'artère cérébelleuse postero inferieure: étude clinico-pathologique de 28 cas. Rev Neurol (Paris). 1989;145:277–86.
7. Hauw AP, Gautier J-C J-J. Arterial pathology in cerebellar infarction. Stroke. 1990;21:1299–305.
8. Amarenco P, Lévy C, Cohen A, Touboul P-J, Roullet E, Bousser M-G. Causes and mechanisms of territorial and nonterritorial cerebellar infarcts in 115 consecutive cases. Stroke. 1994;25:105–12.
9. Fisher CM, Karnes WE, Kubik CS. Lateral medullary infarction: the pattern of vascular occlusion. J Neuropathol Exp Neurol. 1961;20:323–79.
10. Margolis MT, Newton TH. The posterior inferior cerebellar artery. In: Newton MT, Poots TH, editors. Radiology of the skull and brain angiography, vol. 68. Saint-Louis: CV Mosby; 1974. p. 1710–74.
11. Taveras JM, Wood EH. Diagnostic neuroradiology, vol. II. Baltimore: Williams and Wilkins; 1976. p. 783–7, 793–6.
12. Amarenco P, Hauw JJ. Anatomie des arteres cerebelleuses. Rev Neurol (Paris). 1989;145:267–76.
13. Amarenco P, Hauw JJ. Cerebellar infarction in the territory of the anterior and inferior cerebellar artery. A clinicopathological study of 20 cases. Brain. 1990;113:139–55.
14. Goodhart SP, Davison C. Syndrome of the posterior inferior cerebellar arteries and of anterior inferior cerebellar arteries and their branches. Arch Neurol Psychiatry. 1936;35:501–24.
15. Duvernoy HM. Human brainstem vessels. Berlin: Springer; 1978.
16. Hauw JJ, Der Agopian P, Trelles L, Escourolle R. Les infarctus bulbaires. Etude systematique de la topographie lesionnelle dans 49 cas. J Neurol Sci. 1976;28:83–102.
17. Amarenco P, Roullet E, Hommel M, Chaine P, Marteau R. Infarction in the territory of the medial branch of the posterior inferior cerebellar artery. J Neurol Neurosurg Psychiatry. 1990;53:731–5.
18. Kase CS, Norrving B, Levine SR, et al. Cerebellar infarction. Clinico-anatomic correlations. Stroke. 1993;24:76–83.
19. Amarenco P, Hauw J-J, Caplan LR. Cerebellar infarctions (Chapter 16). In: Lechtenberg R, editor. Handbook of cerebellar diseases. New York: Marcel Dekker; 1993. p. 251–90.
20. Duncan GW, Parker SW, Fisher CM. Acute cerebellar infarction in the PICA territory. Arch Neurol. 1975;32(6):364–8.
21. Amarenco P, Hauw J-J. Infarctus cérébelleux oedémateux. Etude clinico-pathologique de 16 cas. Neurochirurgie. 1990;36:234–41.
22. Kumral E, Kisabay A, Ataç C. Lesion patterns and etiology of ischemia in the anterior inferior cerebellar artery territory involvement: a clinical—diffusion weighted—MRI study. Eur J Neurol. 2006;13(4):395–401.
23. Adams RD. Occlusion of anterior inferior cerebellar artery. Arch NeurPsych. 1943;49(5):765–70.
24. Amarenco P, Rosengart A, DeWitt LD, Pessin MS, Caplan LR. Anterior inferior cerebellar artery territory infarcts. Mechanisms and clinical features. Arch Neurol. 1993;50:154–61.
25. Amarenco P, Hauw J. Cerebellar infarction in the territory of the superior cerebellar artery: a clinicopathologic study of 33 cases. Neurology. 1990;40(9):1383–90.
26. Guillain G, Bertrand I, Peron P. Le syndrome de l'artère cérébelleuse supérieure. Rev Neurol. 1928;2:835.
27. Amarenco P, Roullet E, Goujon C, Chkron F, Hauw J, Bousser M. Infarction in the anterior rostral cerebel-

lum (the territory of the lateral branch of the superior cerebellar artery). Neurology. 1991;41(2 Pt 1):253–8.

28. Kumral E, Kısabay A, Ataç C. Lesion patterns and etiology of ischemia in superior cerebellar artery territory infarcts a clinical—diffusion weighted—MRI study. Cerebrovasc Dis. 2005;19(5):283–90.

29. Yamamoto Y, Georgiadis A, Chang H-M, Caplan LR. Posterior cerebral artery territory infarcts in the New England Medical Center (NEMC) posterior circulation registry. Arch Neurol. 1999;56:824–32.

30. Amarenco P, Kase CS, Rosengart A, Pessin MS, Bousser M-G, Caplan LR. Very small (border zone) cerebellar infarcts: distribution, mechanisms, causes and clinical features. Brain. 1993;116:161–86.

31. De Cocker LJL, van Veluw SJ, Fowkes M, Luijten PR, Mali WPTM, Hendrikse J. Very small cerebellar infarcts: integration of recent insights into a functional topographic classification. Cerebrovasc Dis. 2013;36:81–7. https://doi.org/10.1159/000353668.

32. Canaple S, Bogousslavsky J. Multiple large and small cerebellar infarcts. J Neurol Neurosurg Psychiatry. 1999;66:739–45.

33. Duvernoy H, Delon S, Vannson JL. The vascularization of the human cerebellar cortex. Brain Res Bull. 1983;11(4):419–80.

34. Amarenco P. Small deep cerebellar infarcts (Chapter 20). In: Donnan GA, Norrving B, Bamford JM, Bogousslavsky J, editors. Lacunar and other subcortical infarctions. Oxford: Oxford University Press; 1995. p. 208–13.

35. Kim BJ, Sohn H, Sun BJ, Song JK, Kang DW, Kim JS, et al. Im aging characteristics of ischemic strokes related to patent fora men ovale. Stroke. 2013;44:3350–6.

36. Zürcher E, Richoz B, Faouzi M, Michel P. Differences in ischemic anterior and posterior circulation strokes: a clinico-radiological and outcome analysis. J Stroke Cerebrovasc Dis. 2019;28(3):710–8.

37. Amarenco P, Duyckaerts C, Tzourio C, Hénin D, Bousser M-G, Hauw J-J. The prevalence of ulcerated plaques in the aortic arch in patients with stroke. N Engl J Med. 1992;326:221–5.

38. Castaigne P, Lhermitte F, Gautier JC, Escourolle R, DerouesnÉ C, Agopian PD, et al. Arterial occlusions in the vertebro-basilar system. Brain. 1973;96:133–54.

39. Mohr JP, Wolf PA, Michael A. Stroke E-Book: pathophysiology, diagnosis, and management: Elsevier Health Sciences; 2011.

40. Powers WJ, Rabinstein AA, Ackerson T, et al. 2018 Guidelines for the early management of patients with acute ischemic stroke: a guideline for healthcare professionals from the American Heart Association/American Stroke Association. Stroke. 2018;49(3):e46–e110.

41. CADISS trial investigators. Antiplatelet treatment compared with anticoagulation treatment for cervical artery dissection (CADISS): a randomised trial. Lancet Neurol. 2015;14:361–7.

42. Mas JL, Derumeaux G, Guillon B, et al. Patent foramen ovale closure or anticoagulation vs. antiplatelets after stroke. N Engl J Med. 2017;377:1011–21.

43. Kelly PJ, Stein J, Shafqat S, Eskey C, Doherty D, Chang Y, Kurina A, Furie KL. Functional recovery after rehabilitation for cerebellar stroke. Stroke. 2001;32:530–4.

44. Edlow JA, Newman-Toker DE, Savitz SI. Diagnosis and initial management of cerebellar infarction. Lancet Neurol. 2008;7:951–64.

45. Tohgi H, Takahashi S, Chiba K, Hirata Y. Clinical and neuroimaging analysis in 293 patients. The Tohoku Cerebellar Infarction Study Group. Stroke. 1993;24(11):1697–701. Cerebellar infarction.

46. Savoiardo M, Bracchi M, Passerini A, Visciani A. The vascular territories in the cerebellum and brainstem: CT and MR study. Am J Neuroradiol. 1989;8:199–209.

Ocular, Vestibular, and Otologic Syndromes

7

Eun-Jae Lee, Hyo-Jung Kim, and Ji-Soo Kim

Introduction

The brainstem and cerebellum contain numerous neurons and intricate neural circuits that are involved in generation and control of eye movements [1]. Thus, vertebrobasilar strokes may cause various patterns of abnormal eye movements. Defining the patterns and characteristics of eye movement abnormalities observed in vertebrobasilar strokes is important in understanding the roles of each structure and circuit in ocular motor control as well as in making topographic diagnosis [2]. Furthermore, because abnormal eye movements may be the only or predominant manifestation [3, 4], detection of abnormal ocular motility is crucial in identifying these strokes.

In humans, the subclasses of eye movements comprise saccades, smooth pursuit, optokinetic nystagmus, the vestibulo-ocular reflex (VOR), vergence, and gaze holding [1]. Thus, evaluation of eye movements should include all these subclasses of movements in addition to ocular alignment, pupillary and eyelid function, and involuntary eye movements such as nystagmus and saccadic oscillations [5]. Furthermore, each eye movement should be described in the horizontal, vertical, and torsional planes for accurate characterization [5]. Recent developments in brain imaging and eye movement recording have allowed more accurate delineation of the function of each ocular motor structure. In this review, we will detail the abnormal eye movements that may be observed in strokes involving the cerebellum and brainstem.

Medullary Strokes

The medulla contains several structures that control eye movements. These include the vestibular nuclei, perihypoglossal nuclei consisting of the nucleus prepositus hypoglossi (NPH), nucleus intercalatus, and nucleus of Roller, inferior olivary nucleus, inferior cerebellar peduncles (ICP), and cell groups of the paramedian tract (PMT) (Fig. 7.1). The medial vestibular nucleus and NPH also participate in holding the eyes steady during eccentric horizontal gaze as the neural integrator. Thus, strokes involving the medulla show various patterns of nystagmus and vestibular impairments.

E.-J. Lee
Department of Neurology, Asan Medical Center, College of Medicine, University of Ulsan, Seoul, South Korea
e-mail: eunjae.lee@amc.seoul.kr

H.-J. Kim
Research Administration Team, Seoul National University Bundang Hospital, Seongnam, South Korea

J.-S. Kim (✉)
Department of Neurology, Seoul National University College of Medicine, Seoul National University Bundang Hospital, Seongnam, South Korea
e-mail: jisookim@snu.ac.kr

© Springer Nature Singapore Pte Ltd. 2021
J. S. Kim (ed.), *Posterior Circulation Stroke*, https://doi.org/10.1007/978-981-15-6739-1_7

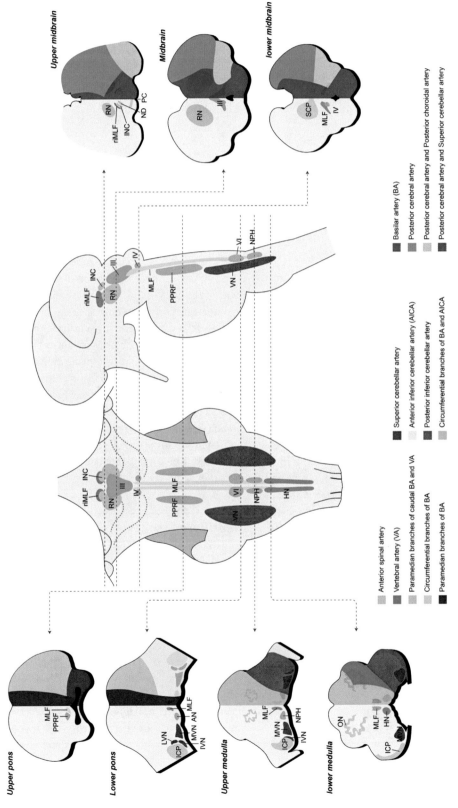

Fig. 7.1 Ocular motor structures in the brainstem. *AN* abducens nucleus, *HN* hypoglossal nucleus, *ICP* inferior cerebellar peduncle, *INC* interstitial nucleus of Cajal, *IVN* inferior vestibular nucleus, *LVN* lateral vestibular nucleus, *MLF* medial longitudinal fasciculus, *MVN* medial vestibular nucleus, *ND* nucleus of Darkschewitsch, *NPH* nucleus prepositus hypoglossi, *ON* olivary nucleus, *PC* posterior commissure, *PPRF* paramedian pontine reticular formation, *riMLF* rostral interstitial MLF, *RN* red nucleus, *SCP* superior cerebellar peduncle, *VN* vestibular nucleus

Lateral Medullary Infarction (LMI)

Infarction involving the dorsolateral medulla (Wallenberg syndrome) commonly affects the inferior and medial vestibular nuclei and usually manifests with nausea/vomiting, vertigo, and imbalance (see Chap. 4 for details) [6].

Typically, horizontal nystagmus beats away from the lesion side (Table 7.1) [7, 8], but patients with an infarction in the middle and rostral portions may have ipsilesional nystagmus [8]. These findings are consistent with an experimental study in monkeys: spontaneous nystagmus beats mostly contralesionally in unilateral lesions involving the vestibular nerve root or the caudal lateral parts of the vestibular nuclei, [9] whereas the nystagmus beats ipsilesionally when the superior vestibular nucleus or the rostral portion of the medial vestibular nucleus is lesioned [9]. The vertical component is usually upbeating, [7, 8] and torsional nystagmus may be ipsi- or contralesional [10]. Later, the spontaneous nystagmus may change its directions [8]. Seesaw and hemi-seesaw nystagmus, rarely observed in LMI, [11, 12] are ascribed to vestibular imbalance in the roll plane due to disruption of the pathways from the utricle or vertical semicircular canals [12]. Horizontal gaze-evoked nystagmus (GEN) is common while positional nystagmus is rare and usually torsional [13]. Horizontal head oscillation at 2–3 Hz for 10–20 s frequently induces nystagmus (head-shaking nystagmus, HSN) that is invariably ipsilesional [8]. Even in patients with contralesional spontaneous nystagmus, horizontal head shaking reverses the direction of spontaneous horizontal nystagmus [13]. HSN may also be unusually strong or perverted; i.e., the nystagmus develops in the plane other than that being stimulated (downbeat or upbeat after horizontal head oscillation) [8]. Since visual fixation markedly suppresses HSN even in patients with vigorous HSN, removal of visual fixation (e.g., Frenzel goggles) is required for proper observation of HSN.

The ocular tilt reaction (OTR), which consists of head tilt, ocular torsion, and skew deviation, is commonly observed during the acute phase and is ipsilesional; i.e., the head is tilted to the lesion side, the upper poles of the eyes rotate toward the ipsilesional shoulder, and the ipsilesional eye lies lower than the contralesional one [13]. The OTR is mostly associated with the ipsilesional tilt of the subjective visual vertical (SVV) [13, 14]. The OTR and SVV tilts are explained by interruption of the otolith-ocular or vertical semicircular canal pathways at the level of the vestibular nucleus [14, 15].

Table 7.1 Comparison of ocular motor findings between lateral and medullary infarct

	Lateral medullary infarct	Medial medullary infarct
Spontaneous nystagmus		
Horizontal	Contralesional (usually)	Ipsilesional, weak
	Ipsilesional (occasionally)	
Vertical	Upbeating (usually)	Upbeating (occasionally)
Torsional	Ipsi or contralesional	Ipsilesional
Miscellaneous	Seesaw or hemi-seesaw (rarely)	Hemi-seesaw (rarely)
Gaze-evoked nystagmus	Contralesional, stronger	Ipsilesional, stronger
Ocular lateropulsion	Ipsipulsion	Contrapulsion
Head-shaking nystagmus	Ipsilesional (horizontal),	Contralesional (occasionally)
	Perverted (downbeat or upbeat)	
Saccades	Normal	Normal
Smooth pursuit	Impaired, ipsilesional	Impaired, ipsilesional
Bedside HIT	Intact (usually)	Normal
	May be impaired in vestibular nucleus lesions (ipsilesional)	May be impaired in NPH lesions (contralesional)
Caloric test	Intact (usually)	Normal
	Ipsilesional caloric paresis in vestibular nucleus lesions	
Ocular tilt reaction	Ipsilesional	Contralesional
	Contralesional (rarely)	

HIT head impulse test, *NPH* nucleus prepositus hypoglossi

Patients may show an ocular motor bias toward the lesion side without limitation of eye motion (ocular ipsipulsion), which consists of a steady-state ocular deviation to the lesion side, saccadic hypermetria to the lesion side and hypometria to the intact side, and oblique misdirection of vertical saccades toward the lesion side [7, 16, 17]. Ocular lateropulsion may occur in lesions involving neural pathways connecting the ION, cerebellar Purkinje cells, fastigial nucleus, and paramedian pontine reticular formation (PPRF) [18]. Ocular ipsipulsion in LMI has been ascribed to damage of the climbing fibers from the contralesional ION to the dorsal vermis [18]. Increased Purkinje cell activity following damage to the climbing fibers after decussation in the lateral medulla would inhibit the ipsilateral fastigial nucleus and create a bias toward ipsilateral saccades (Fig. 7.2).

Medial Medullary Infarction (MMI)

MMI generates distinct patterns of ocular motor abnormalities [19, 20], especially when lesions extend into the tegmentum. Whereas the horizontal nystagmus is typically contralesional in LMI, it mostly beats ipsilesionally in patients with MMI probably by involving the NPH (Table 7.1) [19]. GEN is usually more intense on looking to the lesion side [19]. Upbeat nystagmus occasionally occurs in MMI and has been ascribed to involvement of the perihypoglossal nuclei [21, 22]. However, the evolution of upbeat or torsional upbeat into hemi-seesaw nystagmus suggests an involvement of the VOR pathways from both anterior semicircular canals as a mechanism of upbeat nystagmus [23, 24]. Since the MLF is a midline structure that conveys signals from the vestibular to the ocular motor nuclei, upbeat nystagmus in unilateral lesions may be explained by concurrent damage to decussating fibers from both anterior semicircular canals at the rostral medulla [23]. In the caudal medullary lesions, the nucleus intercalatus and the caudal subgroup of the PMT cells, which are involved in processing of vertical eye position through their projections to the cerebellar

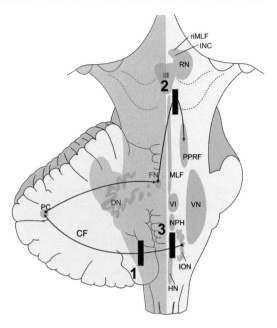

Fig. 7.2 Schematic representation of the involved pathways in ocular lateropulsion. *CF* climbing fibers, *DN* dentate nucleus, *FN* fastigial nucleus, *HN* hypoglossal nucleus, *ICP* inferior cerebellar peduncle, *ION* the inferior olivary nucleus, *MLF* medial longitudinal fasciculus, *NPH* nucleus prepositus hypoglossi, *PC* cerebellar Purkinje cells, *PPRF* paramedian pontine reticular formation, *RN* red nucleus, *UF* uncinate fasciculus, *VN* vestibular nucleus. PC in the cerebellum, which is inhibited by CF from the contralateral ION, decreases the activity of ipsilateral FN, while FN generates contralateral saccades via stimulating contralateral PPRF. Therefore, damage to CF before or after decussation would cause ocular lateropulsion, of which direction is determined by the activity of PC. Ocular ipsipulsion in the Wallenberg syndrome may be ascribed to damaging the CF from the contralesional ION to the PC of dorsal vermis after decussation (1) while ocular contrapulsion in superior cerebellar artery infarction occurs due to damage of the fibers from the contralesional FN to the ipsilesional PPRF near the uncinate fasciculus (2). In medial medullary infarction, disruption of the CF before decussation (3) gives rise to ocular contrapulsion

flocculus, may be other neural substrates for upbeat nystagmus [22, 25]. The OTR is contraversive in isolated unilateral MMI [19, 20, 23]. The contraversive OTR in MMI indicates a unilateral lesion of the graviceptive or vertical semicircular canal pathways from the vestibular nuclei after decussation. In MMI, damage to the climbing fibers before decussation also causes ocular contrapulsion (Fig. 7.2) [19, 20].

Pontine Strokes

The pontine tegmentum contains important structures for conjugate horizontal gazes, which
include the PPRF, abducens nucleus, nucleus
raphe interpositus, and MLF (Fig. 7.1) [1]. Thus,
horizontal gaze palsy is characteristic of pontine
strokes [26, 27]. However, various patterns of vertical eye movement abnormalities, including vertical GEN and impaired vertical smooth pursuit
and the VOR, may also occur because the pontine
ocular motor centers are linked via the MLF to the
midbrain and midbrain–diencephalic junctional
area that mainly control vertical gaze [28].

Nystagmus and Saccadic Intrusions/ Oscillations

Upbeat nystagmus may occur in tegmental infarctions by disrupting the upward VOR pathways
from both anterior semicircular canals, which lie
in the MLFs [25]. Since the MLF carries the
excitatory fibers originating from the contralateral anterior and posterior canals to the ocular
motor nuclei, various patterns of dissociated torsional–vertical nystagmus may occur in strokes
involving the MLF [29, 30]. Upbeat nystagmus
was also reported in a focal infarction between
the basis pontis and tegmentum slightly above
the midpontine level and was ascribed to damage
to the decussating ventral tegmental tracts that is
believed to transmit the upward VOR [22]. Ocular
bobbing, intermittent downward jerk of the eyes
followed by slow return to the primary position,
can be observed in extensive strokes involving
the pontine base and tegmentum [31]. In patients
with extensive pontine lesions, horizontal gaze is
lost, but vertical gaze is preserved; the relatively
accentuated vertical vector of gaze may be manifested as "ocular bobbing."

Internuclear Ophthalmoplegia (INO)

INO is caused by a lesion involving the MLF,
which contains fibers connecting the abducens
interneurons and contralateral medial rectus sub-

nucleus (Fig. 7.3) [32]. INO is characterized by an
impairment of adduction in the ipsilesional eye
and dissociated abducting nystagmus of the contralateral eye on attempted contralesional gaze
[33]. Convergence may be normal or impaired.
Since the MLF also carries the fibers involved in
the vertical VOR and the fibers from the utricle to
the interstitial nucleus of Cajal (INC), INO is usually accompanied by vertical, torsional, or dissociated vertical–torsional nystagmus [29, 34],
contraversive OTR [4, 35], and impaired vertical
VOR [36, 37]. Selective impairment of vertical
VOR originating from the contralateral posterior
semicircular canal may be demonstrated in INO
using the head impulse test [37–39]. The preserved anterior canal function suggests an extra-
route for the ascending VOR pathway from the
anterior canal, possibly the ventral tegmental
tract. Exotropia of the contralesional eye or both
eyes is common in unilateral (wall-eyed monocular INO, WEMINO) or bilateral (wall-eye bilateral INO, WEBINO) INO [40, 41]. In bilateral
INO, vertical smooth pursuit, vertical optokinetic
nystagmus and after-nystagmus, and vertical gaze
holding may also be impaired [36]. Some patients
show impaired fixation and sporadic bursts of
monocular abducting saccades in each eye [42].
INO may occur as an isolated or predominant
symptom of dorsal brainstem infarctions and has
an excellent prognosis [4].

Horizontal Gaze Palsy

The PPRF contains burst neurons for ipsilateral
horizontal saccades [43]. Burst neurons in PPRF
receive inputs from the contralateral frontal eye
field and projects to the ipsilateral abducens
nucleus. Selective damage to the pontine burst
neurons results in isolated ipsilesional saccadic
palsy with contralesional conjugate deviation of
the eyes [44, 45]. In contrast, damage to the abducens nucleus produces ipsilesional palsy of saccades, smooth pursuit, and VOR [46]. A nuclear
lesion gives rise to an ipsilesional conjugate gaze
palsy rather than a unilateral abduction deficit
since the nucleus includes the lateral rectus motor
neurons as well as the interneurons that project to

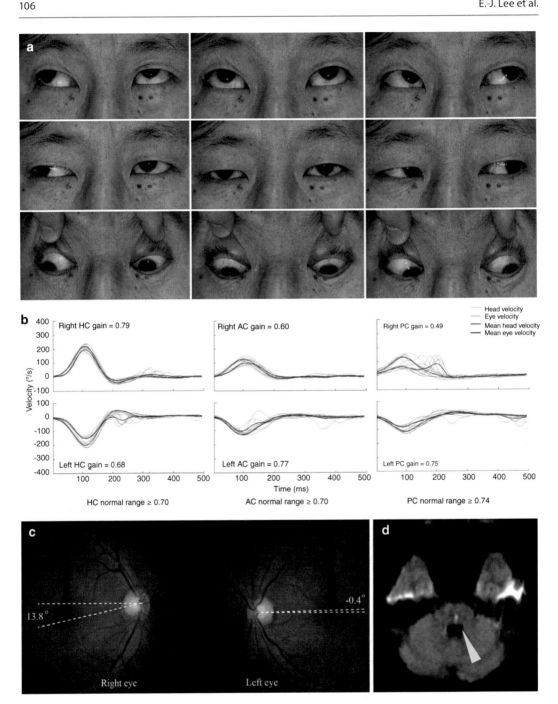

Fig. 7.3 Internuclear ophthalmoplegia. (**a**) Impaired adduction of the left eye on attempted rightward gaze, (**b**) decreased head impulse gain of the vestibulo-ocular reflex for right (contralesional) posterior canal, (**c**) fundus pho-tography showing abnormal extorsion of the right eye and intorsion of the left eye, and (**d**) infarction in the area of left medial longitudinal fasciculus (arrow)

the contralateral medial rectus subnucleus via the MLF [1]. However, saccades toward the lesion side may be relatively preserved in the contralat-eral hemifield. For example, in a lesion affecting right abducens nucleus, the saccades from left-ward gaze to the center are relatively preserved

Table 7.2 Clinical characteristics of abducens nucleus lesion and PPRF lesion

Abducens nucleus lesion	PPRF lesion
– Ipsilesional conjugate horizontal gaze palsy (saccade, smooth pursuit, and VOR)	– Ipsilesional conjugate horizontal saccadic palsy
– Relatively spared saccades toward the lesion side in the contralateral hemifield	– Impaired saccades toward the lesion side in both ipsi- and contralateral hemifields
– Intact convergence and vertical eye movements	– Intact convergence and vertical eye movements
– Horizontal gaze-evoked nystagmus when looking to the contralesional side	– Horizontal gaze-evoked nystagmus when looking to the contralesional side
– Ipsilesional facial palsy (peripheral-type)	

PPRF paramedian pontine reticular formation, *VOR* vestibulo-ocular reflex

because those movements are attained mostly by relaxation of the antagonist muscles (left lateral rectus and right medial rectus), which is mediated by the inhibitory burst neurons in the right medullary reticular formation. Lesions restricted to the abducens nucleus rarely occur, and nuclear lesions usually involve adjacent tegmental structures, especially the MLF, PPRF, and genu of the facial nerve fascicle [47]. Thus, associated ipsilateral facial palsy of the peripheral type is common in nuclear abducens palsy. Clinical characteristics of abducens nucleus lesion and PPRF lesion are summarized in Table 7.2.

One-and-a-Half Syndrome

This syndrome refers to a combination of unilateral conjugate gaze palsy (one) and INO on the same side (a half) [48]. Consequently, the only remaining eye movement is abduction of the contralateral eye (a half). One-and-a-half syndrome is caused by combined damage to the PPRF/abducens nucleus and the MLF. The term paralytic pontine exotropia was coined for patients who had an exotropia of the contralesional eye with one-and-a-half syndrome [49].

Abducens Palsy

Intra-axial damage to the abducens fascicle causes ipsilateral lateral rectus palsy [50]. Fascicular abducens nerve palsy is rarely isolated [51] but is usually accompanied by contralateral hemiplegia or ipsilateral facial weakness [52].

Other Findings

The dorsolateral pontine nuclei (DLPN) and the nucleus reticularis tegmenti pontis (NRTP) participate in the control of smooth pursuit eye movements. Damage to DLPN impairs ipsilesional smooth pursuit [53, 54], and NRTP lesions impair vertical smooth pursuit [55] and vergence eye movements [56]. Although tegmental infarctions usually present with vestibular or ocular motor symptoms [57], infarctions involving other territories may also produce eye movement abnormalities. Anteromedial pontine infarction usually causes a motor deficit with dysarthria and ataxia. However, one-third of patients may show tegmental symptoms and signs, including vertigo, nystagmus, Horner's syndrome, and horizontal gaze palsy [57]. Tegmental symptoms and signs also occur in more than half of the patients with anterolateral infarctions [57].

Massive pontine strokes, usually hemorrhages, cause a rapid onset of coma, pinpoint but reactive pupils [48], ocular bobbing [31], horizontal gaze palsy, and quadriplegia [58]. Inferior olivary pseudohypertrophy and oculopalatal tremor may develop as delayed complications [59, 60].

Midbrain Stroke

The midbrain contains the oculomotor and trochlear nuclei and fascicles, and the mesodiencephalic junction harbors the key structures involved in the premotor control of vertical and torsional eye movements, especially the saccades and gaze holding (Figs. 7.1 and 7.4). Thus, vertical ophthalmoplegia is characteristic of lesions involving the midbrain or mesodiencephalic

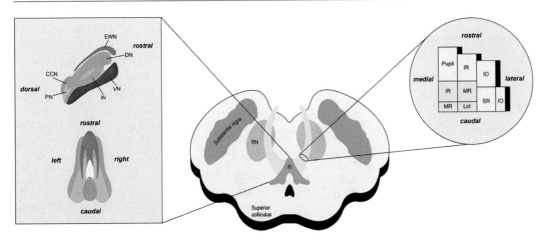

Fig. 7.4 Topography of oculomotor nucleus and fascicles. *CCN* central caudal nucleus, *DN* dorsal nucleus, *EWN* Edinger-Westphal nucleus, *IN* inferior nucleus, *IO* inferior oblique muscle, *IR* inferior rectus muscle, *MR* medial rectus muscle, *PN* posterior nucleus, *RN* red nucleus, *SR* superior rectus, *VN* ventral nucleus

junction and may be supranuclear, nuclear, or fascicular origin. Since this area also contains the neural structures for the control of pupil, eyelid and vergence, and the descending fibers for horizontal eye motion, abnormalities of these eye movements may occur with or without vertical ophthalmoplegia when damaged.

Ocular Dysfunction in Top of the Basilar Syndrome

Occlusion of the rostral tip of the basilar artery gives rise to a characteristic combination of ocular motor abnormalities by damaging the pretectum that contains the rostral interstitial nucleus of the medial longitudinal fasciculus (riMLF), INC, the rostral portion of the mesencephalic reticular formation (MRF), and the posterior commissure (PC), which are involved in the premotor control of vertical and torsional eye movements (pretectal syndrome) (Fig. 7.5; see also Chap. 4) [61].

Both riMLF and INC are important structures modulating vertical and torsional saccades, and lesions in these structures show characteristic oculomotor findings (Table 7.3). The riMLF lies in the prerubral area near the midline and contains the medium lead burst neurons that generate vertical and ipsiversive (top poles of the eyes toward the shoulder on the same side) torsional saccades [62]. Each riMLF projects bilaterally to motoneurons for the elevator muscles (superior rectus and inferior oblique) but ipsilaterally to motoneurons for the depressor muscles (inferior rectus and superior oblique) [63, 64]. Unilateral riMLF lesions result in contralesional ocular torsion, contralesional torsional nystagmus, and loss of ipsitorsional quick phases and vertical gaze [65–68]. Bilateral lesions cause loss of downward or all vertical saccades [69]. On the other hand, the INC, together with the vestibular nuclei, is an element of the neural integrator for vertical and torsional eye motion [70, 71]. It sends eye-position-, saccade-, and pursuit-related signals, combined in variable proportions on each axon, to the extraocular motoneurons [72]. The INC is separated from the riMLF by the fasciculus retroflexus, but fibers from the riMLF pass through the INC, providing axon collaterals to the INC. [63, 64] Unilateral INC lesions produce contralesional OTR and ipsitorsional nystagmus, while bilateral lesions reduce the range of all vertical eye movements without saccadic slowing [73].

The rostral portion of the MRF, adjacent to the INC and riMLF, contains neurons that have low-frequency long-lead burst of activity before vertical saccades [74]. Unilateral inactivation of the rostral MRF produces slow and hypometric upward and downward saccades without postsac-

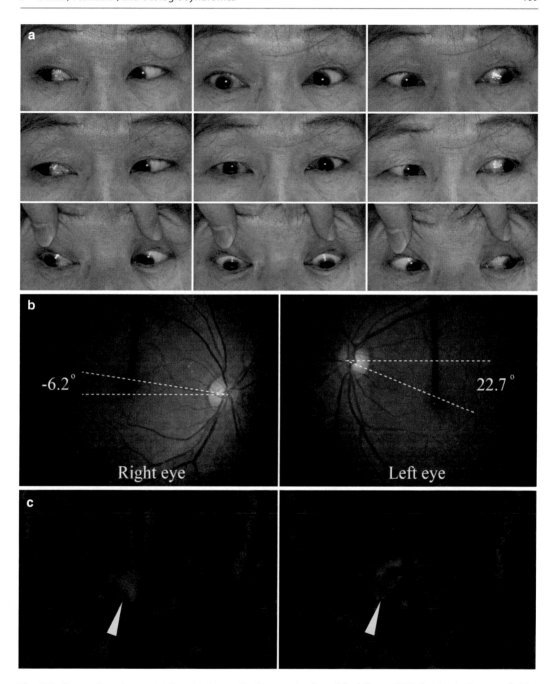

Fig. 7.5 Pretectal syndrome. (**a**) Impaired supraduction of both eyes on attempted upward gaze, (**b**) fundus photography showing abnormal intorsion of the right eye and extorsion of the left eye, (**c**) infarction in the area of right thalamus and midbrain (arrows)

cadic drift [75]. The PC contains several groups of decussating axons from adjacent nuclei of the PC (nPC) and axons from the riMLF and INC that project to corresponding structures in the contralateral midbrain tegmentum [76]. The nPC also contains the neurons that discharge shortly before upward saccades [63]. The PC is a structure critical for upward saccades [77].

Table 7.3 Comparison of ocular motor findings in lesions involving the riMLF vs. INC

	riMLF lesion	INC lesion
Saccade		
Vertical	Decreased amplitudes and velocities	Decreased amplitudes
		Normal velocities
Torsional	Loss of all ipsitorsional components	Decreased contralesional fast phases
Spontaneous nystagmus		
Vertical	No	Downbeat, upbeat (bilateral lesion)
Torsional	Contralesional	Ipsilesional
Gaze-evoked nystagmus	No	Vertical and torsional
Smooth pursuit		Impaired gain
VOR (vertical and torsional)	Loss of ipsitorsional nystagmus	Little effect on VOR gain and phase (unilateral lesion)
	Otherwise normal gain and function	Impaired gain and phase (bilateral lesion)
OTR	Contraversive	Contraversive
Gaze holding	Normal	Impaired

INC interstitial nucleus of Cajal, *OTR* ocular tilt reaction, *riMLF* rostral interstitial medial longitudinal fasciculus, *VOR* vestibulo-ocular reflex

Accordingly, varied combinations of vertical gaze palsy may occur depending on the combination of the structures involved, e.g., upgaze palsy, downgaze palsy, vertical one-and-a-half syndrome, [78] and complete vertical gaze palsy [28, 79]. Dissociated vertical nystagmus may occur in pretectal syndrome [80, 81]. The neurons specifically involved in vergence control are located 1–2 mm dorsal and dorsolateral to the oculomotor nucleus [82, 83]. Pretectal syndrome may cause various ocular motor disorders related to vergence, which include convergence insufficiency, convergence spasm, and convergence nystagmus [84]. Convergence spasm may cause limitation of abduction on voluntary lateral gaze, which resembles abducens nerve palsy (pseudoabducens palsy) [85]. Bilateral ptosis or lid retraction (Collier's sign) may be observed in pretectal syndrome [86].

Third Cranial Nerve Palsy

Anteromedial and anterolateral midbrain infarctions frequently give rise to third cranial nerve palsy by affecting the oculomotor nuclei or fascicles (Figs. 7.1 and 7.4) [87]. Various signs of oculomotor palsy may occur due to the characteristic spatial organization of the oculomotor nuclei and fascicles in the midbrain [88, 89]. Isolated palsy of individual extraocular muscle may occur due to nuclear or fascicular lesions [3, 89, 90]. Rarely, midbrain lesions cause a third cranial nerve palsy mimicking a peripheral palsy due to microvascular ischemia [91].

Trochlear Palsy

The trochlear nucleus is located in the central gray matter of the midbrain, close to the midline, near the MLF and the decussating fibers of the superior cerebellar peduncle. The trochlear nucleus is supplied by paramedian branches at the basilar artery bifurcation, which are susceptible to shear injury from trauma.

Nuclear or fascicular trochlear palsy may be isolated [92, 93] but is more frequently accompanied by various neurologic deficits, including Horner's syndrome, INO, upbeat nystagmus, ataxia, or tinnitus, due to concurrent involvement of the neighboring structures including the descending sympathetic tract, MLF, brachium conjunctivum, ascending trigeminothalamic/spinothalamic tracts, and inferior colliculus [92–94]. Nuclear trochlear lesions give rise to contralesional superior oblique palsy (SOP), but fascicular lesions may cause ipsilesional or contralesional SOP depending upon the lesion location in the brainstem. The lesions are more commonly located posterior to the cerebral aqueduct in patients with ipsilesional SOP than in those with contralesional SOP [93].

Internuclear Ophthalmoplegia

Damage to the MLF in the pontomesencephalic junction causes INO and ataxia due to co-involvement of the decussation of the brachium conjunctivum [95, 96].

Cerebellar Strokes

The cerebellum contains several structures that participate in the control of eye movements. In addition, the cerebellum harbors various fibers that are involved in integrating the proprioceptive and vestibular information [97]. Vertigo/dizziness is the most common symptom of cerebellar strokes and may be isolated mimicking acute peripheral vesetibulopathy [2, 98].

Anterior Inferior Cerebellar Artery (AICA) Infarction

The AICA supplies various peripheral and central vestibular structures, which include the inner ear, lateral pons, middle cerebellar peduncle, and anterior inferior cerebellum [99]. AICA infarction usually results in combined peripheral and central vestibulopathy with various symptoms and signs. Gaze-evoked nystagmus and impaired smooth pursuit are usually associated with unilateral canal paresis and hearing loss [100]. Isolated recurrent attacks of vertigo may precede AICA infarction [101].

Clinical presentation of AICA infarction may mimic more common vestibular disorders such as Meniere's disease or vestibular neuritis. Since lesions may not be detected with imaging, a detailed neurological examination should be performed in patients with acute vertigo [100]. In AICA infarction, spontaneous nystagmus is usually horizontal and beats away from the lesion side [102]. Direction-changing gaze-evoked, especially asymmetrical (Bruns' nystagmus), is frequent. The HINTS (negative head impulse test, direction-changing nystagmus, and skew deviation), which is a surrogate test for strokes in patients with acute spontaneous vertigo, [103] may not be applicable for diagnosis of AICA infarction due to concomitant inner ear damage [104, 105]. Thus, the presence of severe imbalance [101] and central patterns of HSN may be

helpful to identify AICA infarction in patients with negative HINTS [104].

Patients with AICA infarctions are frequently accompanied by sensorineural hearing loss, predominantly of the cochlear origin [100, 106, 107]. The sensorineural hearing loss and caloric paresis during the acute phase usually recover over time [108, 109]. Episodic auditory disturbances including hearing loss with or without tinnitus may be prodromal symptoms of AICA infarction [110].

AICA infarction can cause the OTR in association with a SVV deviation in the direction of the head tilt [111, 112]. Of note, ipsiversive OTR is attributed to inner ear infarction while contraversive OTR is ascribed to brainstem or floccular involvements [97, 112]. These findings suggest that the function of the peripheral vestibular structures probably plays a crucial role in determining the direction of the OTR in patients with AICA infarction [112].

Rarely, AICA infarction gives rise to sudden deafness and vertigo without brainstem or cerebellar signs (i.e., labyrinthine infarction, see below) [113]. Thus, clinicians should be aware of the possibility of AICA infarction even in patients with isolated sudden hearing loss, particularly when the patients are old with multiple vascular risk factors.

Labyrinthine Infarction
The internal auditory artery (IAA), which supplies the cochlea and vestibular labyrinth, is a branch of AICA. Because the IAA is an end artery with minimal collaterals, the labyrinth is especially vulnerable to ischemia [101, 114, 115]. Labyrinthine infarction mostly occurs due to thrombotic narrowing of the AICA itself, or in the basilar artery at the orifice of the AICA [116]. However, labyrinthine infarction may occur due to artery-to-artery or cardiac embolism [117, 118].

Labyrinthine infarction mostly causes a sudden loss of both auditory and vestibular functions. In particular, the apical region of the cochlea is more vulnerable to vascular injury, and low-frequency hearing loss is more common [114, 119]. Isolated vertigo may occur in transient ischemia of the peripheral vestibular labyrinth [115, 120]. The superior part of the vestibular labyrinth may be more vulnerable to ischemia, possibly due to small caliber of the anterior vestibular artery and lack of collaterals [120]. Benign paroxysmal positional vertigo may ensue after anterior vestibular artery infarction and is ascribed to ischemic necrosis of the utricular macule and subsequent release of otoconia into the posterior canal. The posterior canal may be spared in anterior vestibular artery infarction because it is supplied by the posterior vestibular artery, a branch of the common cochlear artery [120, 121].

Middle Cerebellar Peduncular Infarction

The middle cerebellar peduncle (MCP) acts as a conduit for the cortico-ponto-cerebellar connections that carry information regarding eye movements [122]. Common findings of MCP strokes include spontaneous horizontal nystagmus, horizontal GEN, bilaterally impaired horizontal smooth pursuit, unilateral hearing loss or caloric paresis, and the OTR [123]. These findings indicate damage of the inner ear and nearby structures in the brainstem and cerebellum as well as the MCP.

Isolated Floccular Infarction

The cerebellar flocculus participates in the control of smooth pursuit, gaze holding, and eye movements evoked by vestibular stimulation [124]. Although lesions restricted to the flocculus is rare [38], patients with isolated unilateral floccular infarction show several oculomotor and vestibular abnormalities: spontaneous nystagmus beating to the lesion side, contraversive ocular torsion and SVV tilt, increased horizontal VOR gain during low-frequency stimulation, and decreased gain during the higher-velocity/higher-frequency stimulation [125, 126]. Although the mechanism of opposing changes in the gain of the VOR during low- and high-frequency stimulation is unclear, the flocculus appears to modulate the VOR by inhibiting the horizontal VOR during low-frequency stimulation and facilitating it during high-frequency stimulation.

Posterior Inferior Cerebellar Artery (PICA) Infarction

The PICA usually gives rise to medial and lateral branches. The medial PICA irrigates the inferior cerebellar hemisphere and vermis, including the nodulus and uvula [127]. The main structure responsible for vertigo in medial PICA cerebellar infarctions is the nodulus, which is strongly linked to the ipsilateral vestibular nucleus and receives direct afferent fibers from the labyrinth. Functionally, the nodulovestibular Purkinje fibers inhibit the ipsilateral vestibular nucleus [128, 129].

Spontaneous nystagmus and postural instability are variable in their direction and severity in PICA cerebellar infarctions [130]. Unidirectional GEN may be found in patients with unilateral cerebellar strokes, either toward or away from the lesion side [131]. Because GEN is ascribed to damages to the structures including pyramid, uvula, tonsil, and parts of the biventer and inferior semilunar lobules, [131] the presence of GEN suggests lesions involving the midline and lower cerebellar structures. Meanwhile, ipsilesional HSN may also be associated with perverted HSN, of which direction is mostly downbeat [132]. The generation of HSN may be ascribed to damage to the uvula, nodulus, and inferior tonsil [132].

Either paroxysmal or persistent form of positional nystagmus may be observed in patients with lesions involving the nodulus and uvula [133, 134]. Paroxysmal central positional nystagmus (CPN) has its direction mostly aligned with the vector sum of the rotational axes of the semicircular canals that are normally inhibited during the positioning. Paroxysmal CPN is explained by enhanced postrotatory canal signals due to lesion-induced disinhibition. In contrast, the persistent CPN can be simulated when the tilt-estimator circuit in the cerebellum and brainstem malfunctions due to lesions involving the vestibulocerebellum, and the estimated direction of gravity is erroneously biased away from true vertical. Due to overlap of the lesions responsible for either the paroxysmal or persistent form of central positional nystagmus, both types of nystagmus are frequently combined in patients with central positional nystagmus. Characteristics of the nystagmus and associated neuro-otological findings may allow differentiating central from peripheral positional nystagmus [135].

Medial PICA cerebellar infarction can mimic acute peripheral vestibular dysfunction [136]. According to a report dealing with 240 patients with isolated cerebellar infarction, [137] 25 (11%) had isolated vertigo only, mostly in those with an infarction in the medial PICA territory including the nodulus (24/25: 96%). Caloric and head impulse tests may be helpful to distinguish central from peripheral vestibulopathy [138].

Isolated medial PICA territory cerebellar infarction can cause a contraversive partial OTR and SVV tilt [139]. These findings may be ascribed to interruption of the nodular inhibitory projection onto the graviceptive neurons in the ipsilesional vestibular nuclei [139]. Ischemic lesions affecting the nodulus and ventral uvula can also give rise to periodic alternating nystagmus [140]. Rarely, PICA territory cerebellar infarctions can cause acute hearing loss, especially when the PICA is dominant and substitutes for the AICA [141].

Isolated Tonsilar Infarction

The paraflocculus in monkeys consists of three distinct anatomical parts: the ventral and dorsal paraflocculi and the lobulus petrosus [142]. The human cerebellar tonsil, of which demarcation is less clear, corresponds to the simian dorsal paraflocculus and adjacent lobulus petrosus [142]. The relative roles of the paraflocculus versus flocculus are unclear in vestibular function, gaze holding, and smooth pursuit; however, the paraflocculus appears to be more concerned with smooth pursuit, as compared to the flocculus [143–145].

A patient with an acute unilateral tonsilar infarction showed (1) near completely abolished smooth pursuit, more to the lesion side, (2) a low-amplitude ipsilesional beating nystagmus without fixation, (3) gaze-holding deficits, and (4) normal VOR [146]. Ipsilesional spontaneous nystagmus suggests a static vestibular functional

asymmetry. Damage to the Purkinje cells or their inhibitory outflow tracts may have caused disinhibition of the ipsilateral vestibular nuclei. Alternatively, a moderate asymmetry in horizontal pursuit in the patient with a tonsilar lesion could have induced the small spontaneous nystagmus [147]. Of note, a patient with a floccular infarction demonstrated a much stronger spontaneous nystagmus as well as abnormal head impulse responses, suggesting that the flocculus plays a more important role in the control of the VOR than the tonsil [125]. Meanwhile, smooth pursuit is more likely to be severely impaired in tonsilar than in floccular lesions [125, 146].

The horizontal gaze-evoked and rebound nystagmus in the patient with a tonsilar lesion indicates dysfunction of the neural gaze-holding networks, and the small contraversive SVV tilt suggests a tonsilar involvement in controlling the otolithic signals [124, 125].

Isolated Nodular Infarction

The nodulus, which lies in the midline cerebellum, constitutes the vestibulocerebellum along with the flocculus, paraflocculus, and ventral uvula. The nodulus receives vestibular inputs, controls eye movements, and adjusts the posture to gravity [148].

Isolated nodular infarction mostly gives rise to sudden vertigo with unilateral nystagmus and falling in the opposite direction, mimicking acute peripheral vestibulopathy [149, 150]. Severe imbalance and a negative head impulse test are, however, helpful in differentiating nodular infarctions from peripheral vestibular dysfunction. In isolated unilateral nodular infarctions, the direction of spontaneous nystagmus is all ipsilesional and is usually augmented by horizontal head shaking. These findings may be ascribed to impaired gravitoinertial processing of the vestibular signals [151] and disrupted nodular inhibition over the vestibular secondary neurons [152]. Other findings include periodic alternating nystagmus, [140, 153] perverted head-shaking nystagmus, [154] paroxysmal positional nystagmus, [149] and impaired tilt suppression of the postrotatory nystagmus [149].

Superior Cerebellar Artery (SCA) Infarction

The SCA supplies the rostral half of the cerebellum, dentate nucleus, and laterotegmental portion of the rostral pons and caudal midbrain [155]. Each SCA has a short trunk that divides into two main branches, the medial and lateral. Infarctions in the SCA territories are known to rarely cause vertigo [156]. Accordingly, the low frequency of vertigo had been considered a useful finding to discriminate SCA infarction from infarctions in the AICA or PICA territory [156]. However, according to a recent study, [157] about half (19/41) of patients with isolated SCA infarction reported true vertigo, and 27% showed ipsilesional spontaneous nystagmus or GEN. These findings suggest that vertigo and nystagmus are more common than previously thought in SCA infarctions.

Lateral SCA infarctions, which constitute about 50% of SCA infarctions, are characterized by dizziness, nausea, unsteadiness, mild truncal ataxia, and severe limb ataxia [156, 158]. In medial SCA infarctions, the most prominent clinical finding is severe gait ataxia with a sudden fall or veering [159]. Prominent body lateropulsion may be ascribed to dysfunction of the rostral vermis that contributes to the control of gait, muscle tone, and postures. Unilateral rostral cerebellar infarctions can cause contrapulsion of saccades and ipsilateral limb dysmetria [160]. Contralateral saccadic pulsion consists of three elements: (1) contralateral deviation of the eyes during attempted vertical saccades, resulting in oblique trajectories; (2) hypermetria of contralateral saccades; and (3) hypometria of ipsilateral saccades. Asymmetric cerebellar outflows due to blockage of the fastigial outputs in the superior cerebellar peduncle may be responsible for saccadic contrapulsion (Fig. 7.2) [160]. However, a patient with isolated infarction involving unilateral superior cerebellar peduncle presented ipsiversive ocular torsion, mild dysarthria, ipsilesional limb ataxia, and severe truncal ipsipulsion, but no saccadic contrapulsion [161].

References

1. Leigh RJ, Zee D. The neurology of eye movements. 4th ed. New York: Oxford University Press; 2006. p. 261–314.
2. Choi KD, Lee H, Kim JS. Vertigo in brainstem and cerebellar strokes. Curr Opin Neurol. 2013;26(1):90–5.
3. Lee DK, Kim JS. Isolated inferior rectus palsy due to midbrain infarction detected by diffusion-weighted MRI. Neurology. 2006;66(12):1956–7.
4. Kim JS. Internuclear ophthalmoplegia as an isolated or predominant symptom of brainstem infarction. Neurology. 2004;62(9):1491–6.
5. Huh YE, Kim JS. Bedside evaluation of dizzy patients. J Clin Neurol (Seoul, Korea). 2013;9(4):203–13.
6. Kim JS. Pure lateral medullary infarction: clinical-radiological correlation of 130 acute, consecutive patients. Brain J Neurol. 2003;126(Pt 8): 1864–72.
7. Baloh RW, Yee RD, Honrubia V. Eye movements in patients with Wallenberg's syndrome. Ann N Y Acad Sci. 1981;374:600–13.
8. Choi KD, Oh SY, Park SH, Kim JH, Koo JW, Kim JS. Head-shaking nystagmus in lateral medullary infarction: patterns and possible mechanisms. Neurology. 2007;68(17):1337–44.
9. Uemura T, Cohen B. Effects of vestibular nuclei lesions on vestibulo-ocular reflexes and posture in monkeys. Acta Otolaryngol Suppl. 1973;315:1–71.
10. Morrow MJ, Sharpe JA. Torsional nystagmus in the lateral medullary syndrome. Ann Neurol. 1988;24(3):390–8.
11. Porta-Etessam J, Casanova I, Pajuelo B, Di Capua D, del Val J, Garcia ME, et al. See-saw nystagmus in a patient with Wallenberg syndrome. J Neuroophthalmol. 2009;29(1):73–4.
12. Khan SR, Lueck CJ. Hemi-seesaw nystagmus in lateral medullary syndrome. Neurology. 2013;80(13):1261–2.
13. Dieterich M, Brandt T. Wallenberg's syndrome: lateropulsion, cyclorotation, and subjective visual vertical in thirty-six patients. Ann Neurol. 1992;31(4):399–408.
14. Brandt T, Dieterich M. Pathological eye-head coordination in roll: tonic ocular tilt reaction in mesencephalic and medullary lesions. Brain J Neurol. 1987;110(Pt 3):649–66.
15. Kim SH, Kim JS. Effects of head position on perception of gravity in vestibular neuritis and lateral medullary infarction. Front Neurol. 2018;9:60.
16. Kommerell G, Hoyt WF. Lateropulsion of saccadic eye movements. Electro-oculographic studies in a patient with Wallenberg's syndrome. Arch Neurol. 1973;28(5):313–8.
17. Kim JS, Moon SY, Park SH, Yoon BW, Roh JK. Ocular lateropulsion in Wallenberg syndrome. Neurology. 2004;62(12):2287.

18. Helmchen C, Straube A, Buttner U. Saccadic latero-pulsion in Wallenberg's syndrome may be caused by a functional lesion of the fastigial nucleus. J Neurol. 1994;241(7):421–6.

19. Kim JS, Choi KD, Oh SY, Park SH, Han MK, Yoon BW, et al. Medial medullary infarction: abnormal ocular motor findings. Neurology. 2005;65(8):1294–8.

20. Kim JS, Moon SY, Kim KY, Kim HC, Park SH, Yoon BW, et al. Ocular contrapulsion in rostral medial medullary infarction. Neurology. 2004;63(7):1325–7.

21. Kim JS, Kim HG, Chung CS. Medial medullary syndrome. Report of 18 new patients and a review of the literature. Stroke. 1995;26(9):1548–52.

22. Pierrot-Deseilligny C, Milea D. Vertical nystagmus: clinical facts and hypotheses. Brain J Neurol. 2005;128(Pt 6):1237–46.

23. Choi KD, Jung DS, Park KP, Jo JW, Kim JS. Bowtie and upbeat nystagmus evolving into hemi-seesaw nystagmus in medial medullary infarction: possible anatomic mechanisms. Neurology. 2004;62(4):663–5.

24. Lee SU, Park SH, Jeong SH, Kim HJ, Kim JS. Evolution of torsional-upbeat into hemi-seesaw nystagmus in medial medullary infarction. Clin Neurol Neurosurg. 2014;118:80–2.

25. Kim JS, Yoon B, Choi KD, Oh SY, Park SH, Kim BK. Upbeat nystagmus: clinicoanatomical correlations in 15 patients. J Clin Neurol (Seoul, Korea). 2006;2(1):58–65.

26. Buttner-Ennever JA, Buttner U. Neuroanatomy of the ocular motor pathways. Baillieres Clin Neurol. 1992;1(2):263–87.

27. Pierrot-Deseilligny C. Saccade and smooth-pursuit impairment after cerebral hemispheric lesions. Eur Neurol. 1994;34(3):121–34.

28. Bhidayasiri R, Plant GT, Leigh RJ. A hypothetical scheme for the brainstem control of vertical gaze. Neurology. 2000;54(10):1985–93.

29. Oh K, Chang JH, Park KW, Lee DH, Choi KD, Kim JS. Jerky seesaw nystagmus in isolated internuclear ophthalmoplegia from focal pontine lesion. Neurology. 2005;64(7):1313–4.

30. Oh SY, Kim HJ, Kim JS. Vestibular-evoked myogenic potentials in central vestibular disorders. J Neurol. 2016;263(2):210–20.

31. Fisher CM. Ocular bobbing. Arch Neurol. 1964;11:543–6.

32. SPILLER WG. Ophthalmoplegia internuclearis anterior: a case with necropsy. Brain J Neurol. 1924;47(3):345–57.

33. Bender MB, Weinstein E. Effects of stimulation and lesion of the median longitudinal fasciculus in the monkey. Arch Neurol Psychiatr. 1944;52(2):106–13.

34. Dehaene I, Casselman JW, D'Hooghe M, Van Zandijcke M. Unilateral internuclear ophthalmoplegia and ipsiversive torsional nystagmus. J Neurol. 1996;243(6):461–4.

35. Zwergal A, Cnyrim C, Arbusow V, Glaser M, Fesl G, Brandt T, et al. Unilateral INO is associated with ocular tilt reaction in pontomesencephalic lesions: INO plus. Neurology. 2008;71(8):590–3.

36. Ranalli PJ, Sharpe JA. Vertical vestibulo-ocular reflex, smooth pursuit and eye-head tracking dysfunction in internuclear ophthalmoplegia. Brain J Neurol. 1988;111(Pt 6):1299–317.

37. Cremer PD, Migliaccio AA, Halmagyi GM, Curthoys IS. Vestibulo-ocular reflex pathways in internuclear ophthalmoplegia. Ann Neurol. 1999;45(4):529–33.

38. Choi SY, Kim HJ, Kim JS. Impaired vestibular responses in internuclear ophthalmoplegia: association and dissociation. Neurology. 2017;89(24):2476–80.

39. Lee SH, Kim SH, Kim SS, Kang KW, Tarnutzer AA. Preferential impairment of the contralesional posterior semicircular canal in internuclear ophthalmoplegia. Front Neurol. 2017;8:502.

40. Cogan DG, Kubik CS, Smith WL. Unilateral internuclear ophthalmoplegia; report of 8 clinical cases with one postmortem study. AMA Arch Ophthalmol. 1950;44(6):783–96.

41. Cogan DG. Internuclear ophthalmoplegia, typical and atypical. Arch Ophthalmol (Chicago, Ill: 1960). 1970;84(5):583–9.

42. Herishanu YO, Sharpe JA. Saccadic intrusions in internuclear ophthalmoplegia. Ann Neurol. 1983;14(1):67–72.

43. Cohen B, Komatsuzaki A, Bender MB. Electrooculographic syndrome in monkeys after pontine reticular formation lesions. Arch Neurol. 1968;18(1):78–92.

44. Hanson MR, Hamid MA, Tomsak RL, Chou SS, Leigh RJ. Selective saccadic palsy caused by pontine lesions: clinical, physiological, and pathological correlations. Ann Neurol. 1986;20(2):209–17.

45. Johnston JL, Sharpe JA, Morrow MJ. Paresis of contralateral smooth pursuit and normal vestibular smooth eye movements after unilateral brainstem lesions. Ann Neurol. 1992;31(5):495–502.

46. Muri RM, Chermann JF, Cohen L, Rivaud S, Pierrot-Deseilligny C. Ocular motor consequences of damage to the abducens nucleus area in humans. J Neuroophthalmol. 1996;16(3):191–5.

47. Hirose G, Furui K, Yoshioka A, Sakai K. Unilateral conjugate gaze palsy due to a lesion of the abducens nucleus. Clinical and neuroradiological correlations. J Clin Neuroophthalmol. 1993;13(1):54–8.

48. Fisher CM. Some neuro-ophthalmological observations. J Neurol Neurosurg Psychiatry. 1967;30(5):383–92.

49. Sharpe JA, Rosenberg MA, Hoyt WF, Daroff RB. Paralytic pontine exotropia. A sign of acute unilateral pontine gaze palsy and internuclear ophthalmoplegia. Neurology. 1974;24(11):1076–81.

50. Bronstein AM, Morris J, Du Boulay G, Gresty MA, Rudge P. Abnormalities of horizontal gaze. Clinical, oculographic and magnetic resonance imaging

findings. I. Abducens palsy. J Neurol Neurosurg Psychiatry. 1990;53(3):194–9.

51. Donaldson D, Rosenberg NL. Infarction of abducens nerve fascicle as cause of isolated sixth nerve palsy related to hypertension. Neurology. 1988;38(10):1654.

52. Azarmina M, Azarmina H. The six syndromes of the sixth cranial nerve. J Ophthalmic Vis Res. 2013;8(2):160–71.

53. May JG, Keller EL, Suzuki DA. Smooth-pursuit eye movement deficits with chemical lesions in the dorsolateral pontine nucleus of the monkey. J Neurophysiol. 1988;59(3):952–77.

54. Ahn BY, Choi KD, Kim JS, Park KP, Bae JH, Lee TH. Impaired ipsilateral smooth pursuit and gaze-evoked nystagmus in paramedian pontine lesion. Neurology. 2007;68(17):1436.

55. Suzuki DA, Yamada T, Hoedema R, Yee RD. Smooth-pursuit eye-movement deficits with chemical lesions in macaque nucleus reticularis tegmenti pontis. J Neurophysiol. 1999;82(3):1178–86.

56. Rambold H, Neumann G, Helmchen C. Vergence deficits in pontine lesions. Neurology. 2004;62(10):1850–3.

57. Kumral E, Bayulkem G, Evyapan D. Clinical spectrum of pontine infarction. Clinical-MRI correlations. J Neurol. 2002;249(12):1659–70.

58. Kushner MJ, Bressman SB. The clinical manifestations of pontine hemorrhage. Neurology. 1985;35(5):637–43.

59. Moon SY, Park SH, Hwang JM, Kim JS. Oculopalatal tremor after pontine hemorrhage. Neurology. 2003;61(11):1621.

60. Kim JS, Moon SY, Choi KD, Kim JH, Sharpe JA. Patterns of ocular oscillation in oculopalatal tremor: imaging correlations. Neurology. 2007;68(14):1128–35.

61. Wall M, Slamovits TL, Weisberg LA, Trufant SA. Vertical gaze ophthalmoplegia from infarction in the area of the posterior thalamo-subthalamic paramedian artery. Stroke. 1986;17(3):546–55.

62. King WM, Fuchs AF. Reticular control of vertical saccadic eye movements by mesencephalic burst neurons. J Neurophysiol. 1979;42(3):861–76.

63. Moschovakis AK, Scudder CA, Highstein SM. Structure of the primate oculomotor burst generator. I. Medium-lead burst neurons with upward on-directions. J Neurophysiol. 1991;65(2):203–17.

64. Moschovakis AK, Scudder CA, Highstein SM, Warren JD. Structure of the primate oculomotor burst generator. II. Medium-lead burst neurons with downward on-directions. J Neurophysiol. 1991;65(2):218–29.

65. Ranalli PJ, Sharpe JA. Upbeat nystagmus and the ventral tegmental pathway of the upward vestibulo-ocular reflex. Neurology. 1988;38(8):1329–30.

66. Leigh RJ, Seidman SH, Grant MP, Hanna JP. Loss of ipsidirectional quick phases of torsional nystagmus with a unilateral midbrain lesion. J Vestib Res. 1993;3(2):115–21.

67. Riordan-Eva P, Faldon M, Buttner-Ennever JA, Gass A, Bronstein AM, Gresty MA. Abnormalities of torsional fast phase eye movements in unilateral rostral midbrain disease. Neurology. 1996;47(1):201–7.

68. Helmchen C, Rambold H, Kempermann U, Buttner-Ennever JA, Buttner U. Localizing value of torsional nystagmus in small midbrain lesions. Neurology. 2002;59(12):1956–64.

69. Leigh RJ, Zee D. The neurology of eye movements. New York: Oxford University Press; 2006. p. 598–718.

70. Crawford JD, Cadera W, Vilis T. Generation of torsional and vertical eye position signals by the interstitial nucleus of Cajal. Science (New York, NY). 1991;252(5012):1551–3.

71. Fukushima K, Fukushima J, Harada C, Ohashi T, Kase M. Neuronal activity related to vertical eye movement in the region of the interstitial nucleus of Cajal in alert cats. Exp Brain Res. 1990;79(1):43–64.

72. Dalezios Y, Scudder CA, Highstein SM, Moschovakis AK. Anatomy and physiology of the primate interstitial nucleus of Cajal. II. Discharge pattern of single efferent fibers. J Neurophysiol. 1998;80(6):3100–11.

73. Halmagyi GM, Brandt T, Dieterich M, Curthoys IS, Stark RJ, Hoyt WF. Tonic contraversive ocular tilt reaction due to unilateral meso-diencephalic lesion. Neurology. 1990;40(10):1503–9.

74. Handel A, Glimcher PW. Response properties of saccade-related burst neurons in the central mesencephalic reticular formation. J Neurophysiol. 1997;78(4):2164–75.

75. Waitzman DM, Silakov VL, DePalma-Bowles S, Ayers AS. Effects of reversible inactivation of the primate mesencephalic reticular formation. II. Hypometric vertical saccades. J Neurophysiol. 2000;83(4):2285–99.

76. Kokkoroyannis T, Scudder CA, Balaban CD, Highstein SM, Moschovakis AK. Anatomy and physiology of the primate interstitial nucleus of Cajal I. efferent projections. J Neurophysiol. 1996;75(2):725–39.

77. Pasik P, Pasik T, Bender MB. The pretectal syndrome in monkeys. I. Disturbances of gaze and body posture. Brain J Neurol. 1969;92(3):521–34.

78. Bogousslavsky J, Regli F. Upgaze palsy and monocular paresis of downward gaze from ipsilateral thalamo-mesencephalic infarction: a vertical "one-and-a-half" syndrome. J Neurol. 1984;231(1):43–5.

79. Mehler MF. The neuro-ophthalmologic spectrum of the rostral basilar artery syndrome. Arch Neurol. 1988;45(9):966–71.

80. Marshall RS, Sacco RL, Kreuger R, Odel JG, Mohr JP. Dissociated vertical nystagmus and internuclear ophthalmoplegia from a midbrain infarction. Arch Neurol. 1991;48(12):1304–5.

81. Halmagyi GM, Aw ST, Dehaene I, Curthoys IS, Todd MJ. Jerk-waveform see-saw nystagmus due to unilateral meso-diencephalic lesion. Brain J Neurol. 1994;117(Pt 4):789–803.

82. Mays LE, Porter JD, Gamlin PD, Tello CA. Neural control of vergence eye movements: neurons encoding vergence velocity. J Neurophysiol. 1986;56(4):1007–21.

83. Judge SJ, Cumming BG. Neurons in the monkey midbrain with activity related to vergence eye movement and accommodation. J Neurophysiol. 1986;55(5):915–30.

84. Pullicino P, Lincoff N, Truax BT. Abnormal vergence with upper brainstem infarcts: pseudoabducens palsy. Neurology. 2000;55(3):352–8.

85. Caplan LR. "top of the basilar" syndrome. Neurology. 1980;30(1):72–9.

86. Keane JR. The pretectal syndrome: 206 patients. Neurology. 1990;40(4):684–90.

87. Biller J, Shapiro R, Evans LS, Haag JR, Fine M. Oculomotor nuclear complex infarction. Clinical and radiological correlation. Arch Neurol. 1984;41(9):985–7.

88. Ksiazek SM, Slamovits TL, Rosen CE, Burde RM, Parisi F. Fascicular arrangement in partial oculomotor paresis. Am J Ophthalmol. 1994;118(1): 97–103.

89. Castro O, Johnson LN, Mamourian AC. Isolated inferior oblique paresis from brain-stem infarction. Perspective on oculomotor fascicular organization in the ventral midbrain tegmentum. Arch Neurol. 1990;47(2):235–7.

90. Lee HS, Yang TI, Choi KD, Kim JS. Teaching video NeuroImage: isolated medial rectus palsy in midbrain infarction. Neurology. 2008;71(21):e64.

91. Hopf HC, Gutmann L. Diabetic 3rd nerve palsy: evidence for a mesencephalic lesion. Neurology. 1990;40(7):1041–5.

92. Lee SH, Park SW, Kim BC, Kim MK, Cho KH, Kim JS. Isolated trochlear palsy due to midbrain stroke. Clin Neurol Neurosurg. 2010;112(1):68–71.

93. Jeong SH, Kim SH, Lee SH, Park SH, Kim HJ, Kim JS. Central trochlear palsy: report of two patients with Ipsilesional palsy and review of the literature. J Neuroophthalmol. 2016;36(4):377–82.

94. Choi SY, Song JJ, Hwang JM, Kim JS. Tinnitus in fourth nerve palsy: an indicator for an intra-axial lesion. J Neuroophthalmol. 2010;30(4):325–7.

95. Okuda B, Tachibana H, Sugita M, Maeda Y. Bilateral internuclear ophthalmoplegia, ataxia, and tremor from a midbrain infarction. Stroke. 1993;24(3):481–2.

96. Jeong SH, Kim EK, Lee J, Choi KD, Kim JS. Patterns of dissociate torsional-vertical nystagmus in internuclear ophthalmoplegia. Ann N Y Acad Sci. 2011;1233:271–8.

97. Kim SH, Park SH, Kim HJ, Kim JS. Isolated central vestibular syndrome. Ann N Y Acad Sci. 2015;1343:80–9.

98. Lee H. Neuro-otological aspects of cerebellar stroke syndrome. J Clin Neurol (Seoul, Korea). 2009;5(2):65–73.

99. Amarenco P, Hauw JJ. Cerebellar infarction in the territory of the anterior and inferior cerebellar artery.

A clinicopathological study of 20 cases. Brain J Neurol. 1990;113(Pt 1):139–55.

100. Lee H, Sohn SI, Jung DK, Cho YW, Lim JG, Yi SD, et al. Sudden deafness and anterior inferior cerebellar artery infarction. Stroke. 2002;33(12):2807–12.

101. Oas JG, Baloh RW. Vertigo and the anterior inferior cerebellar artery syndrome. Neurology. 1992;42(12):2274–9.

102. Lee H, Kim JS, Chung E-J, Yi H-A, Chung I-S, Lee S-R, et al. Infarction in the territory of anterior inferior cerebellar artery: spectrum of audiovestibular loss. Stroke. 2009;40(12):3745–51.

103. Newman-Toker DE, Kattah JC, Alvernia JE, Wang DZ. Normal head impulse test differentiates acute cerebellar strokes from vestibular neuritis. Neurology. 2008;70(24 Pt 2):2378–85.

104. Huh YE, Koo JW, Lee H, Kim JS. Head-shaking aids in the diagnosis of acute audiovestibular loss due to anterior inferior cerebellar artery infarction. Audiol Neurootol. 2013;18(2):114–24.

105. Choi S-Y, Kee H-J, Park J-H, Kim H-J, Kim J-S. Combined peripheral and central vestibulopathy. J Vestib Res. 2014;24(5, 6):443–51.

106. Rajesh R, Rafeequ M, Girija AS. Anterior inferior cerebellar artery infarct with unilateral deafness. J Assoc Physicians India. 2004;52:333–4.

107. Patzak MJ, Demuth K, Kehl R, Lindner A. Sudden hearing loss as the leading symptom of an infarction of the left anterior inferior cerebellar artery. HNO. 2005;53(9):797–9.

108. Lee H, Yi H-A, Chung I-S, Lee S-R. Long-term outcome of canal paresis of a vascular cause. J Neurol Neurosurg Psychiatry. 2011;82(1):105–9.

109. Kim H-A, Lee B-C, Hong J-H, Yeo C-K, Yi H-A, Lee H. Long-term prognosis for hearing recovery in stroke patients presenting vertigo and acute hearing loss. J Neurol Sci. 2014;339(1):176–82.

110. Lee H, Cho YW. Auditory disturbance as a prodrome of anterior inferior cerebellar artery infarction. J Neurol Neurosurg Psychiatry. 2003;74(12): 1644–8.

111. Lee H, Lee SY, Lee SR, Park BR, Baloh RW. Ocular tilt reaction and anterior inferior cerebellar artery syndrome. J Neurol Neurosurg Psychiatry. 2005;76(12):1742–3.

112. Lee H, Yi HA, Lee SR, Lee SY, Park BR. Ocular torsion associated with infarction in the territory of the anterior inferior cerebellar artery: frequency, pattern, and a major determinant. J Neurol Sci. 2008;269(1–2):18–23.

113. Lee H, Ahn BH, Baloh RW. Sudden deafness with vertigo as a sole manifestation of anterior inferior cerebellar artery infarction. J Neurol Sci. 2004;222(1–2):105–7.

114. Perlman HB, Kimura R, Fernandez C. Experiments on temporary obstruction of the internal auditory artery. Laryngoscope. 1959;69(6):591–613.

115. Grad A, Baloh RW. Vertigo of vascular origin. Clinical and electronystagmographic features in 84 cases. Arch Neurol. 1989;46(3):281–4.

116. Amarenco P, Rosengart A, DeWitt LD, Pessin MS, Caplan LR. Anterior inferior cerebellar artery territory infarcts. Mechanisms and clinical features. Arch Neurol. 1993;50(2):154–61.

117. Choi KD, Chun JU, Han MG, Park SH, Kim JS. Embolic internal auditory artery infarction from vertebral artery dissection. J Neurol Sci. 2006;246(1–2):169–72.

118. Liqun Z, Park KH, Kim HJ, Lee SU, Choi JY, Kim JS. Acute unilateral audiovestibulopathy due to embolic labyrinthine infarction. Front Neurol. 2018;9:311.

119. Lee H, Yi HA, Baloh RW. Sudden bilateral simultaneous deafness with vertigo as a sole manifestation of vertebrobasilar insufficiency. J Neurol Neurosurg Psychiatry. 2003;74(4):539–41.

120. Kim J, Lopez I, DiPatre P, Liu F, Ishiyama A, Baloh R. Internal auditory artery infarction Clinicopathologic correlation. Neurology. 1999;52(1):40–4.

121. Hemenway WG, Lindsay JR. Postural vertigo due to unilateral sudden partial loss of vestibular function. Ann Otol Rhinol Laryngol. 1956;65(3):692–706.

122. Glickstein M, Sultan F, Voogd J. Functional localization in the cerebellum. Cortex. 2011;47(1):59–80.

123. Kim S-H, Kim J-S. Eye movement abnormalities in middle cerebellar peduncle strokes. Acta Neurol Belg. 2019;119(1):37–45.

124. Zee D, Yamazaki A, Butler PH, Gucer G. Effects of ablation of flocculus and paraflocculus of eye movements in primate. J Neurophysiol. 1981;46(4):878–99.

125. Park H-K, Kim J-S, Strupp M, Zee DS. Isolated floccular infarction: impaired vestibular responses to horizontal head impulse. J Neurol. 2013;260(6):1576–82.

126. Yacovino DA, Akly MP, Luis L, Zee DS. The floccular syndrome: dynamic changes in eye movements and vestibulo-ocular reflex in isolated infarction of the cerebellar flocculus. Cerebellum. 2018;17(2):122–31.

127. Amarenco P, Roullet E, Hommel M, Chaine P, Marteau R. Infarction in the territory of the medial branch of the posterior inferior cerebellar artery. J Neurol Neurosurg Psychiatry. 1990;53(9):731–5.

128. Voogd J, Gerrits NM, Ruigrok TJ. Organization of the vestibulocerebellum. Ann N Y Acad Sci. 1996;781:553–79.

129. Fushiki H, Barmack NH. Topography and reciprocal activity of cerebellar Purkinje cells in the uvula-nodulus modulated by vestibular stimulation. J Neurophysiol. 1997;78(6):3083–94.

130. Lee H. Isolated vascular vertigo. J Stroke. 2014;16(3):124–30.

131. Baier B, Dieterich M. Incidence and anatomy of gaze-evoked nystagmus in patients with cerebellar lesions. Neurology. 2011;76(4):361–5.

132. Huh YE, Kim JS. Patterns of spontaneous and head-shaking nystagmus in cerebellar infarction: imaging correlations. Brain J Neurol. 2011;134(Pt 12):3662–71.

133. Choi JY, Kim JH, Kim HJ, Glasauer S, Kim JS. Central paroxysmal positional nystagmus: characteristics and possible mechanisms. Neurology. 2015;84(22):2238–46.

134. Choi JY, Glasauer S, Kim JH, Zee DS, Kim JS. Characteristics and mechanism of apogeotropic central positional nystagmus. Brain J Neurol. 2018;141:762–75.

135. Lee S-H, Kim H-J, Kim J-S. Ocular motor dysfunction due to brainstem disorders. J Neuroophthalmol. 2018;38(3):393–412.

136. Huang CY, Yu YL. Small cerebellar strokes may mimic labyrinthine lesions. J Neurol Neurosurg Psychiatry. 1985;48(3):263–5.

137. Lee H, Sohn SI, Cho YW, Lee SR, Ahn BH, Park BR, et al. Cerebellar infarction presenting isolated vertigo: frequency and vascular topographical patterns. Neurology. 2006;67(7):1178–83.

138. Kim HA, Hong JH, Lee H, Yi HA, Lee SR, Lee SY, et al. Otolith dysfunction in vestibular neuritis: recovery pattern and a predictor of symptom recovery. Neurology. 2008;70(6):449–53.

139. Mossman S, Halmagyi GM. Partial ocular tilt reaction due to unilateral cerebellar lesion. Neurology. 1997;49(2):491–3.

140. Jeong HS, Oh JY, Kim JS, Kim J, Lee AY, Oh SY. Periodic alternating nystagmus in isolated nodular infarction. Neurology. 2007;68(12):956–7.

141. Lee H. Sudden deafness related to posterior circulation infarction in the territory of the nonanterior inferior cerebellar artery: frequency, origin, and vascular topographical pattern. Eur Neurol. 2008;59(6):302–6.

142. Voogd J, Schraa-Tam CK, van der Geest JN, De Zeeuw CI. Visuomotor cerebellum in human and nonhuman primates. Cerebellum. 2012;11(2):392–410.

143. Rambold H, Churchland A, Selig Y, Jasmin L, Lisberger S. Partial ablations of the flocculus and ventral paraflocculus in monkeys cause linked deficits in smooth pursuit eye movements and adaptive modification of the VOR. J Neurophysiol. 2002;87(2):912–24.

144. Nagao S. Different roles of flocculus and ventral paraflocculus for oculomotor control in the primate. Neuroreport. 1992;3(1):13–6.

145. Belton T, McCrea RA. Role of the cerebellar flocculus region in the coordination of eye and head movements during gaze pursuit. J Neurophysiol. 2000;84(3):1614–26.

146. Lee SH, Park SH, Kim JS, Kim HJ, Yunusov F, Zee DS. Isolated unilateral infarction of the cerebellar tonsil: ocular motor findings. Ann Neurol. 2014;75(3):429–34.

147. Sharpe JA. Pursuit paretic nystagmus. Ann Neurol. 1979;6(5):458.

148. Nolte J. The human brain: an introduction to its functional anatomy. St. Louis, MO: Mosby; 2002.

149. Moon IS, Kim JS, Choi KD, Kim M-J, Oh S-Y, Lee H, et al. Isolated nodular infarction. Stroke. 2009;40(2):487–91.

150. Lee H, Cho Y-W. A case of isolated nodulus infarction presenting as a vestibular neuritis. J Neurol Sci. 2004;221(1):117–9.
151. Sheliga BM, Yakushin SB, Silvers A, Raphan T, Cohen B. Control of spatial orientation of the angular Vestibulo-ocular reflex by the nodulus and uvula of the vestibulocerebellum. Ann N Y Acad Sci. 1999;871(1):94–122.
152. Waespe W, Cohen B, Raphan T. Dynamic modification of the vestibulo-ocular reflex by the nodulus and uvula. Science (New York, NY). 1985;228(4696):199–202.
153. Oh Y-M, Choi K-D, Oh S-Y, Kim J. Periodic alternating nystagmus with circumscribed nodular lesion. Neurology. 2006;67(3):399.
154. Kim J, Ahn K, Moon S, Choi K, Park S, Koo J. Isolated perverted head-shaking nystagmus in focal cerebellar infarction. Neurology. 2005;64(3):575–6.
155. Mohr J, Caplan LR. Vertebrobasilar disease. In: Stroke. 4th ed. Philadelphia: Elsevier; 2004. p. 207–74.
156. Kase CS, White JL, Joslyn JN, Williams JP, Mohr JP. Cerebellar infarction in the superior cerebellar artery distribution. Neurology. 1985;35(5):705–11.
157. Lee H, Kim H-A. Nystagmus in SCA territory cerebellar infarction: pattern and a possible mechanism. J Neurol Neurosurg Psychiatry. 2013;84(4):446–51.
158. Chaves C, Caplan LR, Chung C-S, Tapia J, Amarenco P, Teal P, et al. Cerebellar infarcts in the New England Medical Center posterior circulation stroke registry. Neurology. 1994;44(8):1385.
159. Sohn SI, Lee H, Lee SR, Baloh RW. Cerebellar infarction in the territory of the medial branch of the superior cerebellar artery. Neurology. 2006;66(1): 115–7.
160. Ranalli PJ, Sharpe JA. Contrapulsion of saccades and ipsilateral ataxia: a unilateral disorder of the rostral cerebellum. Ann Neurol. 1986;20(3):311–6.
161. Lee S-U, Bae H-J, Kim J-S. Ipsilesional limb ataxia and truncal ipsipulsion in isolated infarction of the superior cerebellar peduncle. J Neurol Sci. 2015;349(1):251–3.

Hemorrhagic Strokes

8

Jong-Won Chung and Chin-Sang Chung

Epidemiology

Intracerebral hemorrhages (ICHs) are most often caused by the rupture of small, penetrating arteries due to hypertensive changes or other vascular abnormalities [1, 2]. Although the incidence of hypertensive ICH has decreased with the improvement in blood pressure control in developed countries, [3] it still accounts for approximately 10–20% of all strokes: [4, 5] 8–15% in Western countries (e.g., the USA, the UK, and Australia) [6, 7] and 18–24% in Japan and Korea [3, 8]. However, the incidence of ICH may be higher in less-well-developed countries.

The incidence of ICH involving posterior circulation is unclear due to lack of data and adequate definitions for categorizing ICH [9]. However, hospital studies have reported that thalamic ICHs account for 10–15% of ICH cases, cerebellar ICHs for 5–15%, and pontine ICHs for approximately 10% [10]. Therefore, ICHs involving posterior circulation are not rare.

Etiology and Pathophysiology

Primary ICH

Hypertensive ICH

Hypertension is the most important risk factor for ICH. It contributes to the decreased elasticity of arteries, thereby increasing the likelihood of rupture in response to acute elevations in intravascular pressure [11]. Chronic hypertension is responsible for the degeneration of the tunica media and smooth muscle in cerebral arteries [2]. Vascular wall resistance to the stress due to elevated blood pressure in hypertension is weakened by the presence of hyaline, and this material in the cerebral vasculature has been linked to minimal resistance of the surrounding cerebral parenchyma. This may explain why the cerebral parenchyma is the only tissue in which increased blood pressure can lead to vascular rupture and hemorrhage [12].

J.-W. Chung · C.-S. Chung (✉)
Department of Neurology, Samsung Medical Center,
School of Medicine, Sungkyunkwan University,
Seoul, South Korea

© Springer Nature Singapore Pte Ltd. 2021
J. S. Kim (ed.), *Posterior Circulation Stroke*, https://doi.org/10.1007/978-981-15-6739-1_8

Amyloid Angiopathy

Cerebral amyloid angiopathy-related ICH accounts for 10–30% of primary ICH in older patients [13, 14]. It is characterized by the deposition of amyloid-β peptide in capillaries, arterioles, and small- and medium-sized arteries in the cerebral cortex, leptomeninges, and cerebellum [15]. The secondary pathological changes associated with advanced cerebral amyloid angiopathy include loss of vascular smooth muscle cells, microaneurysms, concentric splitting of the vessel wall, chronic perivascular or transmural inflammation, and fibrinoid necrosis [16–18]. Cerebral amyloid angiopathy-related hemorrhages occur preferentially in lobular areas, especially in the posterior brain regions (e.g., occipital and temporal lobes), reflecting the distribution of vascular amyloid deposits [19–21].

Secondary ICH

Arteriovenous Malformation

Vascular malformations are an important cause of intracranial hemorrhage, especially in younger patients. Among vascular malformations, arteriovenous malformations are the most frequent causes of ICH. These malformations are often found in border zone regions shared by the distal anterior, middle, and posterior cerebral arteries [22]. Potential risk factors for these malformation-related hemorrhages include (1) malformations with exclusively deep venous drainage (typically defined as drainage through the periventricular, galenic, or cerebellar pathways), (2) malformations associated with aneurysms, (3) malformations located deep within the brain, and (4) infratentorial malformations [23, 24] (Fig. 8.1).

Cavernous Malformation

Cerebral cavernous malformations, the second most common type of central nervous system vascular lesion, constitute abnormally enlarged capillary cavities without intervening brain parenchyma [25, 26]. These lesions may occur anywhere, including the cortical surface, white matter pathways, basal ganglia, brainstem, or the cerebellum. (Fig. 8.2) For patients who initially presented without both an overt intracranial hemorrhage and a brainstem cavernous

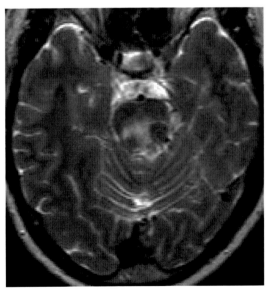
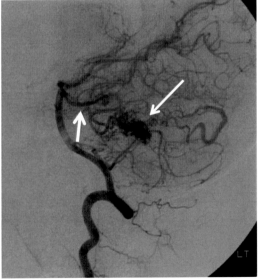

Fig. 8.1 A 42-year-old woman developed dizziness and tingling sensation in the right extremities. Left image: T2-weighted Brain MRI showed a round, dark signal intensity with adjacent high signal intensity signals consistent with acute hemorrhage surrounded by edema. Right image: Angiogram showed arteriovenous malformation (long arrow) that is mainly supplied by enlarged superior cerebellar artery (short arrow). The patient was treated with embolization

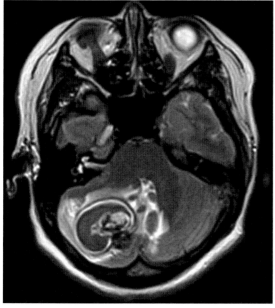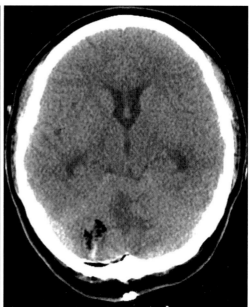

Fig. 8.2 An 18-year-old girl developed sudden dizziness, headache, and gait ataxia. Left image: T2-weighted MRI showed heterogeneous (dark, iso, high) lobulated signals suggesting multistage hemorrhages that were surrounded by edema. Angiogram findings were normal. These findings were consistent with repeated bleeding from cavernous hemangioma. Right image: Follow-up CT showed that the hemorrhages and mass were surgically resected

malformation, the initial 5-year risk of hemorrhage was 3.8%, and the recurrent 5-year hemorrhage risk was 18.4%. In contrast, patients with brainstem cavernous malformations were reported to have significantly higher 5-year rates of initial (8%) and recurrent (30.8%) hemorrhage [27].

Dural Arteriovenous Fistula

Dural arteriovenous fistulae constitute arteriovenous shunts at the level of the meninges that are usually supplied by branches of the external carotid or vertebral arteries. Hemorrhages due to these fistulae show more benign clinical courses than those with other vascular lesions (e.g., intracranial aneurysms) due to the bleeding site being a venous rather than a direct arterial source [28].

Cerebral Venous Thrombosis

Cerebral venous thrombosis is a well-established cause of ICH. Elevated cerebral venous pressure due to venous occlusion results in a spectrum of pathophysiological changes, including dilated venous and capillary beds, development of interstitial brain edema, increased CSF production, decreased CSF absorption, and rupture of cerebral veins leading to hemorrhagic lesions [29]. It is crucial to recognize ICH caused by cerebral venous thrombosis because it is the only variety of ICH that should be treated with anticoagulants.

ICHs Associated with Antithrombotics

Coagulopathy caused by oral anticoagulation therapy is also an important pathophysiology of ICH. Oral anticoagulants can directly interfere with the synthesis of vitamin K-dependent clotting factors, resulting in dysfunctional prothrombin and factors VII, IX, and Xa [30–32]. Oral anticoagulants can trigger preexisting subclinical intracerebral bleeding, especially in patients with underlying hypertension and cerebrovascular disease [33]. Subdural hematoma has also been reported to be a rare complication of anticoagulation therapy [34, 35].

ICHs Associated with Cancer

Cancer-related intracerebral bleeding is an uncommon cause of ICH. The incidence of tumoral hemorrhages has been estimated to be 0.8–4.4% of all ICHs [36]. However, intracere-

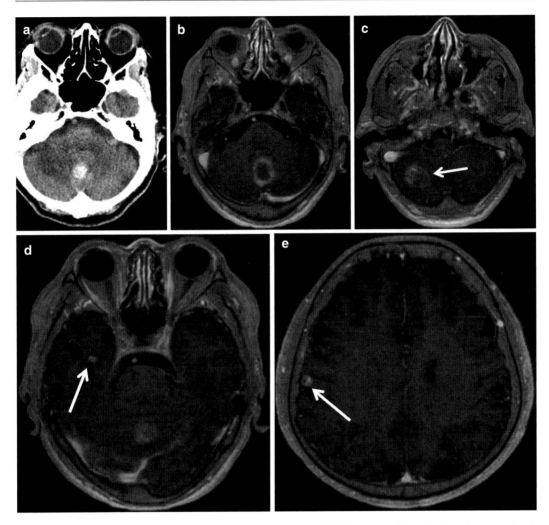

Fig. 8.3 An 88-year-old woman developed dizziness and gait difficulty. She had malignant papillary thyroid carcinoma with multiple lung and bone metastasis. Brain CT showed an acute hemorrhage in the midline cerebellum (**a**), which was identified by MRI (**b**). Gadolinium-enhanced MRI showed additional enhancing hemorrhagic lesion in the right cerebellum (**c**) and small enhancing lesions in the right temporal (**d**) and frontal lobe (**e**). It is likely that the current cerebellar hemorrhage was bleeding from the metastatic cancer

bral hemorrhage is relatively common in cancer patients and has been demonstrated in 3.0–14.6% patients at autopsy [37–39]. There are multiple causes of hemorrhage in cancer patients, including intratumoral bleeding, coagulation disorders, and complications of anticancer treatment (Fig. 8.3).

Reversible Cerebral Vasoconstriction

Reversible cerebral vasoconstriction syndrome is a group of conditions typically preceded by severe thunderclap headaches associated with reversible, segmental, multifocal cerebral artery vasoconstriction. In a large cohort of patients with this syndrome, brain hemorrhages were reported to be frequent (43%) [40].

Aneurysm

Rupture of intracranial arteries causes subarachnoid hemorrhages. Dissecting aneurysms involving intracranial posterior circulation are unusual lesions that affect otherwise healthy young adults. The dissection usually occurs between the intima or internal elastic lamina and the media;

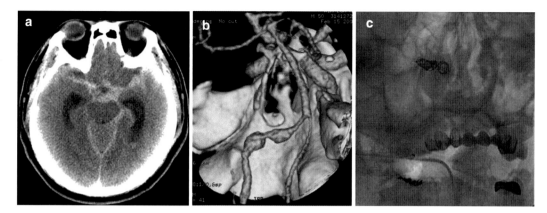

Fig. 8.4 A 45-year-old man developed sudden severe headache after baseball playing. CT showed subarachnoid hemorrhage (**a**). CT angiogram showed dissecting aneu-rysm in the left distal vertebral artery (**b**), which was treated with coil embolization (**c**)

subadventitial dissection can also occur and accounts for the infrequent finding of subarachnoid hemorrhage [41].

Hemorrhagic stroke due to dissection seems to involve posterior circulation more commonly than anterior circulation. Pathology studies have shown that subadventitial dissections are more frequent in the vertebral artery than in the middle cerebral artery; [42, 43] this could explain the relatively high frequency of hemorrhages in patients with posterior circulation dissection (Fig. 8.4).

Diagnosis

Computed tomography (CT) has excellent sensitivity and specificity (nearly 100%) for the detection of acute hemorrhage [44]. Acute hematomas appear as hyperdense areas on a noncontrast CT scan owing to their high protein concentration and high mass density. The density seen on a CT scan varies according to the timing of the scan. CT angiography is used to detect underlying vascular abnormalities and conditions, such as intracranial aneurysms and the "spot sign," an early predictor of hematoma expansion [45]. Traditionally, magnetic resonance imaging (MRI) has been considered to be insensitive to the presence of acute intraparenchymal blood and has been used to detect ischemia. With the use of gradient-echo imaging and susceptible weighted imaging, MRI has a diagnostic accuracy similar to that of noncontrast CT for acute blood and is markedly superior in the detection of chronic hemorrhage [46]. High-resolution vessel wall MRI is being increasingly used to assess vascular wall pathology (see Chap. 9).

Clinical Features

Thalamic Hemorrhage

At the beginning of the nineteenth century, Dejerine and Roussy provided a detailed description of thalamic syndrome [47]. Recent advances in neuroimaging have provided accurate diagnoses and have enabled clinicians to correlate clinical findings with neuroimaging findings. The clinical features of thalamic ICH vary with hematoma location and volume. The classic symptoms include the following: (1) contralateral hemiparesis, as the thalamus is close to the posterior limb of the internal capsule; hemiparesis was reported in 95% of cases; [48, 49] (2) hemisensory syndrome; approximately 85% of patients with thalamic ICH develop prominent sensory loss in the face, limb, and trunk [48] (Fig. 8.5); and (3) ophthalmologic symptoms such as paresis of upward gaze ("peering at the tip of the nose"), miotic

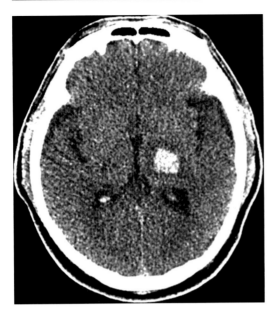

Fig. 8.5 A 60-year-old hypertensive man developed dysarthria, right hemiparesis, and severe sensory deficits. CT showed a thalamic hemorrhage of posterolateral type (Fig. 8.6c)

and unreactive pupils caused by ICH-induced pressure on the dorsal midbrain, [50] and skew deviation and horizontal gaze disturbances accompanied by involvement of the oculomotor tracts at the midbrain level [51].

The clinical syndromes associated with thalamic ICH differ according to the location of the hematoma and are subclassified based on the ruptured arterioles supplying specific thalamic areas (Table 8.1 and Fig. 8.6) [49, 52].

Midbrain Hemorrhage

A nontraumatic, spontaneous, primary midbrain hemorrhage is extremely rare. Midbrain hemorrhages mostly result from secondary extensions of hematomas from thalamic or pontine ICHs. The most frequent cause of an isolated midbrain hemorrhage is an arteriovenous malformation; rarely, it can also be caused by hypertension [53].

Table 8.1 Clinical syndromes of thalamic intracerebral hemorrhage

	Anterior type	Posteromedial type	Posterolateral type	Dorsal type	Global type
Ruptured artery	Branches of the "polar" or tuberothalamic artery	Thalamo-perforating arteries	Thalamo-geniculate arteries	Branches of the posterior choroidal artery	Nonspecific
Consciousness	Alert	Usually acute stupor or coma	Consciousness level parallels hematoma size	Usually alert	Stupor or coma in 3/4 of patients
Behavioral changes	Acute confusion, language dysfunctions, memory impairment, and apathy	Prominent memory dysfunction in case of hematoma limited to the medial thalamus; decorticate posture in the early stage with concomitant midbrain involvement	Hemi-neglect in right-sided lesions and simulating lesions; dysphasia in left-sided lacunar syndrome (sensorimotor stroke > pure motor stroke > pure sensory stroke)	None	Frequent decerebrate postures in the early stage; very similar to the posterolateral type in less severe cases
Sensory manifestation	Rare	Uncommon	Frequent; preceding paresthetic episodes at onset, contralateral hypesthesia, and late thalamic pain syndrome	Preceding paresthesia in 1/3 of patients; frequent sensory dysfunction	Almost always; severe

Table 8.1 (continued)

	Anterior type	Posteromedial type	Posterolateral type	Dorsal type	Global type
Motor manifestation	Usually absent and only slight, if any	Moderate-to-marked contralateral hemiparesis	Frequent moderate-to-marked contralateral hemiparesis mainly due to compression of the cerebral peduncle	Mild-to-moderate contralateral hemiparesis due to compression of the posterior limb of the internal capsule	Severe contralateral hemiparesis
Ocular findings	None	Very frequent	Infrequent extraocular muscle dysfunctions; occasional Horner's syndrome	None	Frequent classic ocular features
Prognosis	Excellent	High fatality	High fatality and morbidity	Very good	Very high fatality

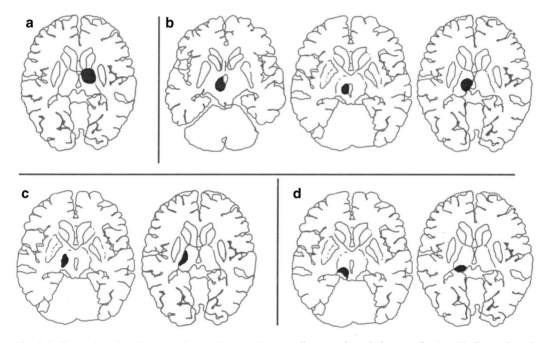

Fig. 8.6 Hemorrhage location according to the vascular supply of the thalamus. (**a**) Anterior type: Thalamo-tuberal arteries of posterior communicating arteries. (**b**) Posteromedial type: Posterior thalamo-subthalamic para-median arteries, thalamo-perforate. (**c**) Posterolateral type: Infero-lateral arteries, thalamo-geniculate. (**d**) Dorsal type: Posterior choroidal arteries

Midbrain ICHs present with progressive symptoms of ipsilateral ataxia or contralateral hemiparesis in combination with ophthalmoplegia (typically an ipsilateral partial/complete third cranial nerve palsy). In rare cases, isolated syndromes can also occur (Table 8.2).

Pontine Hemorrhage

Pontine hemorrhaging accounts for 10% of ICHs [59, 60] and shows a wide spectrum of clinical symptoms and prognosis, with its mortality ranging widely from 30% to 90% [61–63]. This wide

Table 8.2 Clinical syndromes of midbrain intracerebral hemorrhage

Syndromes	Symptoms
Dorsal midbrain syndrome [54]	Vertical gaze palsy, nystagmus retractorius, eyelid retraction, and light-near pupillary dissociation
Dorsal midbrain syndrome + [55]	Dorsal midbrain syndrome with associated bilateral fourth nerve palsy
Weber's syndrome [56]	Ipsilateral third nerve palsy and contralateral hemiparesis
Fascicular third nerve palsy syndrome [57]	Isolated ipsilateral third nerve palsy without hemiparesis
Movement disorder [58]	Contralateral limb dystonia and tremors with "rubral" characteristics

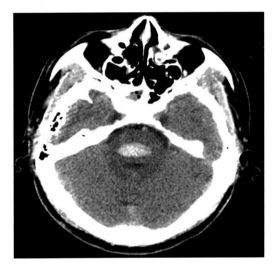

Fig. 8.7 A hypertensive, 53-year-old man suddenly became drowsy. Neurologic examination showed severe dysarthria, quadriparesis, and sensory deficits bilaterally. CT showed a pontine hemorrhage (bilateral-tegmental type, Fig. 8.8C)

range is mainly attributed to the size and location of the hematoma; thus, pontine ICH is classified as either small unilateral-tegmental, basal- or bilateral-tegmental, or massive (Figs. 8.7 and 8.8 and Table 8.3) [63].

Medullary Hemorrhage

Isolated medulla oblongata ICH has rarely been reported in the literature [64, 65]. The common symptoms of medullary ICH are vertigo, headache, and diplopia. Various neuro-otological

symptoms, including spontaneous nystagmus, ocular lateropulsion, and apogeotropic positional nystagmus, have been reported [66].

Cerebellar Hemorrhage

Regarding cerebellar hemorrhage, over 75% of patients complain of dizziness with headache being common at onset, while dysarthria, tinnitus, and hiccups can occur but less frequently [67]. Neurological exam findings differ depending on the involvement of the dentate nucleus, hemispheric white matter, and tegmental pons. Ipsilateral ataxia is found in 70% of all patients and also in patients with peripheral facial palsy, ipsilateral horizontal gaze palsy, sixth cranial nerve palsy, depressed corneal reflex, and miosis. In noncomatose patients, a characteristic triad of ipsilateral appendicular ataxia, horizontal gaze palsy, and peripheral facial palsy appear together when the ipsilateral pontine tegmentum is involved [67]. Ocular bobbing has occasionally been reported after cerebellar hemorrhage, [68] and the overall clinical course during the acute period of cerebellar hemorrhage is reported to be unpredictable [69–71].

Cortical Hemorrhage

The occipital lobe is a relatively rare site for hypertensive hematomas. Occipital hemorrhages are reported to be caused by arteriovenous angioma and cerebral angiopathy [72]. These hemorrhages can cause severe headaches, usually at or around the ipsilateral eye, contralateral homonymous hemianopia, contralateral extinction, dysgraphia, and dyslexia.

Management

Blood Pressure Control

Hypertension is the most common cause of ICH, and its early management is extremely important. Current evidence indicates that early and intensive lowering of blood pressure (BP) is safe and

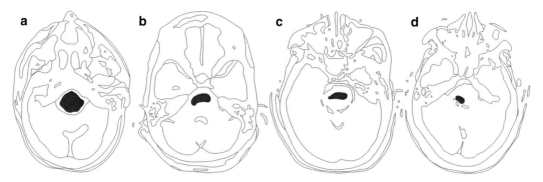

Fig. 8.8 Hemorrhage locations in the pons. (**a**) Massive type, (**b**) basal-tegmental type, (**c**) bilateral-tegmental type, and (**d**) unilateral-tegmental type

Table 8.3 Clinical syndromes of pontine intracerebral hemorrhage

	Small unilateral-tegmental type	Basal-tegmental/ bilateral-tegmental type	Massive type
Ruptured artery	Penetrating branches of the long circumferential arteries	Perforators of the basilar artery	Perforators of the basilar artery
Consciousness	Alert	Usually acute stupor or coma	Coma
Behavioral changes	Uncommon	Uncommon	Uncommon
Sensory manifestation	Facial numbness	Uncommon; hypesthesia	Bilateral hypesthesia
Motor manifestation	Frequent hemiparesis and palatal myoclonus	Pure motor stroke and ataxic hemiparesis	Progressive hemiparesis
Ocular findings	Ipsilateral miosis, "one-and-a-half syndrome," horizontal gaze palsy, internuclear ophthalmoplegia, partial involvement of vertical eye movements, ocular bobbing, and ocular ataxia	Rare; isolated abducens nerve palsy	Miotic pinpoint pupils, absent horizontal eye movements, and ocular bobbing
Prognosis	Excellent	Moderate to high fatality	Very high fatality

feasible and that surviving patients show modestly better functional recovery, with a favorable trend toward a reduction in the mortality and major disability endpoints. However, two large clinical trials, INTERACT II and ATACH II, failed to demonstrate an improved functional outcome with intensive reduction of systolic BP to <140 mmHg, compared to the standard goal of <180 mmHg, in acute primary ICH [73, 74]. Based on currently available data, for ICH patients presenting with a systolic BP between 150 and 220 mmHg and without any contraindications for acute BP treatment, acute lowering to 140 mmHg is safe. For ICH patients presenting with a systolic BP >220 mmHg, it may be reason-

able to consider an aggressive reduction of BP using a continuous intravenous infusion and frequent BP monitoring [75].

ICH Related to Antithrombotics

ICH related to anticoagulation therapy is a medical emergency and is associated with high mortality and an unfavorable outcome. In patients treated with vitamin K antagonists (VKAs), determination of anticoagulant status is performed by measuring the international normalized ratio (INR). Patients with ICH whose INR is elevated because of anticoagulation therapy should have their VKA withheld, receive therapy to replace vitamin K-dependent factors and correct the INR, and receive intravenous vitamin K [75]. Three agents are capable of correcting an elevated INR: activated factor VII, fresh frozen plasma, and prothrombin complex concentrate [76].

In contrast to VKA-ICH, in which INR measurements allow the assessment of anticoagulation status, coagulation testing in patients treated with novel oral anticoagulants is not available. Data from experimental settings suggest that prothrombin complex concentrate, fresh frozen plasma, and activated factor VII are all effective in preventing hematoma expansion with rivaroxaban and dabigatran [77–79]. For specific antidotes, idarucizumab is recommended as frontline therapy in patients receiving dabigatran who present with major or life-threatening bleeding, and andexanet alfa is a first choice for reversing life-threatening bleeding under FXa-inhibitor therapy [80]. The PATCH trial randomized patients with spontaneous acute ICH taking antiplatelet therapy (aspirin, clopidogrel, and dipyridamole) to either receive platelet transfusion therapy or standard therapy and reported an increased likelihood of death or unfavorable outcomes in the platelet transfusion group [81]. For ICH-related coagulation therapy, cessation of antiplatelet therapy is considered sufficient.

Control of Increased Intracranial Pressure

Increased intracranial pressure (ICP) is associated with worse outcomes following ICH, suggesting that ICP monitoring may benefit high-risk patients [82]. Current AHA/ASA guidelines recommend ICP monitoring and treatment for patients with a Glasgow Coma Scale score of ≤8, those with clinical evidence of transtentorial herniation, and those with significant intraventricular hemorrhage or hydrocephalus. A cerebral perfusion pressure of 50–70 mmHg may be reasonable. Corticosteroids are not recommended for the treatment of increased ICP in ICH [75].

Surgical Management of ICH

Two large clinical trials, STICH and STICH II, were undertaken to determine whether early surgery reduces mortality and improves the neurological outcomes for supratentorial ICH compared to those with conservative management. Early hematoma evacuation was not found to be beneficial [83, 84]. Although a randomized clinical trial has not been performed, craniotomy for posterior fossa hemorrhage patients with cerebellar hemorrhages >3 cm in diameter is recommended for patients with neurological deterioration or with brainstem compression and/or hydrocephalus from ventricular obstruction. In contrast to cerebellar hemorrhage, evacuation of brainstem hemorrhages may be harmful [75].

Prognosis

ICH involving posterior cerebral circulation demonstrates diverse prognoses depending on the location of the ICH and size of the hematoma. Several studies have reported the factors associated with prognosis according to the location of the ICH (Table 8.4)

Table 8.4 Poor prognostic factors of ICH involving posterior circulation

Thalamic ICH [49, 85]	Pontine ICH [86]	Cerebellar ICH
Low level of consciousness at onset	Low level of consciousness at onset	Low level of consciousness at onset
Severe motor weakness and appearance of decerebrate posturing	Dilated pupils	Delayed surgical decompression
Systemic complications	Abnormal respiration	Severe hydrocephalus
Global and posteromedial types	Larger hematoma	Identifiable underlying causes, such as arteriovenous malformation and coagulopathy
Larger hematoma	Systolic blood pressure of <100 mmHg	Volume of cerebellar hematoma

Table 8.4 (continued)

Thalamic ICH [49, 85]	Pontine ICH [86]	Cerebellar ICH
Extension of hematoma, involving the midbrain and basal ganglia	Hydrocephalus	Obliteration of the quadrigeminal cistern
Markedly enlarged ventricles and severe mass effect, causing a midline shift		
Presence of dense blood clots in the third ventricle		

ICH intracerebral hemorrhage

References

1. Qureshi AI, Mendelow AD, Hanley DF. Intracerebral haemorrhage. Lancet. 2009;373(9675):1632–44.
2. Qureshi AI, Tuhrim S, Broderick JP, Batjer HH, Hondo H, Hanley DF. Spontaneous intracerebral hemorrhage. N Engl J Med. 2001;344(19):1450–60.
3. Hong KS, Bang OY, Kang DW, Yu KH, Bae HJ, Lee JS, et al. Stroke statistics in Korea: part I. epidemiology and risk factors: a report from the korean stroke society and clinical research center for stroke. J Stroke. 2013;15(1):2–20.
4. Feigin VL, Lawes CM, Bennett DA, Barker-Collo SL, Parag V. Worldwide stroke incidence and early case fatality reported in 56 population-based studies: a systematic review. Lancet Neurol. 2009;8(4):355–69.
5. Sacco S, Marini C, Toni D, Olivieri L, Carolei A. Incidence and 10-year survival of intracerebral hemorrhage in a population-based registry. Stroke. 2009;40(2):394–9.
6. Kannel WB, Wolf PA, Verter J, McNamara PM. Epidemiologic assessment of the role of blood pressure in stroke. The Framingham study. JAMA. 1970;214(2):301–10.
7. Broderick J, Connolly S, Feldmann E, Hanley D, Kase C, Krieger D, et al. Guidelines for the management of spontaneous intracerebral hemorrhage in adults: 2007 update: a guideline from the American Heart Association/American Stroke Association Stroke Council, High Blood Pressure Research Council, and the Quality of Care and Outcomes in Research Interdisciplinary Working Group. Stroke. 2007;38(6):2001–23.
8. Toyoda K. Epidemiology and registry studies of stroke in Japan. J Stroke. 2013;15(1):21–6.
9. An SJ, Kim TJ, Yoon BW. Epidemiology, risk factors, and clinical features of Intracerebral hemorrhage: An update. J Stroke. 2017;19(1):3–10.
10. Auer RN, Sutherland GR. Primary intracerebral hemorrhage: pathophysiology. Can J Neurol Sci. 2005;32(Suppl 2):S3–12.
11. Plesea IE, Camenita A, Georgescu CC, Enache SD, Zaharia B, Georgescu CV, et al. Study of cerebral vascular structures in hypertensive intracerebral haemorrhage. Romanian J Morphol Embryol. 2005;46(3):249–56.
12. Sutherland GR, Auer RN. Primary intracerebral hemorrhage. J Clin Neurosci. 2006;13(5):511–7.
13. Jellinger KA. Alzheimer disease and cerebrovascular pathology: an update. J Neural Transm (Vienna). 2002;109(5–6):813–36.
14. Knudsen KA, Rosand J, Karluk D, Greenberg SM. Clinical diagnosis of cerebral amyloid angiopathy: validation of the Boston criteria. Neurology. 2001;56(4):537–9.
15. Scott O, Shi D, Andriashek D, Clark B, Goez HR. Clinical clues for autoimmunity and neuroinflammation in patients with autistic regression. Dev Med Child Neurol. 2017;59(9):947–51.
16. Mandybur TI. Cerebral amyloid angiopathy: the vascular pathology and complications. J Neuropathol Exp Neurol. 1986;45(1):79–90.
17. Vonsattel JP, Myers RH, Hedley-Whyte ET, Ropper AH, Bird ED, Richardson EP Jr. Cerebral amyloid angiopathy without and with cerebral hemorrhages: a comparative histological study. Ann Neurol. 1991;30(5):637–49.
18. Yamada M, Itoh Y, Shintaku M, Kawamura J, Jensson O, Thorsteinsson L, et al. Immune reactions associated with cerebral amyloid angiopathy. Stroke. 1996;27(7):1155–62.
19. Rosand J, Muzikansky A, Kumar A, Wisco JJ, Smith EE, Betensky RA, et al. Spatial clustering of hemorrhages in probable cerebral amyloid angiopathy. Ann Neurol. 2005;58(3):459–62.
20. Vinters HV, Gilbert JJ. Cerebral amyloid angiopathy: incidence and complications in the aging brain. II. The distribution of amyloid vascular changes. Stroke. 1983;14(6):924–8.
21. Tian J, Shi J, Bailey K, Mann DM. Relationships between arteriosclerosis, cerebral amyloid angiopathy and myelin loss from cerebral cortical white matter in Alzheimer's disease. Neuropathol Appl Neurobiol. 2004;30(1):46–56.
22. Solomon RA, Connolly ES Jr. Arteriovenous malformations of the brain. N Engl J Med. 2017;376(19):1859–66.
23. da Costa L, Wallace MC, Ter Brugge KG, O'Kelly C, Willinsky RA, Tymianski M. The natural history and predictive features of hemorrhage from brain arteriovenous malformations. Stroke. 2009;40(1):100–5.
24. Dinc N, Platz J, Tritt S, Quick-Weller J, Eibach M, Wolff R, et al. Posterior fossa AVMs: increased risk of bleeding and worse outcome compared to supratentorial AVMs. J Clin Neurosci. 2018;53:171–6.
25. Maraire JN, Awad IA. Intracranial cavernous malformations: lesion behavior and management strategies. Neurosurgery. 1995;37(4):591–605.

26. Moriarity JL, Clatterbuck RE, Rigamonti D. The natural history of cavernous malformations. Neurosurg Clin N Am. 1999;10(3):411–7.

27. Horne MA, Flemming KD, Su IC, Stapf C, Jeon JP, Li D, et al. Clinical course of untreated cerebral cavernous malformations: a meta-analysis of individual patient data. Lancet Neurol. 2016;15(2):166–73.

28. King WA, Martin NA. Intracerebral hemorrhage due to dural arteriovenous malformations and fistulae. Neurosurg Clin N Am. 1992;3(3):577–90.

29. Schaller B, Graf R. Cerebral venous infarction: the pathophysiological concept. Cerebrovasc Dis. 2004;18(3):179–88.

30. Makris M, Greaves M, Phillips WS, Kitchen S, Rosendaal FR, Preston EF. Emergency oral anticoagulant reversal: the relative efficacy of infusions of fresh frozen plasma and clotting factor concentrate on correction of the coagulopathy. Thromb Haemost. 1997;77(3):477–80.

31. Hirsh J, Dalen J, Anderson DR, Poller L, Bussey H, Ansell J, et al. Oral anticoagulants: mechanism of action, clinical effectiveness, and optimal therapeutic range. Chest. 2001;119(1 Suppl):8S–21S.

32. Yeh CH, Hogg K, Weitz JI. Overview of the new oral anticoagulants: opportunities and challenges. Arterioscler Thromb Vasc Biol. 2015;35(5):1056–65.

33. Hart RG. What causes intracerebral hemorrhage during warfarin therapy? Neurology. 2000;55(7):907–8.

34. Kanter R, Kanter M, Kirsch W, Rosenberg G. Spontaneous posterior fossa subdural hematoma as a complication of anticoagulation. Neurosurgery. 1984;15(2):241–2.

35. Stendel R, Schulte T, Pietila TA, Suess O, Brock M. Spontaneous bilateral chronic subdural haematoma of the posterior fossa. Case report and review of the literature. Acta Neurochir. 2002;144(5):497–500.

36. Licata B, Turazzi S. Bleeding cerebral neoplasms with symptomatic hematoma. J Neurosurg Sci. 2003;47(4):201–10; discussion 10

37. Barth H, Fritsch G, Haaks T. Intracerebral hematoma as an acute manifestation of intracranial tumors. Nervenarzt. 1994;65(12):854–8.

38. Kondziolka D, Bernstein M, Resch L, Tator CH, Fleming JF, Vanderlinden RG, et al. Significance of hemorrhage into brain tumors: clinicopathological study. J Neurosurg. 1987;67(6):852–7.

39. Wakai S, Yamakawa K, Manaka S, Takakura K. Spontaneous intracranial hemorrhage caused by brain tumor: its incidence and clinical significance. Neurosurgery. 1982;10(4):437–44.

40. Topcuoglu MA, Singhal AB. Hemorrhagic reversible cerebral vasoconstriction syndrome: features and mechanisms. Stroke. 2016;47(7):1742–7.

41. Berger MS, Wilson CB. Intracranial dissecting aneurysms of the posterior circulation. Report of six cases and review of the literature. J Neurosurg. 1984;61(5):882–94.

42. Day AL, Gaposchkin CG, Yu CJ, Rivet DJ, Dacey RG Jr. Spontaneous fusiform middle cerebral artery aneurysms: characteristics and a proposed mechanism of formation. J Neurosurg. 2003;99(2):228–40.

43. Endo S, Nishijima M, Nomura H, Takaku A, Okada E. A pathological study of intracranial posterior circulation dissecting aneurysms with subarachnoid hemorrhage: report of three autopsied cases and review of the literature. Neurosurgery. 1993;33(4):732–8.

44. Hsieh PC, Awad IA, Getch CC, Bendok BR, Rosenblatt SS, Batjer HH. Current updates in perioperative management of intracerebral hemorrhage. Neurol Clin. 2006;24(4):745–64.

45. Wada R, Aviv RI, Fox AJ, Sahlas DJ, Gladstone DJ, Tomlinson G, et al. CT angiography "spot sign" predicts hematoma expansion in acute intracerebral hemorrhage. Stroke. 2007;38(4):1257–62.

46. Kato H, Izumiyama M, Izumiyama K, Takahashi A, Itoyama Y. Silent cerebral microbleeds on T2*-weighted MRI: correlation with stroke subtype, stroke recurrence, and leukoaraiosis. Stroke. 2002;33(6):1536–40.

47. Jahngir MU, Qureshi AI. Dejerine Roussy syndrome. Treasure Island, FL: StatPearls; 2019.

48. Steinke W, Sacco RL, Mohr JP, Foulkes MA, Tatemichi TK, Wolf PA, et al. Thalamic stroke. Presentation and prognosis of infarcts and hemorrhages. Arch Neurol. 1992;49(7):703–10.

49. Chung CS, Caplan LR, Han W, Pessin MS, Lee KH, Kim JM. Thalamic haemorrhage. Brain. 1996;119(Pt 6):1873–86.

50. Fisher CM. The pathologic and clinical aspects of thalamic hemorrhage. Trans Am Neurol Assoc. 1959;84:56–9.

51. Tijssen CC. Contralateral conjugate eye deviation in acute supratentorial lesions. Stroke. 1994;25(7):1516–9.

52. Kumral E, Kocaer T, Ertubey NO, Kumral K. Thalamic hemorrhage. A prospective study of 100 patients. Stroke. 1995;26(6):964–70.

53. Durward QJ, Barnett HJ, Barr HW. Presentation and management of mesencephalic hematoma. Report of two cases. J Neurosurg. 1982;56(1):123–7.

54. Lee AG, Brown DG, Diaz PJ. Dorsal midbrain syndrome due to mesencephalic hemorrhage. Case report with serial imaging. J Neuroophthalmol. 1996;16(4):281–5.

55. Bhola R, Olson RJ. Dorsal midbrain syndrome with bilateral superior oblique palsy following brainstem hemorrhage. Arch Ophthalmol. 2006;124(12):1786–8.

56. Morel-Maroger A, Metzger J, Bories J, Gardeur D, Verger JB, Noel MC. Non-lethal brain stem hematomas in hypertensive patients. Rev Neurol (Paris). 1982;138(5):437–45.

57. Mizushima H, Seki T. Midbrain hemorrhage presenting with oculomotor nerve palsy: case report. Surg Neurol. 2002;58(6):417–20.

58. Walker M, Kim H, Samii A. Holmes-like tremor of the lower extremity following brainstem hemorrhage. Mov Disord. 2007;22(2):272–4.

59. Goto N, Kaneko M, Hosaka Y, Koga H. Primary pontine hemorrhage: clinicopathological correlations. Stroke. 1980;11(1):84–90.

60. Wessels T, Moller-Hartmann W, Noth J, Klotzsch C. CT findings and clinical features as markers for patient outcome in primary pontine hemorrhage. AJNR Am J Neuroradiol. 2004;25(2):257–60.

61. Murata Y, Yamaguchi S, Kajikawa H, Yamamura K, Sumioka S, Nakamura S. Relationship between the clinical manifestations, computed tomographic findings and the outcome in 80 patients with primary pontine hemorrhage. J Neurol Sci. 1999;167(2):107–11.

62. Jeong JH, Yoon SJ, Kang SJ, Choi KG, Na DL. Hypertensive pontine microhemorrhage. Stroke. 2002;33(4):925–9.

63. Chung CS, Park CH. Primary pontine hemorrhage: a new CT classification. Neurology. 1992;42(4):830–4.

64. Mastaglia FL, Edis B, Kakulas BA. Medullary haemorrhage: a report of two cases. J Neurol Neurosurg Psychiatry. 1969;32(3):221–5.

65. Barinagarrementeria F, Cantu C. Primary medullary hemorrhage. Report of four cases and review of the literature. Stroke. 1994;25(8):1684–7.

66. Lee SU, Kim HJ, Kang BS, Kim JS. Isolated medullary hemorrhage: clinical features in eleven consecutive patients. J Stroke. 2017;19(1):111–4.

67. Ott KH, Kase CS, Ojemann RG, Mohr JP. Cerebellar hemorrhage: diagnosis and treatment. A review of 56 cases. Arch Neurol. 1974;31(3):160–7.

68. Bosch EP, Kennedy SS, Aschenbrener CA. Ocular bobbing: the myth of its localizing value. Neurology. 1975;25(10):949–53.

69. Fisher CM, Picard EH, Polak A, Dalal P, Pojemann RG. Acute hypertensive cerebellar hemorrhage: diagnosis and surgical treatment. J Nerv Ment Dis. 1965;140:38–57.

70. Brillman J. Acute hydrocephalus and death one month after non-surgical treatment for acute cerebellar hemorrhage. Case report. J Neurosurg. 1979;50(3):374–6.

71. St Louis EK, Wijdicks EF, Li H, Atkinson JD. Predictors of poor outcome in patients with a spontaneous cerebellar hematoma. Can J Neurol Sci. 2000;27(1):32–6.

72. Flugel KA, Fuchs HH, Huk W. Spontaneous intracerebral hematomas: occipital lobe hemorrhages. Fortschr Med. 1982;100(25):1201–9.

73. Anderson CS, Heeley E, Huang Y, Wang J, Stapf C, Delcourt C, et al. Rapid blood-pressure lowering in patients with acute intracerebral hemorrhage. N Engl J Med. 2013;368(25):2355–65.

74. Qureshi AI, Palesch YY, Barsan WG, Hanley DF, Hsu CY, Martin RL, et al. Intensive blood-pressure lowering in patients with acute cerebral hemorrhage. N Engl J Med. 2016;375(11):1033–43.

75. Hemphill JC 3rd, Greenberg SM, Anderson CS, Becker K, Bendok BR, Cushman M, et al. Guidelines for the management of spontaneous intracerebral hemorrhage: a guideline for healthcare professionals from the American Heart Association/American Stroke Association. Stroke. 2015;46(7):2032–60.

76. Neal M, Crowther M, Douketis J, Verhovsek M, Stidley C, Garcia D. Reversal of vitamin K antagonist-associated coagulopathy: a survey of current practice. Thromb Res. 2008;122(6):864–6.

77. Zhou W, Schwarting S, Illanes S, Liesz A, Middelhoff M, Zorn M, et al. Hemostatic therapy in experimental intracerebral hemorrhage associated with the direct thrombin inhibitor dabigatran. Stroke. 2011;42(12):3594–9.

78. Zhou W, Zorn M, Nawroth P, Butehorn U, Perzborn E, Heitmeier S, et al. Hemostatic therapy in experimental intracerebral hemorrhage associated with rivaroxaban. Stroke. 2013;44(3):771–8.

79. Grottke O, Aisenberg J, Bernstein R, Goldstein P, Huisman MV, Jamieson DG, et al. Efficacy of prothrombin complex concentrates for the emergency reversal of dabigatran-induced anticoagulation. Crit Care. 2016;20(1):115.

80. Steffel J, Verhamme P, Potpara TS, Albaladejo P, Antz M, Desteghe L, et al. The 2018 European Heart Rhythm Association practical guide on the use of non-vitamin K antagonist oral anticoagulants in patients with atrial fibrillation. Eur Heart J. 2018;39(16):1330–93.

81. Eke O, Shanechi M, Gottlieb M. Efficacy of platelet transfusion for acute intracerebral hemorrhage among patients on antiplatelet therapy. CJEM. 2018;20(S2):S78–81.

82. Diringer MN. Intracerebral hemorrhage: pathophysiology and management. Crit Care Med. 1993;21(10):1591–603.

83. Mendelow AD, Gregson BA, Fernandes HM, Murray GD, Teasdale GM, Hope DT, et al. Early surgery versus initial conservative treatment in patients with spontaneous supratentorial intracerebral haematomas in the International Surgical Trial in Intracerebral Haemorrhage (STICH): a randomised trial. Lancet. 2005;365(9457):387–97.

84. Mendelow AD, Gregson BA, Rowan EN, Murray GD, Gholkar A, Mitchell PM, et al. Early surgery versus initial conservative treatment in patients with spontaneous supratentorial lobar intracerebral haematomas (STICH II): a randomised trial. Lancet. 2013;382(9890):397–408.

85. Lee SH, Park KJ, Kang SH, Jung YG, Park JY, Park DH. Prognostic factors of clinical outcomes in patients with spontaneous thalamic hemorrhage. Med Sci Monit. 2015;21:2638–46.

86. Jang JH, Song YG, Kim YZ. Predictors of 30-day mortality and 90-day functional recovery after primary pontine hemorrhage. J Korean Med Sci. 2011;26(1):100–7.

Imaging Diagnosis

9

Yunsun Song and Seung Chai Jung

Introduction

Although imaging methods for the evaluation of posterior circulation stroke are similar to those in anterior circulation stroke, there are substantial differences in the choice of imaging modality and interpretation of radiological features. Computed tomography (CT), magnetic resonance imaging (MRI), catheter digital subtraction angiography (DSA), and ultrasound (USG) including Doppler are commonly used to evaluate posterior circulation stroke. However, midbrain, pons, medulla, and cerebellum, which take up the majority of posterior circulation, are surrounded by air- and bone-filled structures. Although brain parenchyma in the posterior fossa has smaller volume, more area is closely abutted on air, bones, or fluid collection when compared with anterior circulation. Therefore, CT has more demerits than MRI for brain parenchyma. Time-of-flight MR angiography (TOF-MRA) is more vulnerable in susceptibility artifact (more in posterior fossa) than CT angiography (CTA). However, loss of angiographic information during postprocessing can occur on CTA because intracranial vertebrobasilar artery runs along the skull base. Therefore, the interpretation of steno-occlusion should be cautioned. Vessel wall MRI, which provides direct vessel wall information beyond luminal imaging such as CTA, MRA, and DSA, has merits to delineate vessels in posterior fossa because intracranial vertebrobasilar artery is located away from the brain parenchyma and has relatively larger diameters to anterior circulation. DSA has limited roles in the screening and diagnosis because of the radiation exposure and invasive procedure-related complications. However, DSA is still a gold standard and offers superb resolution and additional hemodynamic information relative to CTA and MRA in both anterior and posterior circulation evaluation. Ultrasound including Doppler has advantage of bed-side imaging modality to offer flow information but can show disadvantage of limited view relative to carotid arteries. This chapter will describe general characteristics and radiological peculiarity of each imaging modality in posterior circulation stroke to anterior circulation stroke.

Brain Imaging

CT

Modern multirow detector CT can generate reconstructed two-dimensional (2D) images in diverse imaging planes from the volume data by continuous spiral acquisition with short scanning time. However, the sequential axial acquisition for noncontrast CT is still used for the brain imaging widely because the sequential acquisition

Y. Song · S. C. Jung (✉)
Department of Radiology and Research Institute of Radiology, Asan Medical Center, University of Ulsan College of Medicine, Seoul, South Korea

may provide better image quality when compared with the spiral acquisition [1, 2].

CT has advantage of being more widely available and accessible and disadvantage of radiation exposure when compared with MRI [3, 4]. Although the technology in MRI is advanced, CT still remains the excellent screening imaging modality to detect and diagnose acute hemorrhage, including epidural, subdural, subarachnoid, and intraventricular hemorrhage even in posterior fossa, and to show pressure effects on basal cisterns and hydrocephalus well [5, 6]. Increased intracellular water or cytotoxic edema occurs in brain parenchyma in acute ischemic stroke, leading to decreased attenuation, loss of gray-white matter differentiation, swelling, and mass effect on CT [7]. CT has lower sensitivity to detect or depict acute ischemic stroke when compared to MRI. The overall sensitivity is 12% in the first 3 h and 57–71% in the first 24 h and worse in posterior fossa and deep infarcts [8].

Although CT is the conventional imaging modality to detect and diagnose cerebral ischemic or hemorrhagic stroke in wide use for about 20 years, it has not been as helpful in evaluating patients with posterior circulation ischemia relative to those of anterior circulation ischemia. Brain parenchyma, including midbrain, pons, cerebellums, and medulla in the posterior fossa, has smaller volume but is mostly surrounded by air, bones, or fluid collection relative to the supratentorial area, which make it vulnerable to artifacts and degrade image quality [5, 9] (Fig. 9.1).

The Alberta Stroke Program Early CT Score (ASPECTS) offers a useful assessment of early acute ischemic changes in the MCA territory [10, 11] while those in posterior circulation are not well-established on noncontrast CT but may be useful on CTA source images [12]. Puetz et al. introduced posterior circulation Acute Stroke Prognosis Early CT score (pc-ASPECTS) on CTA source images or noncontrast CT for basilar artery occlusion and allocated scores according to posterior circulation regions as follows: 2 for pontine or midbrain and 1 each for left and right thalamus, left and right cerebellum, and left and right posterior cerebral artery territory [12] (Fig. 9.2). A score of 10 is normal, and the score

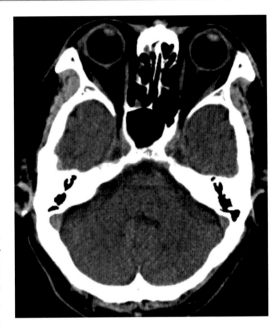

Fig. 9.1 CT shows a streak across pons due to beam hardening artifact. CT is vulnerable to a bone related artifact, which degrades image quality

is calculated by subtracting the sum of each early ischemic region showing hypo-attenuation from 10. The same ASPECTS scoring system is applied to DWI [5].

Among posterior circulation, temporo-occipital lobes, which belong to posterior cerebral artery territories, are comparable in the imaging information to other anterior circulation territories [5]. Noncontrast CT can show the presence of dolichoectatic aneurysmal change and the hyperdense basilar artery sign representing a thrombus or occlusion [5, 13] with a sensitivity of 71%, a specificity of 98%, a positive predictive value of 83%, and a negative predictive value of 95% [13].

Magnetic Resonance Imaging

MRI can be a more useful imaging modality in vertebrobasilar ischemia when compared with CT because of superior detection or diagnosis of acute ischemic stroke and robustness to bone- or air-related artifact in posterior fossa [9]. However, the disadvantage in the scan time, availability,

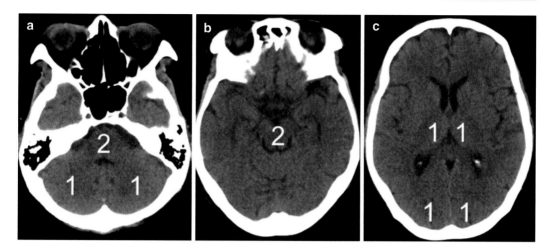

Fig. 9.2 The posterior circulation Acute Stroke Prognosis Early CT score (pc-ASPECTS). The score is calculated by subtracting the sum of each early ischemic region showing hypo-attenuation from 10. The assigned scores depend on the posterior circulation regions as follows: 2 for pon-tine or midbrain and 1 each for left and right thalamus, left and right cerebellum, and left and right posterior cerebral artery territory on noncontrast CT or CTA source images (**a–c**). Therefore, 10-point is normal and 0-point means early ischemic changes in the entire above regions

and contraindications due to MR compatibility limit the application of MRI to acute ischemic stroke [3, 9, 14]. Fast MR protocols for hyperacute to acute ischemic stroke patients have been recently introduced [15–17]. In addition, a study showed the feasibility of MRI as routine screening imaging modality under the quality improvement processes with Screening with MRI for Accurate and Rapid Stroke Treatment (SMART) [18], and another study showed hyperacute MRI protocol can reduce the number of endovascular stroke interventions by 50% avoiding futile treatment [19]. Therefore, MRI may be considered to be one of the important imaging modalities for acute ischemic stroke patients, especially posterior circulation stroke. However, New England Medical Center Posterior Circulation Registry (NEMC-PCR) revealed a discrepancy between clinical and MRI abnormalities that occurred in one-third of patients. Clinical findings were more extensive than expected from the imaging in 20% among patients with posterior circulation infarcts, and imaging abnormalities were presented without relation to clinical symptoms or signs in 12.5% patients [5]. Therefore, imaging is necessary to combine with adequate history taking, and thorough neurologic examination and follow-up imaging should be occasionally consid-ered even in the case of negative on initial imaging.

MRI protocols for acute ischemic stroke generally consist of diffusion-weighted imaging (DWI), perfusion-weighted imaging (PWI), T2-weighted imaging (T2W) or fluid-attenuated inversion recovery imaging (FLAIR), T2*-weighted gradient-echo imaging (GRE) or susceptibility-weighted imaging (SWI), and MR angiography (MRA) [5, 14].

DWI

DWI is the most powerful imaging method to detect and delineate hyperacute to acute infarct even in small size. DWI plays a role as the gold standard in the imaging diagnosis of acute infarct with a sensitivity of 73–92% within the first 3 h and a sensitivity of approximately 100% within the first 6 h after the symptom onset [4]. DWI can present early ischemic change at 30 min after the symptom onset, whereas FLAIR tends to present early ischemic hyperintensity by 6 h after the symptom onset [20].

Ischemia beyond benign oligemia results in a net transfer of water from extracellular to intracellular compartment, reduced extracellular space volume, and increased intracellular viscosity where water mobility is decreased [21]. DWI can present the degree of free diffusion of water molecules, indicating apparent diffusion coefficient [22, 23]. Apparent diffusion coefficient values gradually recover to normal within 5–10 days and then rise up in the chronic stage while DWI high signal intensity lasts due to T2 shine-through [23]. DWI lesion can reverse spontaneously or following recanalization in one-third of patients after endovascular treatment or a half after intravenous thrombolysis [24] even though the reversal does not imply the normalization of brain tissue [25].

DWI plays an even more important role in detecting a posterior circulation infarct rather than those in anterior circulation because CT has a limited value in posterior fossa [9, 26, 27] (Fig. 9.3). DWI became an essential investigation in patients with dizziness or vertigo, particularly

[26]. However, DWI can be occasionally negative for small infarct lesions in patients with clinically definite posterior circulation infarcts, especially brain stem lesions [28]. Oppenheim et al. showed that false-negative on DWI was 5.8% among patients who last stroke symptoms more than 24 h and underwent DWI within 48 h after stroke onset (n = 139) [29]. False-negative DWI occurred more common in posterior circulation than in anterior circulation stroke (19 vs 2%) [29]. Of the 6 false-negative vertebrobasilar stroke lesions, five lesions were located in brain stem. Among patients with vertebrobasilar stroke, 31% showed a false-negative on DWI during the first 24 h, who showed positive results on follow-up imaging [29]. Chalela et al. prospectively compared CT and MRI for assessment of patients with suspected acute stroke (n = 356) [30]. DWI showed a higher false-negative rate in brain stem (adjusted odds ratio, 7.3; 95% confidence

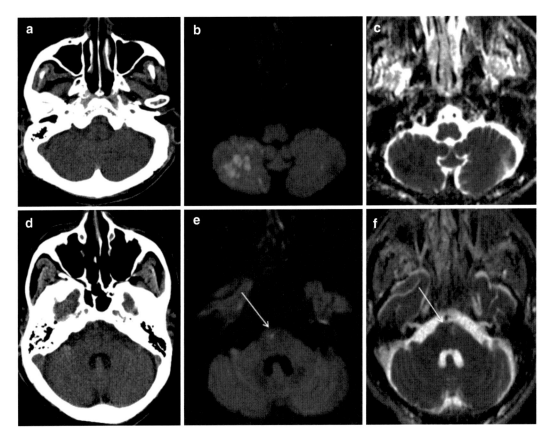

Fig. 9.3 CT has a limited value to detect and delineate acute infarcts in posterior fossa relative to DWI

interval, 2.2 to 25.0) [30]. Initial DWI showed a false-negative of 12% among patients with acute vestibular syndrome and who underwent imaging within 48 h after symptom onset [31]. Therefore, high suspicion based on adequate history taking and thorough neurologic examination and awareness in the limitation of imaging may not miss the precise diagnosis [9]. In addition, follow-up imaging should be considered when the patient is clinically suspected as posterior circulation stroke in spite of negative results on initial imaging (Fig. 9.4).

DWI lesion volume did not correlate with the NIHSS score and was no predictor of outcome [32, 33] while a study postulated that the ASPECT score in posterior circulation using DWI is a powerful marker for predicting the functional outcome [34]. Therefore, further investigation is necessary.

FLAIR and GRE

FLAIR can present hyperintense vessel signs representing slow flows including leptomeningeal collaterals [35], acute ischemic hyperintensity that may represent established infarct [36], and chronic ischemic lesions including old infarcts. FLAIR is not sensitive to detect ischemic lesions within the first few hours relative to

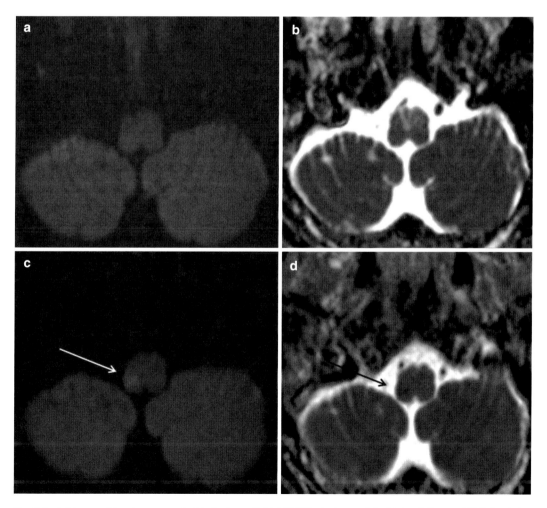

Fig. 9.4 A 74-year-old male presented with dizziness. Initial DWI looked normal (**a**, **b**), but follow-up DWI after 1 day showed acute infarct in right lateral medulla (**c**, **d**)

DWI. Cytotoxic edema can be detected within minutes on DWI, but vasogenic edema, which is detected on FLAIR well, is induced slowly. Therefore, the mismatch between DWI and FLAIR may be used to estimate infarct age [20, 36, 37].

Hemorrhage in MRI depends on the age of the blood and sequences [36]. GRE detects hemorrhagic lesions based on the paramagnetic effect due to deoxyhemoglobin or hemosiderin [36]. GRE can delineate hemorrhagic transformation better than noncontrast CT [38] and intraluminal thrombus. SWI shows better hemorrhagic detection than conventional GRE [39]. The detection depends on the imaging sequences and strength of magnetic fields. Therefore, the direct comparison between CT and MR or GRE and SWI or GRE in 1.5- and 3-tesla machine should be done with caution.

Vascular Imaging

CTA

CTA has become a majority among imaging modalities for the evaluation of a steno-occlusion. Recent randomized control studies demonstrated that the appropriate patients' selection and rapid revascularization become the most fundamental and definite contributors for a good prognosis for patients with ischemic stroke [40–45]. CTA can provide sufficient information for the steno-occlusion, and those with multiphase acquisitions give us the collateral and/or perfusion information [46, 47]. The rapid acquisition and excellent accessibility of CTA can lead to the early decision for the intra-arterial thrombectomy or aspiration and can make it rapid revascularization.

CTA generates images with the first intra-arterial pass of iodinated contrast agents and can present postprocessed images based on various techniques. Multiplanar reformation (MPR), maximum intensity projection (MIP), and volume rending were representative techniques for the evaluation of steno-occlusion. MPR can display various 2D imaging planes without loss of information [48] (Fig. 9.5a, b). MIP selects contrast tissues with the highest attenuation, including enhanced vessels, bone, and calcification, and then they are incorporated into 2D images [49]. However, other high attenuation structures such as a dense calcification or stent are able to obscure the assessment of steno-occlusion, and three-dimensional (3D) relationships between vessels and other structures are not visualized [49] (Fig. 9.5c). Volume rending is the principal technique used for all clinical applications including steno-occlusion or aneurysm [49], which can provide a good 3D impression but may lose detailed vascular information during postprocessing (Fig. 9.5d). The postprocessed images cannot be enough in accurate measurements and make a loss of detailed anatomic structures. Therefore, the evaluation combined with source images may be warranted in the quantitative measurement or detailed imaging interpretation.

Iodinated contrast media can induce contrast-induced nephropathy in patients with decreased renal function. However, the 2018 AHA/ASA guideline for the early management of patients with acute ischemic stroke describes that it is reasonable to perform CTA in patients with suspected intracranial large vessel occlusion before testing a serum creatinine concentration [50]. The recommendation is based on the observation that the risk of contrast-induced nephropathy is relatively low secondary to CTA, especially in patients without a history of renal impairment [50].

CTA provides the anatomical information for steno-occlusion primarily, which is similar to contrast-enhanced MRA (CE-MRA), while TOF-MRA offers the flow information primarily. Therefore, CTA and CE-MRA have theoretical advantages over TOF-MRA when blood flow is changed in steno-occlusion or turbulent flow in a tortuous arterial course or abruptly dilated arterial segment [5].

Good collateral flow is a well-known marker to correlate with better prognosis in acute ischemic stroke. Multiphase CTA, recently introduced, gives us information on collateral flows in the whole brain as well as steno-occlusion in

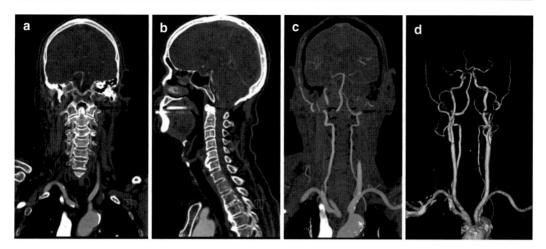

Fig. 9.5 Three postprocessing techniques in CTA. Coronal MPR (**a**) and sagittal MPR (**b**), coronal MIP (**c**), and volume rendering (**d**)

the intracranial and neck arteries in a time-resolved manner and quick acquisition [47], which may have similar ability to predict tissue fate in acute ischemic stroke compared with CT perfusion [46].

Both CTA and CE-MRA are useful imaging methods to evaluate steno-occlusion from extracranial arteries to intracranial arteries, including the vertebrobasilar artery system [9, 28, 51, 52]. In general, CTA, TOF-MRA, and CE-MRA show similar accuracy with high sensitivity and specificity for the evaluation of intracranial arterial steno-occlusion [53–57]. However, there may be some differences depending on vascular locations or disease. Ultrasound is mostly used as a screening method at bed-side level with inferior diagnostic performance to CTA and MRA in the vertebrobasilar artery system [9, 58–60]. The specific comparisons among vascular imaging modalities will be described in MRA.

CTA can provide detailed clot information such as location, length, burden, and permeability of the thrombus [61]. More proximal arterial occlusion, longer length, higher burden, and lower permeability in the thrombus can result in a lower recanalization rate [61]. Residual flow or permeability within the thrombus indicates increased attenuation. The clot with higher permeability is more likely to be recanalized [62].

MRA

Magnetic resonance angiography (MRA), including contrast-enhanced MRA (CE-MRA) and time-of-flight MRA (TOF-MRA), is widely used for assessing intracranial and cervical steno-occlusion or aneurysm since the 1980s [63]. TOF-MRA is the most useful screening imaging modality to evaluate intracranial vessels and can cover neck vessels. TOF-MRA adopts a flow-related enhancement phenomenon to generate the images without an exogenous contrast agent at saturated background tissue [64]. However, TOF-MRA is susceptible to artifacts associated with various flow phenomena and spatial anatomic distortion, and thus it is likely to overestimate steno-occlusion [64, 65] (Fig. 9.6). Recent TOF-MRA is 3D imaging and adopts multiple overlapping thin slab acquisition and tilted optimized nonsaturation excitation to overcome slow flow-related saturation artifact [64]. The saturation artifact occurs with repeated excitation radiofrequency (RF) pulses and leads to signal loss. The signal loss can cause artefactual steno-occlusion and can overestimate the degree of stenosis [53, 66]. CE-MRA commonly covers from the intracranial to the neck vessels with short scanning time. CE-MRA often provides a poor spatial resolution of intracranial vessels owing to the large coverage and has narrow time window for

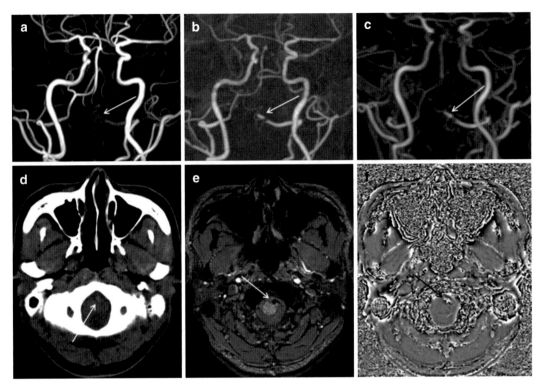

Fig. 9.6 A 43-year-old female was diagnosed as left vertebral artery dissection. TOF-MRA poorly delineated focal aneurysmal dilatation just distal to focal severe stenosis in left vertebral artery with weak antegrade flow (**a**) while CTA (**b**) and CE-MRA (**c**) depicted those well. Noncontrast CT (**d**) showed slightly increased attenuation in left vertebral artery, whereas SWI (**e**) with phase information (**f**) presented intramural hematoma in vertebral artery dissection well

appropriate arterial phase enhancement relative to TOF-MRA but is less likely to overestimate the degree and extent in the stenosis [4, 67] and can make small vessels more visible [68] in neck vessels.

Khan et al. systematically reviewed vertebral artery stenosis in 11 studies [59]. CTA showed the highest sensitivity (100%) and specificity (95.2%) for detecting ≥50% stenosis followed by CE-MRA (sensitivity, 93.9%; specificity, 94.8%), TOF-MRA (sensitivity, 71.4%; specificity, 95.1%), and ultrasound (sensitivity, 70.2%; specificity, 97.7%) [59]. Another study prospectively compared CE-MRA, CTA, and ultrasound in the evaluation of vertebral artery stenosis using DSA as a reference standard (n = 46) [60]. CE-MRA showed the highest sensitivity of 83–89% followed by CTA (58–68%) and ultrasound (44%), while CE-MRA presented the lowest specificity of 87–91% followed by CTA (92–93%) and ultrasound (95%)

for detecting ≥50% stenosis in whole vertebral artery. For detecting ≥50% stenosis in vertebral artery origin, CE-MRA showed the highest sensitivity of 82–91%, followed by CTA (82%) and ultrasound (67%), but CE-MRA presented the lowest specificity of 89–92%, followed by CTA (93%) and ultrasound (98%) [60]. However, Jumaa et al. postulated that CTA had higher sensitivity (61.9%) and lower specificity (77.8%) rather than MRA (sensitivity, 55%; specificity, 85.7%) in spite of the lack of statistical significance [69]. CE-MRA is superior to TOF-MRA for detecting and evaluating steno-occlusion or aneurysm in vertebral arteries [28]. However, CE-MRA has a limitation in the evaluation of vertebral artery origin steno-occlusion because of artifacts related with aortic pulsation and breathing [27]. CTA may provide better delineation of vertebral artery origin rather than MRA. Both MRA and CTA can detect vertebral artery dissection well, but MRA can present low specificity relative to CTA [9, 70]. CTA may delineate more wall information in the dissection relative to MRA [71].

Both MRA and CTA are sufficient to depict intracranial posterior circulation, including the vertebrobasilar system and posterior cerebral artery well [28]. The SONIA study ($n = 407$) showed that the positive predictive value and negative predictive value in TOF-MRA were 59% and 91%, respectively, for detecting ≥50% stenosis in pooled intracranial artery while vertebral artery showed a positive predictive value of 61% and negative predictive value of 88% and basilar artery showed a positive predictive value of 60% and negative predictive value of 89% [72]. Another study showed that TOF-MRA had a sensitivity of 78–85%, a specificity of 95%, a positive predictive value of 75–79%, and a negative predictive value of 95–97% for detecting ≥50% stenosis in pooled intracranial artery using DSA as the reference standard. In the study, discordant proportions between TOF-MRA and DSA were 8.1% in internal carotid artery, 7.4% in middle cerebral artery, and 4.1% in vertebrobasilar artery, respectively [73]. Although TOF-MRA can be dependable in the exclusion of intracranial arterial steno-occlusion based on the high negative predictive value, it may not be enough to measure intracranial artery stenosis accurately because of the low positive predictive value. TOF-MRA can overestimate stenosis due to the disadvantage of flow-related artifact. However, the flow-related artifact can provide hemodynamic information, which is not offered by CE-MRA or CTA. In addition, TOF-MRA is robust to evaluate stenosis due to calcified plaques such as cavernous internal carotid artery or intracranial vertebral artery, in which CTA can overestimate the stenosis [65] (Fig. 9.7).

Vessel Wall MRI

Vessel wall MRI provides direct wall information beyond indirect luminal imaging such as CTA, MRA, and DSA. Vessel wall MRI has been widely used for further investigation following luminal imaging and clinically established one of imaging modality for the evaluation of steno-occlusion.

Vessel wall MRI needs sufficient resolution, perpendicular imaging planes to the arterial long axis, and an appropriate imaging contrast [21, 74, 75]. Vessel wall MRI has to provide a resolution of less than 0.7 mm^3 to present vessel wall information even in intracranial arteries having small diameters as well as extracranial arteries [76–78]. In particular, vertebrobasilar arteries have the advantage of using vessel wall MRI because those have larger diameter and are surrounded by CSF space when compared with anterior circulation. Vessel wall MRI can play an appropriate role in 3-tesla machines [64, 74]. The perpendicular imaging planes to the arterial long axis can make vessel walls characterize most accurately, in particular eccentricity or wall thickness. Furthermore, the imaging planes are useful to distinguish true lesions from pseudo-lesions such as normal meninges or veins, which surround vessel walls closely [79]. Therefore, the imaging planes perpendicular to the arterial course have to be able to obtain during the scanning or after postprocessing along with other orthogonal imaging planes. Accordingly, 3D acquisition of vessel wall MRI has been preferred. The appropriate multicontrast imaging includes precontrast and postcontrast T1-weighted imaging with sufficient black-blood and black-CSF state. According to the purpose or circumstances of the study, T2-weighted imaging, proton-density imaging, and susceptibility-weighted imaging can be added in the vessel wall sequences.

The useful vessel wall MRI sequences are as follows: precontrast and postcontrast T1-weighted imaging, T2-weighted imaging, proton-density imaging, and susceptibility-weighted imaging. Precontrast T1-weighted imaging plays a crucial role in the evaluation of vessel walls to provide basic morphology and signal intensity. Postcontrast T1-weighted imaging can present the most remarkable finding. The vessel wall enhancement is considered to be an indicator of disease activity. Postcontrast T1-weighted imaging is acquired with injection of a contrast agent based on gadolinium [64]. Proton-density imaging offers vessel information having the highest signal-to-noise ratio, which makes it useful to demarcate outer arterial walls, in particular intracranial vessels [80]. T2-weighted imaging

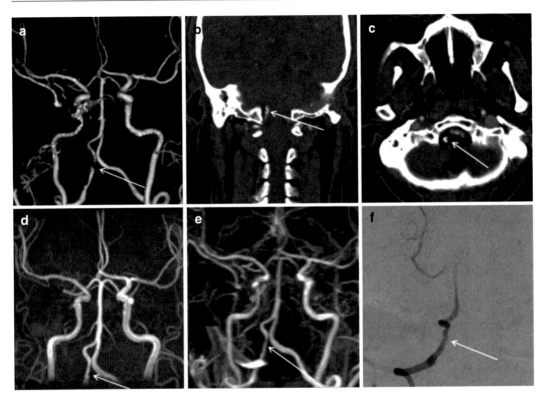

Fig. 9.7 CTA shows focal severe stenosis in right vertebral artery on volume rendering images (**a**) with dense calcified plaque on CTA source images (**b**, **c**). TOF-MRA presents basic morphology and signal intensity in vessel walls.

(**d**), CE-MRA (**e**), and DSA (**f**) present only focal mild stenosis. CTA can have a demerit in the evaluation of the degree of steno-occlusion with dense calcified plaques

presents basic morphology and signal intensity in vessel walls.

Susceptibility-weighted imaging gives us helpful information in terms of hemorrhage or calcification in vessel walls. Susceptibility-weighted imaging is 3D high-resolution gradient-echo sequence with phase information and flow compensated state, which can provide higher performance in the detection of hemorrhage or calcification than conventional T2* gradient-echo imaging [81]. Therefore, it can detect intramural hematoma, intraplaque hemorrhage, or calcified plaque even in small anatomic regions like vessel walls [81, 82].

Black-blood techniques commonly include methods to suppress luminal blood black and surrounding CSF black to improve the contrast of vessel walls [74, 75]. Their sequences are based on the suppression of moving protons like blood or CSF. Representative and widely used black-blood techniques are double inversion recovery, motion-sensitized driven equilibrium (MSDE), or improved motion-sensitized driven equilibrium (iMSDE) and delay alternating with nutation for tailored excitation (DANTE). Double inversion recovery is less likely to be used in the recent vessel wall MRI because 2D imaging commonly adopts the techniques [75]. MSDE or iMSDE suppresses the signal from moving spins using preparation radiofrequency pulses, which are made up of flip angles of 90° and 180°. It has merits to reduce preparation time and cover a larger extent when compared with double inversion recovery. Although it can reduce the signal and provide insufficient black-blood and black-CSF state and field inhomogeneity [74, 75, 83], it is widely used with technological improvement. DANTE is also a widely used black-blood technique, which adopts a chain of nonselective pulses with low flip angles, which is interleaved with gradient pulses with short repetition times.

The pulse induces the attenuation of flowing tissue signals, but DANTE is known to be less than MSDE in the attenuation of static tissue signal [84].

Simultaneous acquisition of intracranial and neck vessel walls is useful to evaluate overall atherosclerotic plaques or the extent of craniocervical dissection, which become clinically available with large coverage and short scan time in recent MR machines [85].

Atherosclerosis

Vessel wall MRI can give us useful information to estimate the stroke mechanism as well as the etiology of the steno-occlusion in posterior circulation stroke and is helpful to differentiate the vascular disease such as dissection, moyamoya disease, and vasculitis, which can be confused with atherosclerosis. In addition, vessel wall MRI is able to demonstrate atherosclerotic plaques even in nonstenotic lesion on luminal imaging [86, 87] (Fig. 9.8).

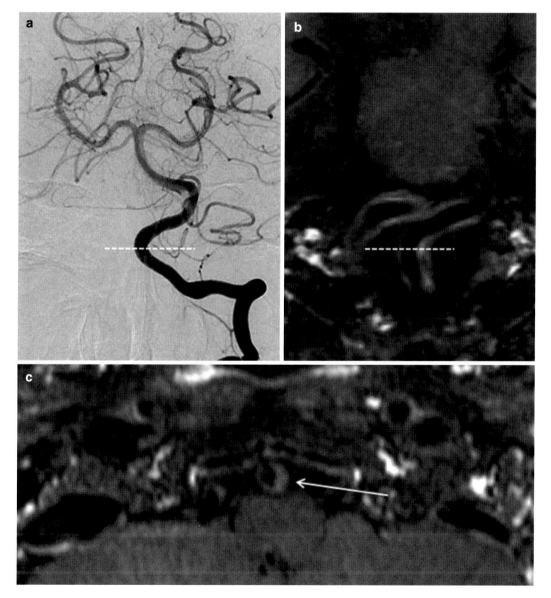

Fig. 9.8 DSA looks normal in left vertebral artery (**a**) while vessel wall MRI shows eccentric wall thickening with contrast enhancement on coronal and axial postcontrast T1-weighted imaging (**b**, **c**). Vessel wall MRI provides the direct wall information beyond the luminography

Atherosclerotic plaques consist of lipid core, fibrous tissue, intraplaque hemorrhage, and calcium [88]. Vessel wall MRI can provide each component in the plaques intracranial arteries as well as extracranial carotid arteries. The plaque analysis gives us useful information to differentiate vulnerable plaques from stable plaques using vessel wall MRI [88, 89].

Typical morphology of the atherosclerotic plaque is asymmetric wall thickening, so-called eccentricity, whereas vasculitis shows smooth concentric wall thickening [90] (Fig. 9.9). However, concentric wall thickening is also reported in atherosclerotic plaques [91]. The remodeling index, which is described in coronary artery atherosclerosis, is also useful information

to characterize and differentiate intracranial and cervical atherosclerotic plaques [92]. The remodeling index is calculated as follows: maximum outer wall area/ ([proximal normal arterial area + distal normal arterial area]/2). Positive remodeling is defined as the index ≥ 1.0, while negative remodeling is as < 1.0 [92]. Positive remodeling is more likely to be seen in symptomatic and/or vulnerable plaques [86, 93–95].

Plaques vulnerability is known to associate with intraplaque hemorrhage, large lipid-rich necrotic core with fissuring or rupture of the fibrotic cap, and plaque enhancement on vessel wall MRI [88, 96, 97]. Intraplaque hemorrhage is commonly seen as hyperintensity on T1-weighted imaging. It is considered that the rupture of neovessels or plaque

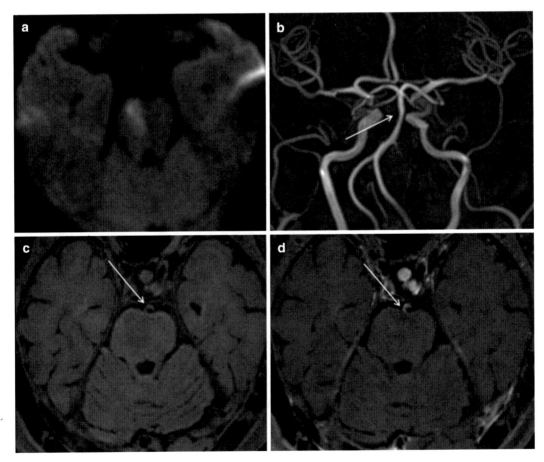

Fig. 9.9 A 73-year-old female presented with left side weakness. Acute infarct in right pons was seen on DWI (**a**). TOF-MRA showed focal mild stenosis in upper to mid basilar artery (**b**). Vessel wall MRI showed eccentric wall thickening with contrast enhancement, indicating atherosclerotic plaque, in right lateral wall of basilar artery on axial precontrast T1-weighted imaging (**c**) and postcontrast T1-weighted imaging (**d**)

rupture causes intraplaque hemorrhage [97]. Intraplaque hemorrhage can present various signal intensity depending on techniques used for T1-weighted imaging [98] and the stage of hemorrhage [99]. Intramural hematoma in dissection can also present similar signal intensity [100]. Therefore, intraplaque hemorrhage is necessary to be interpreted cautiously, and T2-weighted or susceptibility-weighted imaging can be helpful. The fibrotic cap is a layer of fibrotic connective tissue containing macrophages and smooth muscle cells within a collagen–proteoglycan matrix and separates lipid-rich necrotic core from the arterial lumen. Larger lipid-rich necrotic core and thinner or disrupted fibrotic cap were found to be associated with a risk of cerebrovascular event. The intact thick fibrotic cap may represent low risk of plaque rupture [97]. Lipid core is shown hypo- to isointensity on T1- and T2-weighted imaging without contrast enhancement. The signal intensity is different to subcutaneous fat showing hyperintensitiy on T1- and T2-weighted imaging because the main contributor to MR signal is not lipid but water protons and the main component is not triglycerides (mainly in extravascular lipid) but cholesterol and cholesteryl esters in lipid core [88, 96]. The fibrous cap is shown as iso- to hyperintensity on T1- and T2-weighted imaging with contrast enhancement. Therefore, hyperintensity with enhancement and hypointensity without enhancement in the vessel walls can be seen from lumen to wall, representing fibrous cap and lipid core, respectively [96, 101]. Calcification is shown as a dark signal across all sequences [102].

Plaque enhancement is the most remarkable finding among vessel wall MRI features. Plaque enhancement is more likely to be seen in recent and/or symptomatic ischemic stroke and may indicate severe inflammatory activity [103–105]. The degree of enhancement in symptomatic plaques is known to decrease over time [104]. Plaque enhancement is shown to be associated with neovascularity, inflammatory activity, and/or enhanced endothelial permeability [106, 107]. However, it is not specific for atherosclerotic plaques since nonspecific inflammatory conditions such as vasculitis can present vessel wall enhancement [74].

Vessel wall MRI is helpful in disclosing stroke mechanism by delineating detailed plaque morphology, composition, and distribution. In a study, they showed that high-resolution 3D proton-density imaging with 0.2 mm^3 can identify relevant culprit perforating arteries in lateral pontine infarct [108].

Dissection

Dissection is one of the major vascular pathologies in young patients with cerebral ischemic stroke [109]. Therefore, dissection is a reasonable differential diagnosis for the steno-occlusion without a definite clue on luminal imaging in ischemic stroke patients with minimal vascular risk factors. Vessel wall MRI is quite helpful in depicting the dissecting pathology directly. The direct radiological features include intimal flap, double lumen, intramural hematoma, aneurysmal dilatation, and subsequent geometric change, which is delineated by vessel wall MRI [110, 111]. Additionally, dissection can show wall enhancement. The wall enhancement is considered to be associated with inflammation [112], sluggish blood flow via false lumens, or vasa vasorum enhancement [113] even though the pathology is not completely understood. A study using positron emission tomography (PET)-CT demonstrated pathological uptake at the corresponding site of vessel wall enhancement in the dissection, and the enhancement was disappeared within weeks, which was thought to be a generalized transient inflammatory arteriopathy [112].

Dissection shows a subsequent geometric change from the occurrence to various chronic stages [114–117]. Dissection begins with intimal tear, and blood flow penetrates into arterial walls, which is seen as intimal flap and double lumen. Thrombus in the vessel walls is seen as intramural hematoma, which can make aneurysmal dilatation like positive remodeling in atherosclerotic plaques. The radiological features in acute to subacute stage change over time [110, 111, 117]. Vessel wall can show various chronic stages, including occlusion, dissecting aneurysm, incomplete normalization, and complete normalization [118].

Intramural hematoma can present similar signal intensity to intraplaque hemorrhage on vessel wall MRI [100]. The differentiation between intramural hematoma and intraplaque hemorrhage is sometimes difficult, which leads to confusion between atherosclerosis and dissection. Therefore, the precise diagnosis may rely on clinical features and brain parenchymal and vascular imaging beyond target vessels, and subsequent geometric change. Dissection shows more clear and rapid subsequent geometric change, including spontaneous normalization relative to atherosclerotic plaques [114]. In unruptured intracranial artery dissections, the subsequent change in geometry was shown from 2 weeks to 2 months in 83.9%, and among which, improvement and complete normalization were shown in 61.5% and 18.3%, respectively [114]. Spontaneous improvement was seen in 37.4–75% of patients with unruptured intracranial vertebral artery dissection [119, 120]. The improvement rate is more likely to be higher in dissection rather than intracranial atherosclerosis (<30%) [121, 122] (Fig. 9.10).

Catheter Digital Subtraction Angiography

Catheter digital subtraction angiography (DSA) plays an important role as the gold standard in vascular imaging, even though it is the oldest technique since 1927 [123]. DSA is widely used and is an advanced technique both in subtraction and magnification as Seldinger introduces the percutaneous catheterization in 1953 [124]. Modern DSA provides excellent spatial (less than 0.2 mm^2) and contrast resolution. DSA is the most invasive method among vascular imaging, and available only at highly specialized centers [125, 126]. DSA carries the risk of procedural complications and exposure to the radiation and contrast agent. A large population retrospective research (n = 19,826) reported that neurological decline, permanent disability, and death rate were 2.63%, 0.14%, and 0.06% in diagnostic DSA, respectively [127]. In a meta-analysis study, permanent and transient neurologic complication was higher in a group with transient ischemic attack (TIA) and stroke (0.7% and 3.0%) compared to a group with subarachnoid hemorrhage,

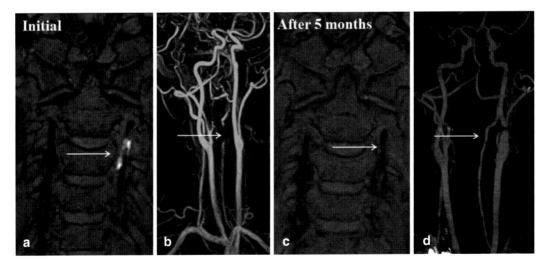

Fig. 9.10 A 25-year-old female was diagnosed as a dissection in left cervical vertebral artery. Vessel wall MRI showed an intramural hematoma and aneurysmal dilatation indicating dissection in the left cervical vertebral artery on coronal precontrast T1-weighted imaging (**a**), but CE-MRA showed severe stenosis in the corresponding location (**b**). After 5 months, vessel wall MRI (**c**) and CTA (**d**) looked normal, indicating complete normalization

cerebral aneurysm, and arteriovenous malforma-tion (0.07% and 0.8%) when they experience DSA [126]. Therefore, modern DSA is mainly used when more detailed information is neces-sary to guide therapies or about small vessels. Use of DSA must be balanced between the procedure-related risk and the risk of an incorrect diagnosis [128, 129].

Although the degree of stenosis is one of the oldest parameters, it is still the most important in the evaluation of vascular lesions [128] and DSA shows good agreements for measuring intracranial artery stenosis [130]. The degree of stenosis is defined as follows: percent steno-sis = $[(1 - (D(stenosis)/D(normal)))] \times 100$ [130].

Hemodynamic information is another impor-tant advantage in DSA. The hemodynamic infor-mation on vascular flow is poor in other vascular imaging such as CTA, MRA, and vessel wall MR. However, when contrast agent insufficiently fills peripheral vessels to a stenosis, those cannot be seen on DSA. Therefore, CTA can be better than DSA to delineate the distal vessels because CTA can concentrate contrast agent to distal ves-sels beyond the stenosis [54]. However, CTA has a demerit to DSA for the evaluation and measure-ment of small arteries [131]. DSA needs multiple intravascular injections of contrast media to each artery, and bilateral vertebral arterial injection is sometimes necessary for complete assessment of posterior circulation stenosis.

In some cases, vascular imaging can be chal-lenging to evaluate the vascular disease including vertebrobasilar artery steno-occlusion because each modality has merits and demerits depending on techniques, postprocessing, and susceptible artifact, and thus interpretation by a neuroradio-logical expert is necessary.

Ultrasound

Ultrasound for patients with a suspicion of poste-rior circulation stroke provides not only imaging but also additional information on cerebral hemo-dynamics. Ultrasound in parallel with other modalities (CT, MRI) may offer further under-standing on the pathophysiology of stroke. It can also be a very quick, cheap, and noninvasive first-line approach as well as an ideal follow-up modality as it can be performed directly at the bed-side. However, it has demerits in the limited view and insufficient anatomic information rela-tive to carotid arteries in posterior circulation. The US examination of the posterior circulation should include a complete examination of the vertebrobasilar system. It encompasses innomi-nate and subclavian arteries, both extra- and intracranial vertebral artery segments, basilar trunk, and posterior cerebral arteries along with a documentation of cervical collateral pathways [132].

Doppler Ultrasound

Several modes of ultrasound are now commonly used in the posterior circulation. B-mode (bright-ness mode) ultrasound uses 7.5–10 MHz emis-sion frequencies to produce real-time two-dimensional (2D) image of the vessels. Doppler mode makes use of the Doppler effect to measure and visualize blood flow. Pulsed-wave (P-W) and continuous-wave (C-W) Doppler present the flow velocity information of the arter-ies on a timeline. In the P-W Doppler system, a single transducer crystal emits pulses of short bursts of ultrasound energy. Between the pulses, the same crystal acts as the receiver of ultrasound signals [133]. The P-W Doppler is most often combined with B-mode images in a duplex sys-tem. The duplex system improves the identifica-tion of the artery and more reliably detects abnormality [134]. On the other hand, the C-W Doppler system consists of a double element transducer, and it continuously transmits and receives ultrasonic signals [133]. C-W Doppler is helpful in determining the presence and direction of flow in the interosseous (V2) and atlas loop (V3) of the vertebral arteries [134]. Color Doppler flow imaging (CDFI) provides real-time information about blood flow, which is displayed as color images superimposed on B-mode images of the surrounding tissues [132]. CDFI allows better visualization of the proximal vertebral artery and the atlas loop than conventional duplex ultrasonography [135]. Power Doppler imaging

(PDI) uses a display of the amplitude of the Doppler signal rather than the velocity and direction of the flow. It provides better visualization of blood vessels lying in regions anatomically difficult for ultrasound imaging [136]. It also improves the evaluation of the stenosis and visualization of the intravascular surface and plaque morphology [134]. PDI is useful in evaluating vertebral artery as an adjunct to CDFI and P-W Doppler imaging [137].

Transcranial Doppler

Transcranial Doppler (TCD) ultrasound, using a pulsed Doppler system with low transmitter frequency (1.5–2 MHz) to penetrate the skull, is able to record blood flow velocities of the intracranial vessels [138, 139]. Insonation through the foramen magnum (transforminal window) from the top of the neck below the occiput allows detection of blood flow velocities in the basilar artery and the intracranial segments of the vertebral arteries. Transtemporal window is found between the angle of the eye and the pinna above the zygomatic ridge and allows the study of flow through the distal basilar artery, posterior cerebral arteries, and posterior communicating arteries. In conventional TCD, grayscale images of the vessel wall are not routinely obtained because of its limited spatial resolution. The Doppler signal obtained is assigned to a specific artery based on indirect parameters: the depth of the sample volume, the position of the transducer, and the flow direction [140]. Transcranial color duplex ultrasonography, on the other hand, enables the visualization of the intracranial posterior circulation vessels by color-coding of blood flow velocity [141]. It allows the operator to identify the target vessel more accurately and measure the angle of insonation to correct the flow velocity measurement [132, 134, 142]. More recently, the advent of power motion-mode TCD (PMD-TCD) has improved the ability to insonate and visualize the posterior circulation arteries and provides multi-gate flow information simultaneously in power M-mode display [142, 143]. PMD-TCD showed a satisfactory agreement (sensitivity 73%, specificity 96%) with digital subtraction angiography (DSA) in evaluating the patients with acute posterior cerebral ischemia [143]. PMD-TCD also has a role in depicting flow signatures that are complementary to the standard single-gate TCD spectral findings [143]. Microemboli in the posterior cerebral circulation can also be visualized as high-intensity transient signals (HITS), also called microembolic signals (MES), superimposed on the background Doppler spectra [138, 144, 145]. In one study, 13% of the acute posterior circulation cerebral ischemia patients had MES on the TCD monitoring at the basilar artery. The presence of MES can suggest possible mechanisms of the stroke [144].

Application

The ultrasound evaluation of the posterior circulation system should be initiated from the innominate and subclavian arteries [132, 146]. A microconvex array transducer using 3.5–11.5 MHz provided a better visualization of the proximal segments of the supra-aortic arteries and the aortic arch. The cervical segments of the subclavian arteries are usually well visualized by duplex sonography and C-W Doppler [134]. Even though ultrasound imaging of the vertebral arteries is more difficult and less often performed than that of the carotid system, many studies show the feasibility and usefulness of the ultrasound evaluation when performed by experienced operators. The intraforaminal course (V2) of the vertebral artery is the easiest to examine because of the straight course of the artery; therefore, it is recommended to begin the examination from this segment. It can be assessed with a probe parallel to the carotid and angled laterally and oriented to the direction of transverse processes. The origin of the vertebral artery (V0) is a common site of atherosclerotic stenosis, which is difficult to investigate. The insufficient visualization of this segment is reported in 6–14% on the right side and in 14–40% on the left side [147]. Following the artery from the V1/V2 segment junction to the subclavian artery is a good way to assess the origin. Examination of the atlas loop (V3) is performed by placing the probe below the mastoid process, lateral to the sternocleidomastoid muscle, and maintaining the probe directed toward the contralateral orbit [148]. The distal V2 and V3 segments, however, cannot always be satisfactorily imaged.

For the vertebral system, just like a carotid system, peak systolic velocity (PSV) increase can be a good estimator for evaluating the stenosis. A moderate stenosis (50–69%) will show a focal PSV increase (>140 cm/s at the origin, or a stenotic/prestenotic PSV ratio > 2), while a severe stenosis (>70%) will also show indirect hemodynamic signs (prestenotic flow signal with a low diastolic velocity and increased peripheral resistance; post-stenotic flow signal with a delayed systolic flow rise and dampened waveform), contralateral vertebral artery compensation [88]. A unique finding in the posterior circulation system, which is not seen in the carotid system, is the cervical collateral pathways. Distal vertebral artery flow can be reconstituted via ascending cervical artery (from thyrocervical trunk), deep cervical artery (from costocervical trunk), and/or occipital artery (from external carotid artery) when the occlusion is located proximally.

Ultrasound also helps to identify the cause of the stroke such as atherosclerotic plaques (Fig. 9.11), typical sign of dissection (i.e., irregular stenosis or ectasia, an intramural hematoma, a double lumen) (Fig. 9.12), arteritis, vasospasm, Bow-Hunter's syndrome, and subclavian steal phenomenon.

In subclavian steal syndrome, the flow pattern varies depending on the severity of the subclavian artery stenosis and the collateral patterns.

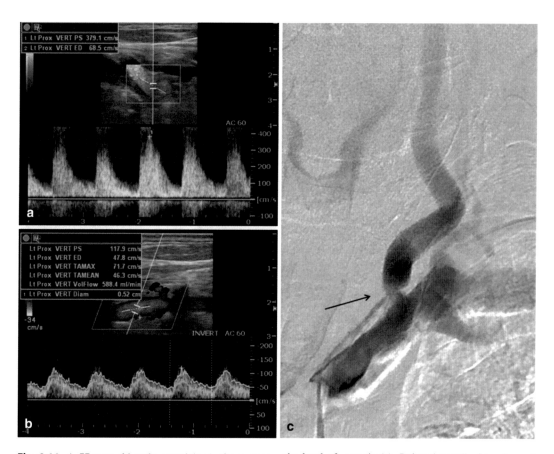

Fig. 9.11 A 77-year-old male complained of recurrent dizziness in whom acute embolic infarctions in the pons were noted on diffusion MRI (not shown). Doppler ultrasonography demonstrated focal stenosis in the origin of the left vertebral artery (VA), markedly increased in peak systolic velocity (379.1 cm/s) and spectral broadening at the level of stenosis (**a**). Delayed systolic flow rise and dampened waveform were noted in the intraforaminal segment of the ipsilateral VA (**b**). Digital subtraction angiography revealed focal severe stenosis at the VA ostium with dense calcified plaques that also encircled the subclavian artery (**c**)

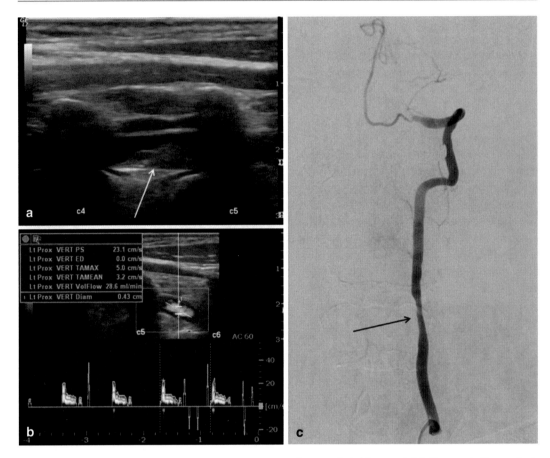

Fig. 9.12 A 59-year-old male presented with sudden onset dizziness and truncal ataxia. Diffusion MRI showed multiple embolic infarctions in the posterior circulation area (not shown). Brightness mode of the Doppler ultrasonography demonstrated irregular focal stenosis in the intraforaminal segment (V2) of the left vertebral artery (VA) between C4 and C5 transverse processes. Intramural hematoma with thickened irregular vessel wall was noted at the stenosis (white arrow) (**a**). Prestenotic flow analysis between C5 and C6 levels showed a high-resistance flow pattern without a diastolic flow component (**b**). Left vertebral angiography revealed focal tapering stenosis (black arrow) at the corresponding segment as well as near occlusion of distal V3 segment, which was considered as a tandem dissecting lesion (**c**)

Incomplete steal usually causes a decrease in systolic blood flow velocity, and in more severe cases, bidirectional blood flow occurs in the ipsilateral vertebral artery [138]. Complete flow reversal is noted in cases of complete steal. TCD can be used in conjunction with duplex vertebral sonography in the diagnosis of this condition [138, 148]. TCD findings may be potentiated by exercise of the arm on the affected side or a hyperemia test in which the brachial artery is compressed and then released to accentuate subclavian steal [138, 148] (Fig. 9.13).

After complete examination of the extracranial vertebral arteries, insonation of the intracranial arteries is performed using TCD through transforaminal window. Both intracranial vertebral arteries are evaluated and then followed to the basilar artery. Visualization of the distal basilar artery and the posterior cerebral arteries is difficult but often can be visualized via transtemporal window. According to a color-coded TCD study [149], adequate quality insonation was successfully achieved in the intracranial vertebral arteries (98%), basilar artery (92%), and P1

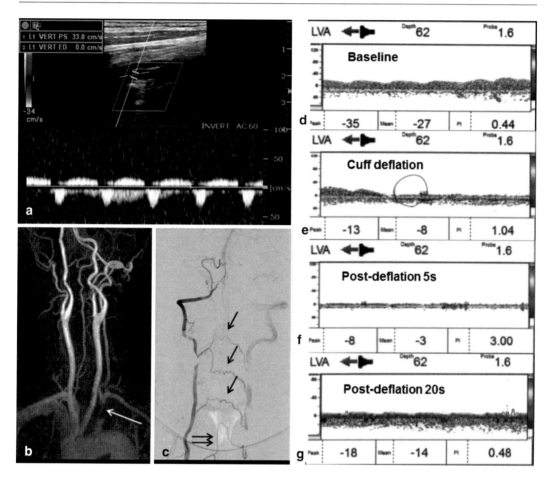

Fig. 9.13 A 61-year-old female complained of dizziness and left arm discomfort. Spectral analysis of the left VA (V2 segment) showed systolic flow reversal and antegrade diastolic flow that suggests subclavian steal syndrome (**a**). Contrast-enhanced MRA demonstrated occlusion of the left proximal subclavian artery (arrow) (**b**). Right vertebral artery angiography showed prominent retrocorporeal anastomosis at C2, C3, and C4 levels (arrows) and anterior spinal artery (double arrow) to reconstitute left VA flows (antegrade flow to the brain and retrograde flow to the arm) (**c**). A typical retrograde left distal VA flow was not visualized due to the hypoplastic right V4 segment. Transcranial Doppler findings of the left intracranial VA was performed during a hyperemic test. A delayed and dampened systolic flow was noted on baseline examination (**d**). After the measurement, a cuff over the left brachial artery was inflated with an affected arm exercised for 2 min. Rapid deflation of the cuff (circle) leads to a sudden decrease of the flow for a while (**e, f**). Recovery of the baseline flow was demonstrated after 20 s (**g**)

segment of the posterior cerebral arteries (84%). The Stroke Outcomes and Neuroimaging of Intracranial Atherosclerosis (SONIA) Trial found that TCD allows reliable exclusion with a substantial negative predictive value (> 0.8) of the presence of intracranial stenosis (50 to 99%) when using mean velocity criteria of 110 cm/s for vertebral artery and 130 cm/s for basilar trunk [72].

Ultrasound has some limitations. First, adequate visualization of the entire vertebral artery cannot always be possible. The origin and the V1 segment is sometimes not accessible because of anatomical difficulties such as deep and posterior origin of the vertebral arteries, direct origin from the aortic arch, tortuous course, or short neck stature. Vertebral processes preclude the whole assessment of the V2 segment; therefore, short segmental lesion can be missed. Therefore, both direct and indirect signs of steno-occlusive lesion must be interpreted together to improve sensitivity and accuracy [4].

Second, there are no established criteria for estimating vertebral artery stenosis like the carotid stenosis criteria of the Society of Radiologists in Ultrasound [150]. Third, the quality of the exam highly depends on the operator, so it is recommended to be performed by well-trained and experienced sonographers.

Perfusion Imaging

CTP

CTP is to provide rapid qualitative and quantitative cerebral perfusion. CTP is obtained using continuous cine imaging for the contrast enhancement during the first pass of an iodinated contrast media bolus through cerebral vasculatures [151, 152]. The degree of contrast enhancement and concentration of the contrast media show a linear relationship with a transient hyperattenuation that is directly proportional to the amount of the contrast media in a given region [151, 152]. It commonly takes 1 to 2-min scan time with a 35 to 50-mL contrast media and a 4 to 5-mL/s injection rate [47, 151, 152] using a tube voltage of 80 kV [153], which differ on the detailed parameters such as a coverage, section thickness, and inter-slice gap. The radiation dose is generally lower to head and neck CTA [47] or similar to noncontrast brain CT [154, 155]. The images are acquired at every second during the first 30–45 s followed by every 2–3 s during the next 30–45 s to generate accurate early-phase concentration curves [153]. The poor cardiac output, atrial fibrillation, and/or steno-occlusive lesions could contribute to the delayed cerebral tissue saturation [153]. Perfusion maps such as CBV, CBF, MTT, and TTP are generated through a postprocessing method, including non-deconvolution-based or deconvolution-based model of the time-attenuation curve [152, 156]. Tmax (time to the peak of the residual function) can be derived from the deconvolution-based model instead of TTP [157, 158]. CBV is defined as the total volume of flowing blood in a given volume in the brain, with units of milliliters of blood per 100 g of brain tissue. CBF is defined as the volume of blood moving through a given volume of brain per unit time, with units of milliliters of blood per 100 g of brain tissue per minute. MTT is defined as the average transit time of blood through a given brain region, measured in seconds [156].

CTP showed additional diagnostic values in acute ischemic posterior circulation stroke when compared with noncontrast CT and/or CTA [159, 160]. CTP combined to noncontrast CT and CTA presented significant improved diagnostic performance with a sensitivity of 76.6%, a specificity of 91.1%, a positive predictive value of 95.4%, a negative predictive value of 62.1% [160], and an area under the curve of 0.86 (noncontrast CT, 0.64; noncontrast CT + CTA source images, 0.68) [159]. A systematic review also demonstrated that CTP (sensitivity, 76%; specificity, 93%) is better than noncontrast CT (sensitivity, 23%; specificity, 97%) and similar to CTA (sensitivity, 42%; specificity, 98%) in the diagnostic accuracy for detection of acute posterior circulation stroke [161]. The largest analysis ($n = 436$) for the diagnostic performance of CTP in acute posterior circulation stroke postulated that the extent of focal hypoperfusion is independently associated with long-term outcome [162]. Infarct core can be defined as decreased CBV and CBF with severely delayed MTT, TTP, and Tmax, whereas penumbra can be estimated by preserved CBV and CBF with delayed MTT, TTP, and Tmax roughly [157]. A decrease in CBF by 30–50% [41, 42, 153, 157, 163] or CBV with less than 2–2.5 g/100 mL [8, 153, 164] relative to the normal cerebral hemisphere for the infarct core and a delay in Tmax more than 6 s for the penumbra [42, 165, 166] have been commonly used, but the quantitative thresholds have been mainly established in anterior circulation stroke.

MRP

Dynamic susceptibility contrast (DSC), dynamic contrast-enhanced (DCE), and arterial spin labeling (ASL) imaging have been widely and clinically used as MR protocols for PWI. Most of PWI in acute ischemic stroke indicates DSC-PWI.

Arterial spin labeling (ASL) is perfusion imaging that is able to provide quantitative CBF values without contrast agent. ASL uses endogenous blood tracer by magnetically labeling blood at the cervical carotid artery levels instead of gadolinium-based contrast media. The labeled blood distributes in cerebral capillary beds, which is acquired as quantitative CBF perfusion imaging [167]. Hypoperfused regions on ASL-CBF may represent the penumbra in patients of acute ischemic stroke. ASL showed high agreement with DSC-PWI in the detection of the penumbra, but it tends to overestimate the penumbra [167–169]. However, ASL limits in the clinical use due to the long scan time and poor availability and has been used mainly in the research field.

DSC-PWI begins with intravenous injection of a gadolinium-based paramagnetic contrast agent. The first pass of the contrast media bolus causes a nonlinear signal loss on T2* images, which represents susceptibility artifact. The tissue signal changes can generate a hemodynamic time-to-signal intensity curve, which can be used to generate CBV, CBF, TTP, MTT, and Tmax [36, 170].

Hypoperfused cerebral tissue includes benign oligemia and ischemic tissue, and the infarct core and penumbra belong to the ischemic tissue [171]. The infarct core is defined as brain tissue likely to be irreversibly infarcted at the time of imaging, and the penumbra is defined as at-risk ischemic brain tissue likely to be infarcted in the absence of early robust recanalization [3]. Both DSC-PWI and CTP have been widely used to delineate the penumbra region in real clinical or research arena even though those can overestimate ischemic tissue and tend to include benign oligemic region, especially MTT, TTP, or Tmax [171]. A threshold or definition for the penumbra is still in debate even though a delay in Tmax more than 6 s is used for the threshold in previous trials [36].

CTP is based on the linear relationship between contrast media and CT attenuation, whereas DSC-PWI shows a nonlinear relationship between the contrast agent and the MR signal. Therefore, the quantification is more easily achieved in CTP, which is confirmed by comparison with positron emission tomography as a reference standard [3, 172]. The major advantage of DSC-PWI can include other effective MR sequences including DWI, FLAIR, or GRE to evaluate various radiological features of ischemic lesions when compared with CTP [3, 36]. The major disadvantage of DSC-PWI over CTP is that the parametric maps provide semiquantitative values rather than absolute values [36]. CTP has a demerit of the susceptibility to bone- or air-related artifact in posterior fossa [23]. Both CTP and DSC-PWI rely on similar basic tracer kinetic concepts and challenges from the acquisition, postprocessing, and interpretation of parametric maps [3].

Although both CTP and DSC-PWI are useful methods to offer cerebral perfusion data including infarct core and penumbra, perfusion imaging is not essential in the assessment of acute ischemic stroke patients. The 2018 AHA/ASA guideline for the early management of patients with acute ischemic stroke recommends that multimodal CT and MRI including perfusion imaging should not delay administration of IV alteplase, and perfusion imaging is not recommended in patients with less than 6 h for the evaluation of indication for mechanical thrombectomy either. However, perfusion imaging is recommended to aid the selection of patients for mechanical thrombectomy within 6–24 h of last known normal and large vessel occlusion in anterior circulation [50].

Both CTP and DSC-PWI can present various mismatch combined with the infarct core. The mismatch can be divided into target mismatch (PWI > DWI) (Fig. 9.14), no target mismatch (PWI = DWI) (Fig. 9.15), and inverse mismatch (PWI < DWI) (Fig. 9.16) [8]. Large artery occlusion results in the target mismatch, in which a growth of infarct core is expected if no revascularization is achieved. An established infarct with large artery occlusion or prevented further infarct growth by sufficient collateral flows may belong to the no target mismatch. Inverse mismatch can be seen in early revascularization phase of large vessel infarcts or lacunar infarcts. DWI lesions without perfusion abnormalities can be seen in transient ischemic attack or small cortical or perforator infarcts. Decreased PWI without DWI

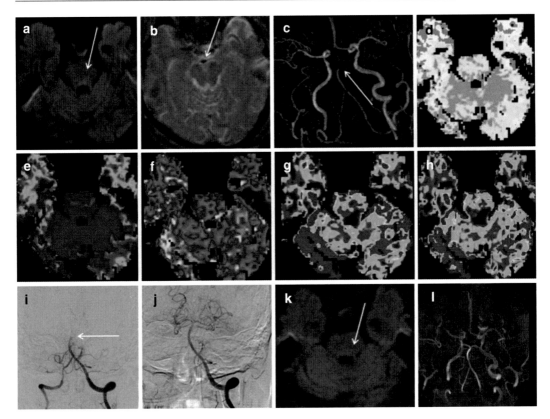

Fig. 9.14 A 84-year-old male was admitted with drowsy mentality. DWI showed small acute infarct in left posterior pons (**a**), and GRE depicted a clot in upper basilar artery (**b**). CE-MRA showed occlusion of upper basilar artery and bilateral proximal posterior cerebral arteries (**c**). Perfusion MR showed extensive delayed perfusion area involving entire pons and bilateral cerebellar hemispheres, and bilateral medial temporal lobes on Tmax (**d**), TTP (**e**), and MTT (**f**) with preserved CBV (**g**) and CBF (**h**). Therefore, MRI showed a large DWI–PWI mismatch. Preprocedural DSA showed occlusion of upper basilar artey (**i**), and postprocedural DSA showed recanalization of basilar artery and bilateral proximal posterior cerebral arteries after mechanical thrombectomy (**j**). Follow-up DWI showed no more additional infarct compared to the initial DWI (**k**), and follow-up TOF-MRA showed patent flow in the posterior circulation (**l**)

lesions can be seen mainly in stroke mimickers such as migraine, reversible cerebral vasoconstriction syndrome, and posterior reversible encephalopathy syndrome. Diffusion lesions with increased PWI can be seen in ictal/postictal seizure and migraine aura [8]. The quantitative definition for infarct core to penumbra mismatch on perfusion imaging is still challenging and in debate. A mismatch with larger than 20% has been used as eligibility criteria in some clinical trials [36, 42, 173, 174]. However, the DEFUSE 3 trial used a mismatch ≥ 1.8 [165] and the DAWN trial used a mismatch between a clinical deficit and infarct volume [163]. There is still a limitation in the direct application of the perfusion thresholds for infarct core and penumbra because of heterogeneity due to poor standardization with high variable imaging protocols and algorithms for postprocessing, and low interobserver reproducibility [8].

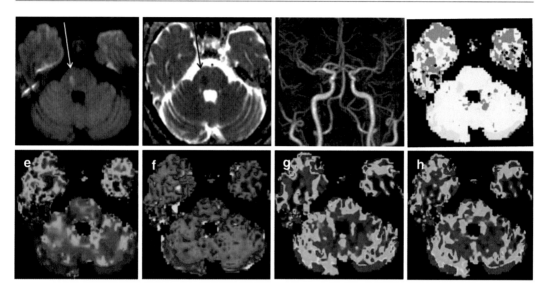

Fig. 9.15 A 61-year-old male presented with gait ataxia. DWI (**a**) and ADC (**b**) showed small acute infarct in right pons (arrows). TOF-MRA looked normal (**c**). Perfusion MR also looked normal on Tmax (**d**), TTP (**e**), MTT (**f**), CBV (**g**), and CBF (**h**). There was only DWI lesion without perfusion abnormality

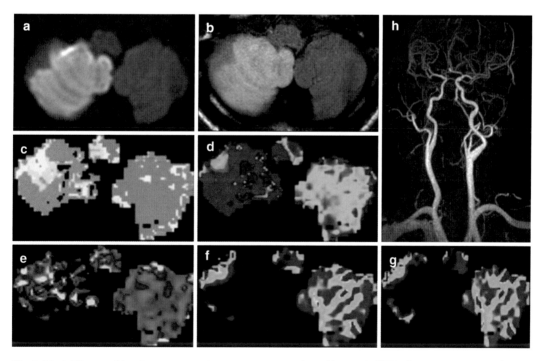

Fig. 9.16 A 78-year-old male presented with dizziness. DWI (**a**) and FLAIR (**b**) showed acute infarct in right cerebellar hemisphere representing posterior inferior cerebellar artery territory. There was no DWI–PWI mismatch on Tmax (**c**), TTP (**d**), MTT (**e**), CBV (**f**), and CBF (**g**). CE-MRA showed severe stenosis at right intradural VA (**h**)

References

1. van Straten M, Venema HW, Majoie CB, Freling NJ, Grimbergen CA, den Heeten GJ. Image quality of multisection CT of the brain: thickly collimated sequential scanning versus thinly collimated spiral scanning with image combining. AJNR Am J Neuroradiol. 2007;28(3):421–7.
2. Pace I, Zarb F. A comparison of sequential and spiral scanning techniques in brain CT. Radiol Technol. 2015;86(4):373–8.
3. Wintermark M, Rowley HA, Lev MH. Acute stroke triage to intravenous thrombolysis and other therapies with advanced CT or MR imaging: pro CT. Radiology. 2009;251(3):619–26.
4. Rudkin S, Cerejo R, Tayal A, Goldberg MF. Imaging of acute ischemic stroke. Emerg Radiol. 2018;25(6):659–72.
5. Caplan LR. Vertebrobasilar ischemia and hemorrhage: clinical findings, diagnosis and management of posterior circulation disease. 2nd ed. Cambridge/New York: Cambridge University Press; 2015. p. xiv, 594p
6. Tsai FY, Teal JS, Heishima GB, Zee CS, Grinnell VS, Mehringer CM, et al. Computed tomography in acute posterior fossa infarcts. AJNR Am J Neuroradiol. 1982;3(2):149–56.
7. Pavlina AA, Radhakrishnan R, Vagal AS. Role of imaging in acute ischemic stroke. Semin Ultrasound CT MR. 2018;39(5):412–24.
8. Vilela P, Rowley HA. Brain ischemia: CT and MRI techniques in acute ischemic stroke. Eur J Radiol. 2017;96:162–72.
9. Nouh A, Remke J, Ruland S. Ischemic posterior circulation stroke: a review of anatomy, clinical presentations, diagnosis, and current management. Front Neurol. 2014;5:30.
10. Pexman JH, Barber PA, Hill MD, Sevick RJ, Demchuk AM, Hudon ME, et al. Use of the Alberta stroke program early CT score (ASPECTS) for assessing CT scans in patients with acute stroke. AJNR Am J Neuroradiol. 2001;22(8):1534–42.
11. Barber PA, Demchuk AM, Zhang J, Buchan AM. Validity and reliability of a quantitative computed tomography score in predicting outcome of hyperacute stroke before thrombolytic therapy. ASPECTS study group. Alberta stroke programme early CT score. Lancet. 2000;355(9216):1670–4.
12. Puetz V, Sylaja PN, Coutts SB, Hill MD, Dzialowski I, Mueller P, et al. Extent of hypoattenuation on CT angiography source images predicts functional outcome in patients with basilar artery occlusion. Stroke. 2008;39(9):2485–90.
13. Goldmakher GV, Camargo EC, Furie KL, Singhal AB, Roccatagliata L, Halpern EF, et al. Hyperdense basilar artery sign on unenhanced CT predicts thrombus and outcome in acute posterior circulation stroke. Stroke. 2009;40(1):134–9.
14. Kohrmann M, Schellinger PD. Acute stroke triage to intravenous thrombolysis and other therapies with advanced CT or MR imaging: pro MR imaging. Radiology. 2009;251(3):627–33.
15. Meshksar A, Villablanca JP, Khan R, Carmody R, Coull B, Nael K. Role of EPI-FLAIR in patients with acute stroke: a comparative analysis with FLAIR. AJNR Am J Neuroradiol. 2014;35(5):878–83.
16. Nael K, Khan R, Choudhary G, Meshksar A, Villablanca P, Tay J, et al. Six-minute magnetic resonance imaging protocol for evaluation of acute ischemic stroke: pushing the boundaries. Stroke. 2014;45(7):1985–91.
17. Chung MS, Lee JY, Jung SC, Baek S, Shim WH, Park JE, et al. Reliability of fast magnetic resonance imaging for acute ischemic stroke patients using a 1.5-T scanner. Eur Radiol. 2019;29(5):2641–50.
18. Shah S, Luby M, Poole K, Morella T, Keller E, Benson RT, et al. Screening with MRI for accurate and rapid stroke treatment: SMART. Neurology. 2015;84(24):2438–44.
19. Wisco D, Uchino K, Saqqur M, Gebel JM, Aoki J, Alam S, et al. Addition of hyperacute MRI AIDS in patient selection, decreasing the use of endovascular stroke therapy. Stroke. 2014;45(2):467–72.
20. Allen LM, Hasso AN, Handwerker J, Farid H. Sequence-specific MR imaging findings that are useful in dating ischemic stroke. Radiographics. 2012;32(5):1285–97; discussion 97-9
21. González RG. Acute ischemic stroke: imaging and intervention. Berlin/New York: Springer; 2005. p. xii, 268p
22. Le Bihan D, Breton E, Lallemand D, Grenier P, Cabanis E, Laval-Jeantet M. MR imaging of intravoxel incoherent motions: application to diffusion and perfusion in neurologic disorders. Radiology. 1986;161(2):401–7.
23. Muir KW, Buchan A, von Kummer R, Rother J, Baron J-C. Imaging of acute stroke. Lancet Neurol. 2006;5(9):755–68.
24. Soize S, Tisserand M, Charron S, Turc G, Ben Hassen W, Labeyrie MA, et al. How sustained is 24-hour diffusion-weighted imaging lesion reversal? Serial magnetic resonance imaging in a patient cohort thrombolyzed within 4.5 hours of stroke onset. Stroke. 2015;46(3):704–10.
25. Ringer TM, Neumann-Haefelin T, Sobel RA, Moseley ME, Yenari MA. Reversal of early diffusion-weighted magnetic resonance imaging abnormalities does not necessarily reflect tissue salvage in experimental cerebral ischemia. Stroke. 2001;32(10):2362–9.
26. Lee SH, Kim JS. Acute diagnosis and Management of Stroke Presenting Dizziness or vertigo. Neurol Clin. 2015;33(3):687–98, xi
27. Schulz UG, Fischer U. Posterior circulation cerebrovascular syndromes: diagnosis and management. J Neurol Neurosurg Psychiatry. 2017;88(1):45–53.

28. Markus HS, van der Worp HB, Rothwell PM. Posterior circulation ischaemic stroke and transient ischaemic attack: diagnosis, investigation, and secondary prevention. Lancet Neurol. 2013;12(10):989–98.

29. Oppenheim C, Stanescu R, Dormont D, Crozier S, Marro B, Samson Y, et al. False-negative diffusion-weighted MR findings in acute ischemic stroke. AJNR Am J Neuroradiol. 2000;21(8):1434–40.

30. Chalela JA, Kidwell CS, Nentwich LM, Luby M, Butman JA, Demchuk AM, et al. Magnetic resonance imaging and computed tomography in emergency assessment of patients with suspected acute stroke: a prospective comparison. Lancet. 2007;369(9558):293–8.

31. Kattah JC, Talkad AV, Wang DZ, Hsieh YH, Newman-Toker DE. HINTS to diagnose stroke in the acute vestibular syndrome: three-step bedside oculomotor examination more sensitive than early MRI diffusion-weighted imaging. Stroke. 2009;40(11):3504–10.

32. Engelter ST, Wetzel SG, Radue EW, Rausch M, Steck AJ, Lyrer PA. The clinical significance of diffusion-weighted MR imaging in infratentorial strokes. Neurology. 2004;62(4):574–80.

33. Linfante I, Llinas RH, Schlaug G, Chaves C, Warach S, Caplan LR. Diffusion-weighted imaging and National Institutes of Health Stroke Scale in the acute phase of posterior-circulation stroke. Arch Neurol. 2001;58(4):621–8.

34. Tei H, Uchiyama S, Usui T, Ohara K. Posterior circulation ASPECTS on diffusion-weighted MRI can be a powerful marker for predicting functional outcome. J Neurol. 2010;257(5):767–73.

35. Lee KY, Latour LL, Luby M, Hsia AW, Merino JG, Warach S. Distal hyperintense vessels on FLAIR: an MRI marker for collateral circulation in acute stroke? Neurology. 2009;72(13):1134–9.

36. Vert C, Parra-Farinas C, Rovira A. MR imaging in hyperacute ischemic stroke. Eur J Radiol. 2017;96:125–32.

37. Thomalla G, Cheng B, Ebinger M, Hao Q, Tourdias T, Wu O, et al. DWI-FLAIR mismatch for the identification of patients with acute ischaemic stroke within 4·5 h of symptom onset (PRE-FLAIR): a multicentre observational study. Lancet Neurol. 2011;10(11):978–86.

38. Arnould MC, Grandin CB, Peeters A, Cosnard G, Duprez TP. Comparison of CT and three MR sequences for detecting and categorizing early (48 hours) hemorrhagic transformation in hyperacute ischemic stroke. AJNR Am J Neuroradiol. 2004;25(6):939–44.

39. Cheng AL, Batool S, McCreary CR, Lauzon ML, Frayne R, Goyal M, et al. Susceptibility-weighted imaging is more reliable than T2*-weighted gradient-recalled echo MRI for detecting microbleeds. Stroke. 2013;44(10):2782–6.

40. Jovin TG, Chamorro A, Cobo E, de Miquel MA, Molina CA, Rovira A, et al. Thrombectomy within 8 hours after symptom onset in ischemic stroke. N Engl J Med. 2015;372(24):2296–306.

41. Saver JL, Goyal M, Bonafe A, Diener HC, Levy EI, Pereira VM, et al. Stent-retriever thrombectomy after intravenous t-PA vs. t-PA alone in stroke. N Engl J Med. 2015;372(24):2285–95.

42. Campbell BC, Mitchell PJ, Kleinig TJ, Dewey HM, Churilov L, Yassi N, et al. Endovascular therapy for ischemic stroke with perfusion-imaging selection. N Engl J Med. 2015;372(11):1009–18.

43. Goyal M, Demchuk AM, Menon BK, Eesa M, Rempel JL, Thornton J, et al. Randomized assessment of rapid endovascular treatment of ischemic stroke. N Engl J Med. 2015;372(11):1019–30.

44. Berkhemer OA, Fransen PS, Beumer D, van den Berg LA, Lingsma HF, Yoo AJ, et al. A randomized trial of intraarterial treatment for acute ischemic stroke. N Engl J Med. 2015;372(1):11–20.

45. Badhiwala JH, Nassiri F, Alhazzani W, Selim MH, Farrokhyar F, Spears J, et al. Endovascular thrombectomy for acute ischemic stroke: a meta-analysis. JAMA. 2015;314(17):1832–43.

46. d'Esterre CD, Trivedi A, Pordeli P, Boesen M, Patil S, Hwan Ahn S, et al. Regional comparison of multiphase computed tomographic angiography and computed tomographic perfusion for prediction of tissue fate in ischemic stroke. Stroke. 2017;48(4):939–45.

47. Menon BK, d'Esterre CD, Qazi EM, Almekhlafi M, Hahn L, Demchuk AM, et al. Multiphase CT angiography: a new tool for the imaging triage of patients with acute ischemic stroke. Radiology. 2015;275(2):510–20.

48. Lell MM, Anders K, Uder M, Klotz E, Ditt H, Vega-Higuera F, et al. New techniques in CT angiography. Radiographics. 2006;26:S45–62.

49. Fishman EK, Ney DR, Heath DG, Corl FM, Horton KM, Johnson PT. Volume rendering versus maximum intensity projection in CT angiography: what works best, when, and why. Radiographics. 2006;26(3):905–22.

50. Powers WJ, Rabinstein AA, Ackerson T, Adeoye OM, Bambakidis NC, Becker K, et al. 2018 guidelines for the early management of patients with acute ischemic stroke: a guideline for healthcare professionals from the American Heart Association/American Stroke Association. Stroke. 2018;49(3):e46–e110.

51. Randoux B, Marro B, Koskas F, Duyme M, Sahel M, Zouaoui A, et al. Carotid artery stenosis: prospective comparison of CT, three-dimensional gadolinium-enhanced MR, and conventional angiography. Radiology. 2001;220(1):179–85.

52. Schellinger PD, Richter G, Kohrmann M, Dorfler A. Noninvasive angiography (magnetic resonance and computed tomography) in the diagnosis of ischemic cerebrovascular disease. Techniques and clinical applications. Cerebrovasc Dis. 2007;24(Suppl 1):16–23.

53. Carvalho M, Oliveira A, Azevedo E, Bastos-Leite AJ. Intracranial arterial stenosis. J Stroke Cerebrovasc Dis. 2014;23(4):599–609.
54. Bash S, Villablanca JP, Jahan R, Duckwiler G, Tillis M, Kidwell C, et al. Intracranial vascular stenosis and occlusive disease: evaluation with CT angiography, MR angiography, and digital subtraction angiography. AJNR Am J Neuroradiol. 2005;26(5):1012–21.
55. Skutta B, Furst G, Eilers J, Ferbert A, Kuhn FP. Intracranial stenoocclusive disease: double-detector helical CT angiography versus digital subtraction angiography. AJNR Am J Neuroradiol. 1999;20(5):791–9.
56. Duffis EJ, Jethwa P, Gupta G, Bonello K, Gandhi CD, Prestigiacomo CJ. Accuracy of computed tomographic angiography compared to digital subtraction angiography in the diagnosis of intracranial stenosis and its impact on clinical decision-making. J Stroke Cerebrovasc Dis. 2013;22(7):1013–7.
57. Nguyen-Huynh MN, Wintermark M, English J, Lam J, Vittinghoff E, Smith WS, et al. How accurate is CT angiography in evaluating intracranial atherosclerotic disease? Stroke. 2008;39(4):1184–8.
58. Nederkoorn PJ, van der Graaf Y, Hunink MG. Duplex ultrasound and magnetic resonance angiography compared with digital subtraction angiography in carotid artery stenosis: a systematic review. Stroke. 2003;34(5):1324–32.
59. Khan S, Cloud GC, Kerry S, Markus HS. Imaging of vertebral artery stenosis: a systematic review. J Neurol Neurosurg Psychiatry. 2007;78(11):1218–25.
60. Khan S, Rich P, Clifton A, Markus HS. Noninvasive detection of vertebral artery stenosis: a comparison of contrast-enhanced MR angiography, CT angiography, and ultrasound. Stroke. 2009;40(11):3499–503.
61. Leiva-Salinas C, Jiang B, Wintermark M. Computed tomography, computed tomography angiography, and perfusion computed tomography evaluation of acute ischemic stroke. Neuroimaging Clin N Am. 2018;28(4):565–72.
62. Mishra SM, Dykeman J, Sajobi TT, Trivedi A, Almekhlafi M, Sohn SI, et al. Early reperfusion rates with IV tPA are determined by CTA clot characteristics. AJNR Am J Neuroradiol. 2014;35(12):2265–72.
63. Pipe JG. Limits of time-of-flight magnetic resonance angiography. Top Magn Reson Imaging. 2001;12(3):163–74.
64. Kim JS, Caplan LR, Wong KS. Intracranial atherosclerosis: pathophysiology, diagnosis, and treatment. Basel/New York: Karger; 2016. p. vii, 226p.
65. Raghavan P, Mukherjee S, Gaughen J, Phillips CD. Magnetic resonance angiography of the extracranial carotid system. Top Magn Reson Imaging. 2008;19(5):241–9.
66. Carr JC, Carroll TJ. Magnetic resonance angiography: principles and applications. New York: Springer; 2012. p. xvii, 412p.
67. Jung H, et al. Contrast-enhanced MR angiography for the diagnosis of intracranial vascular disease: optimal dose of gadopentetate dimeglumine. Am J Roentgenol. 1995;165(5):1251–5.
68. Yang JJ, et al. Comparison of pre- and postcontrast 3D time-of-flight MR angiography for the evaluation of distal intracranial branch occlusions in acute ischemic stroke. Am J Radiol. 2002;23:557–67.
69. Jumaa M, Popescu A, Tsay J, Vaughan C, Vora N, Jankowitz B, et al. Evaluation of vertebral artery origin stenosis: a retrospective comparison of three techniques. J Neuroimag. 2012;22(1):14–6.
70. Provenzale JM, Sarikaya B. Comparison of test performance characteristics of MRI, MR angiography, and CT angiography in the diagnosis of carotid and vertebral artery dissection: a review of the medical literature. AJR Am J Roentgenol. 2009;193(4):1167–74.
71. Vertinsky AT, Schwartz NE, Fischbein NJ, Rosenberg J, Albers GW, Zaharchuk G. Comparison of multidetector CT angiography and MR imaging of cervical artery dissection. AJNR Am J Neuroradiol. 2008;29(9):1753–60.
72. Feldmann E, Wilterdink JL, Kosinski A, Lynn M, Chimowitz MI, Sarafin J, et al. The stroke outcomes and neuroimaging of intracranial atherosclerosis (SONIA) trial. Neurology. 2007;68(24):2099–106.
73. Choi CG, Lee DH, Lee JH, Pyun HW, Kang DW, Kwon SU, et al. Detection of intracranial atherosclerotic steno-occlusive disease with 3D time-of-flight magnetic resonance angiography with sensitivity encoding at 3T. AJNR Am J Neuroradiol. 2007;28(3):439–46.
74. Dieleman N, van der Kolk AG, Zwanenburg JJ, Harteveld AA, Biessels GJ, Luijten PR, et al. Imaging intracranial vessel wall pathology with magnetic resonance imaging: current prospects and future directions. Circulation. 2014;130(2):192–201.
75. Choi YJ, Jung SC, Lee DH. Vessel Wall imaging of the intracranial and cervical carotid arteries. J Stroke. 2015;17(3):238–55.
76. Jain KK. Some observations on the anatomy of the middle cerebral artery. Can J Surg. 1964;7(2):134–9.
77. Kamath S. Observations on the length and diameter of vessels forming the circle of Willis. J Anat. 1981;133(Pt 3):419–23.
78. Akgun V, Battal B, Bozkurt Y, Oz O, Hamcan S, Sari S, et al. Normal anatomical features and variations of the vertebrobasilar circulation and its branches: an analysis with 64-detector row CT and 3T MR angiographies. ScientificWorldJournal. 2013;2013:620162.
79. Mineyko A, Kirton A, Ng D, Wei XC. Normal intracranial periarterial enhancement on pediatric brain MR imaging. Neuroradiology. 2013;55(9):1161–9.
80. Suh CH, Jung SC, Lee HB, Cho SJ. High-resolution magnetic resonance imaging using compressed sensing for intracranial and Extracranial arteries: comparison with conventional parallel imaging. Korean J Radiol. 2019;20(3):487–97.
81. Kim TW, Choi HS, Koo J, Jung SL, Ahn KJ, Kim BS, et al. Intramural hematoma detection by susceptibility-weighted imaging in intracra-

nial vertebral artery dissection. Cerebrovasc Dis. 2013;36(4):292–8.

82. Gao PH, Yang L, Wang G, Guo L, Liu X, Zhao B. Symptomatic unruptured isolated middle cerebral artery dissection: clinical and magnetic resonance imaging features. Clin Neuroradiol. 2016;26(1):81–91.

83. Zhu C, Graves MJ, Yuan J, Sadat U, Gillard JH, Patterson AJ. Optimization of improved motion-sensitized driven-equilibrium (iMSDE) blood suppression for carotid artery wall imaging. J Cardiovasc Magn Reson. 2014;16:61.

84. Li L, Chai JT, Biasiolli L, Robson MD, Choudhury RP, Handa AI, et al. Black-blood multicontrast imaging of carotid arteries with DANTE-prepared 2D and 3D MR imaging. Radiology. 2014;273(2):560–9.

85. Zhang L, Zhang N, Wu J, Liu X, Chung YC. High resolution simultaneous imaging of intracranial and extracranial arterial wall with improved cerebrospinal fluid suppression. Magn Reson Imaging. 2017;44:65–71.

86. Lee WJ, Choi HS, Jang J, Sung J, Kim TW, Koo J, et al. Non-stenotic intracranial arteries have atherosclerotic changes in acute ischemic stroke patients: a 3T MRI study. Neuroradiology. 2015;57(10):1007–13.

87. Zhu XJ, Jiang WJ, Liu L, Hu LB, Wang W, Liu ZJ. Plaques of nonstenotic basilar arteries with isolated Pontine infarction on three-dimensional high isotropic resolution magnetic resonance imaging. Chin Med J. 2015;128(11):1433–7.

88. Oppenheim C, Naggara O, Touze E, Lacour JC, Schmitt E, Bonneville F, et al. High-resolution MR imaging of the cervical arterial wall: what the radiologist needs to know. Radiographics. 2009;29(5):1413–31.

89. Fleg JL, Stone GW, Fayad ZA, Granada JF, Hatsukami TS, Kolodgie FD, et al. Detection of high-risk atherosclerotic plaque: report of the NHLBI working group on current status and future directions. J Am Coll Cardiol Img. 2012;5(9):941–55.

90. Swartz RH, Bhuta SS, Farb RI, Agid R, Willinsky RA, Terbrugge KG, et al. Intracranial arterial wall imaging using high-resolution 3-tesla contrast-enhanced MRI. Neurology. 2009;72(7):627–34.

91. Yang WJ, Chen XY, Zhao HL, Niu CB, Xu Y, Wong KS, et al. In vitro assessment of histology verified intracranial atherosclerotic disease by 1.5T magnetic resonance imaging: concentric or eccentric? Stroke. 2016;47(2):527–30.

92. Zhu XJ, Du B, Lou X, Hui FK, Ma L, Zheng BW, et al. Morphologic characteristics of atherosclerotic middle cerebral arteries on 3T high-resolution MRI. AJNR Am J Neuroradiol. 2013;34(9):1717–22.

93. Xu WH, Li ML, Gao S, Ni J, Zhou LX, Yao M, et al. In vivo high-resolution MR imaging of symptomatic and asymptomatic middle cerebral artery atherosclerotic stenosis. Atherosclerosis. 2010;212(2):507–11.

94. Zhao DL, Deng G, Xie B, Ju S, Yang M, Chen XH, et al. High-resolution MRI of the vessel wall in patients with symptomatic atherosclerotic stenosis of the middle cerebral artery. J Clin Neurosci. 2015;22(4):700–4.

95. Teng Z, Peng W, Zhan Q, Zhang X, Liu Q, Chen S, et al. An assessment on the incremental value of high-resolution magnetic resonance imaging to identify culprit plaques in atherosclerotic disease of the middle cerebral artery. Eur Radiol. 2016;26(7):2206–14.

96. Mandell DM, Mossa-Basha M, Qiao Y, Hess CP, Hui F, Matouk C, et al. Intracranial Vessel Wall MRI: principles and expert consensus recommendations of the American Society of Neuroradiology. AJNR Am J Neuroradiol. 2017;38(2):218–29.

97. Saba L, Yuan C, Hatsukami TS, Balu N, Qiao Y, DeMarco JK, et al. Carotid artery wall imaging: perspective and guidelines from the ASNR vessel wall imaging study group and expert consensus recommendations of the American Society of Neuroradiology. AJNR Am J Neuroradiol. 2018;39(2):E9–E31.

98. Saito A, Sasaki M, Ogasawara K, Kobayashi M, Hitomi J, Narumi S, et al. Carotid plaque signal differences among four kinds of T1-weighted magnetic resonance imaging techniques: a histopathological correlation study. Neuroradiology. 2012;54(11):1187–94.

99. Chu B, Kampschulte A, Ferguson MS, Kerwin WS, Yarnykh VL, O'Brien KD, et al. Hemorrhage in the atherosclerotic carotid plaque: a high-resolution MRI study. Stroke. 2004;35(5):1079–84.

100. Wang Y, Lou X, Li Y, Sui B, Sun S, Li C, et al. Imaging investigation of intracranial arterial dissecting aneurysms by using 3 T high-resolution MRI and DSA: from the interventional neuroradiologists' view. Acta Neurochir. 2014;156(3):515–25.

101. Mossa-Basha M, de Havenon A, Becker KJ, Hallam DK, Levitt MR, Cohen WA, et al. Added value of vessel wall magnetic resonance imaging in the differentiation of Moyamoya vasculopathies in a non-Asian cohort. Stroke. 2016;47(7):1782–8.

102. Turan TN, Rumboldt Z, Granholm AC, Columbo L, Welsh CT, Lopes-Virella MF, et al. Intracranial atherosclerosis: correlation between in-vivo 3T high resolution MRI and pathology. Atherosclerosis. 2014;237(2):460–3.

103. Qiao Y, Zeiler SR, Mirbagheri S, Leigh R, Urrutia V, Wityk R, et al. Intracranial plaque enhancement in patients with cerebrovascular events on high-spatial-resolution MR images. Radiology. 2014;271(2):534–42.

104. Skarpathiotakis M, Mandell DM, Swartz RH, Tomlinson G, Mikulis DJ. Intracranial atherosclerotic plaque enhancement in patients with ischemic stroke. AJNR Am J Neuroradiol. 2013;34(2):299–304.

105. Vakil P, Vranic J, Hurley MC, Bernstein RA, Korutz AW, Habib A, et al. T1 gadolinium enhancement of intracranial atherosclerotic plaques associated with symptomatic ischemic presentations. AJNR Am J Neuroradiol. 2013;34(12):2252–8.

106. Sluimer JC, Kolodgie FD, Bijnens AP, Maxfield K, Pacheco E, Kutys B, et al. Thin-walled microvessels in human coronary atherosclerotic plaques show incomplete endothelial junctions relevance of compromised structural integrity for intraplaque microvascular leakage. J Am Coll Cardiol. 2009;53(17):1517–27.

107. Qiao Y, Etesami M, Astor BC, Zeiler SR, Trout HH 3rd, Wasserman BA. Carotid plaque neovascularization and hemorrhage detected by MR imaging are associated with recent cerebrovascular ischemic events. AJNR Am J Neuroradiol. 2012;33(4):755–60.

108. Lee SH, Jung SC, Kang DW, Kwon SU, Kim JS. Visualization of culprit perforators in anterolateral Pontine infarction: high-resolution magnetic resonance imaging study. Eur Neurol. 2017;78(5–6):229–33.

109. Sikkema T, Uyttenboogaart M, Eshghi O, De Keyser J, Brouns R, van Dijk JM, et al. Intracranial artery dissection. Eur J Neurol. 2014;21(6):820–6.

110. Park KJ, Jung SC, Kim HS, Choi CG, Kim SJ, Lee DH, et al. Multi-contrast high-resolution magnetic resonance findings of spontaneous and unruptured intracranial vertebral artery dissection: qualitative and quantitative analysis according to stages. Cerebrovasc Dis. 2016;42(1–2):23–31.

111. Habs M, Pfefferkorn T, Cyran CC, Grimm J, Rominger A, Hacker M, et al. Age determination of vessel wall hematoma in spontaneous cervical artery dissection: a multi-sequence 3T cardiovascular magnetic resonance study. J Cardiovasc Magn Reson. 2011;13:76.

112. Pfefferkorn T, Saam T, Rominger A, Habs M, Gerdes LA, Schmidt C, et al. Vessel wall inflammation in spontaneous cervical artery dissection: a prospective, observational positron emission tomography, computed tomography, and magnetic resonance imaging study. Stroke. 2011;42(6):1563–8.

113. Sakurai K, Miura T, Sagisaka T, Hattori M, Matsukawa N, Mase M, et al. Evaluation of luminal and vessel wall abnormalities in subacute and other stages of intracranial vertebrobasilar artery dissections using the volume isotropic turbo-spin-echo acquisition (VISTA) sequence: a preliminary study. J Neuroradiol. 2013;40(1):19–28.

114. Mizutani T. Natural course of intracranial arterial dissections. J Neurosurg. 2011;114(4):1037–44.

115. Ahn SS, Kim BM, Suh SH, Kim DJ, Kim DI, Shin YS, et al. Spontaneous symptomatic intracranial vertebrobasilar dissection: initial and follow-up imaging findings. Radiology. 2012;264(1):196–202.

116. Nagahata M, Manabe H, Hasegawa S, Takemura A. Morphological change of Unruptured vertebral artery dissection on serial MR examinations. Evaluation of the arterial outer contour by Basiparallel anatomical scanning (BPAS)-MRI. Interv Neuroradiol. 2006;12(Suppl 1):133–6.

117. Krings T, Choi IS. The many faces of intracranial arterial dissections. Interv Neuroradiol. 2010;16(2):151–60.

118. Jung SC, Kim HS, Choi CG, Kim SJ, Kwon SU, Kang DW, et al. Spontaneous and unruptured chronic intracranial artery dissection: high-resolution magnetic resonance imaging findings. Clin Neuroradiol. 2018;28(2):171–81.

119. Kim BM, Kim SH, Kim DI, Shin YS, Suh SH, Kim DJ, et al. Outcomes and prognostic factors of intracranial unruptured vertebrobasilar artery dissection. Neurology. 2011;76(20):1735–41.

120. Arauz A, Marquez JM, Artigas C, Balderrama J, Orrego H. Recanalization of vertebral artery dissection. Stroke. 2010;41(4):717–21.

121. Tan TY, Kuo YL, Lin WC, Chen TY. Effect of lipid-lowering therapy on the progression of intracranial arterial stenosis. J Neurol. 2009;256(2):187–93.

122. Kwon SU, Cho YJ, Koo JS, Bae HJ, Lee YS, Hong KS, et al. Cilostazol prevents the progression of the symptomatic intracranial arterial stenosis: the multicenter double-blind placebo-controlled trial of cilostazol in symptomatic intracranial arterial stenosis. Stroke. 2005;36(4):782–6.

123. Moniz E. L'encephalographie arterielle, son impartance dans la localisaton des tumeurs cerebrales. Rev Neurol. 1927;2:72–90.

124. Seldinger SI. Catheter replacement of the needle in percutaneous arteriography; a new technique. Acta Radiol. 1953;39(5):368–76.

125. Theodotou BC, Whaley R, Mahaley MS. Complications following transfemoral cerebral angiography for cerebral ischemia. Report of 159 angiograms and correlation with surgical risk. Surg Neurol. 1987;28(2):90–2.

126. Cloft HJ, Joseph GJ, Dion JE. Risk of cerebral angiography in patients with subarachnoid hemorrhage, cerebral aneurysm, and arteriovenous malformation: a meta-analysis. Stroke. 1999;30(2):317–20.

127. Kaufmann TJ, Huston J 3rd, Mandrekar JN, Schleck CD, Thielen KR, Kallmes DF. Complications of diagnostic cerebral angiography: evaluation of 19,826 consecutive patients. Radiology. 2007;243(3):812–9.

128. Chimowitz MI, Lynn MJ, Howlett-Smith H, Stern BJ, Hertzberg VS, Frankel MR, et al. Comparison of warfarin and aspirin for symptomatic intracranial arterial stenosis. NEJM. 2005;352:1305–16.

129. Warfarin-Aspirin Symptomatic Intracranial Disease Trial I. Design, progress and challenges of a double-blind trial of warfarin versus aspirin for symptomatic intracranial arterial stenosis. Neuroepidemiology. 2003;22(2):106–17.

130. Samuels OB, Joseph GJ, Lynn MJ, Smith HA, Chimowitz MI. A standardized method for measuring intracranial arterial stenosis. AJNR Am J Neuroradiol. 2000;21(4):643–6.

131. Villablanca JP, Rodriguez FJ, Stockman T, Dahliwal S, Omura M, Hazany S, et al. MDCT angiography for detection and quantification of small intra-

cranial arteries: comparison with conventional catheter angiography. AJR Am J Roentgenol. 2007;188(2):593–602.

132. Bartels E. Color-coded duplex ultrasonography of the cerebral vessels: atlas and manual. Stuttgart: Schattauer; 1999.

133. Maulik D. Spectral Doppler: basic principles and instrumentation. In: Maulik D, editor. Doppler ultrasound in obstetrics and gynecology. Berlin, Heidelberg: Springer Berlin Heidelberg; 2005. p. 19–34.

134. Caplan LR. Vertebrobasilar ischemia and hemorrhage: clinical findings, diagnosis and management of posterior circulation disease. 2nd ed. Cambridge: Cambridge University Press; 2015.

135. Bartels E, Flugel KA. Advantages of color Doppler imaging for the evaluation of vertebral arteries. J Neuroimag. 1993;3(4):229–33.

136. Jargiello T, Pietura R, Rakowski P, Szczerbo-Trojanowska M, Szajner M, Janczarek M. Power Doppler imaging in the evaluation of extracranial vertebral artery compression in patients with vertebrobasilar insufficiency. Eur J Ultrasound. 1998;8(3):149–55.

137. Ries S, Steinke W, Devuyst G, Artemis N, Valikovics A, Hennerici M. Power Doppler imaging and color Doppler flow imaging for the evaluation of normal and pathological vertebral arteries. J Neuroimag. 1998;8(2):71–4.

138. Sarkar S, Ghosh S, Ghosh SK, Collier A. Role of transcranial Doppler ultrasonography in stroke. Postgrad Med J. 2007;83(985):683–9.

139. Babikian VL, Wechsler LR. Transcranial doppler ultrasonography: Mosby-year book; 1993.

140. Arnolds BJ, von Reutern GM. Transcranial Doppler sonography. Examination technique and normal reference values. Ultrasound Med Biol. 1986;12(2):115–23.

141. Bartels E. Transcranial color-coded duplex ultrasonography in routine cerebrovascular diagnostics. Pers Med. 2012;1(1):325–30.

142. Purkayastha S, Sorond F. Transcranial Doppler ultrasound: technique and application. Semin Neurol. 2012;32(4):411–20.

143. Tsivgoulis G, Sharma VK, Hoover SL, Lao AY, Ardelt AA, Malkoff MD, et al. Applications and advantages of power motion-mode Doppler in acute posterior circulation cerebral ischemia. Stroke. 2008;39(4):1197–204.

144. Hwang J, Kim SJ, Hong JM, Bang OY, Chung CS, Lee KH, et al. Microembolic signals in acute posterior circulation cerebral ischemia: sources and consequences. Stroke. 2012;43(3):747–52.

145. Diehl RR, Sliwka U, Rautenberg W, Schwartz A. Evidence for embolization from a posterior cerebral artery thrombus by transcranial Doppler monitoring. Stroke. 1993;24(4):606–8.

146. Rautenberg W, Hennerici M. Pulsed Doppler assessment of innominate artery obstructive diseases. Stroke. 1988;19(12):1514–20.

147. László Csiba CB. Manual of neurosonology. In: Baracchini C, Csiba L, editors. Manual of neurosonology. Cambridge: Cambridge University Press; 2016. p. iii.

148. Kalaria VG, Jacob S, Irwin W, Schainfeld RM. Duplex ultrasonography of vertebral and subclavian arteries. J Am Soc Echocardiogr. 2005;18(10):1107–11.

149. Martin PJ, Evans DH, Naylor AR. Transcranial color-coded sonography of the basal cerebral circulation. Reference data from 115 volunteers. Stroke. 1994;25(2):390–6.

150. Grant EG, Benson CB, Moneta GL, Alexandrov AV, Baker JD, Bluth EI, et al. Carotid artery stenosis: grayscale and Doppler ultrasound diagnosis—Society of Radiologists in ultrasound consensus conference. Ultrasound Q. 2003;19(4):190–8.

151. Hoeffner EG, Case I, Jain R, Gujar SK, Shah GV, Deveikis JP, et al. Cerebral perfusion CT: technique and clinical applications. Radiology. 2004;231(3):632–44.

152. de Lucas EM, Sanchez E, Gutierrez A, Mandly AG, Ruiz E, Florez AF, et al. CT protocol for acute stroke: tips and tricks for general radiologists. Radiographics. 2008;28(6):1673–87.

153. Heit JJ, Wintermark M. Perfusion computed tomography for the evaluation of acute ischemic stroke: strengths and pitfalls. Stroke. 2016;47(4):1153–8.

154. Diekmann S, Siebert E, Juran R, Roll M, Deeg W, Bauknecht HC, et al. Dose exposure of patients undergoing comprehensive stroke imaging by multidetector-row CT: comparison of 320-detector row and 64-detector row CT scanners. AJNR Am J Neuroradiol. 2010;31(6):1003–9.

155. Tong E, Wintermark M. CTA-enhanced perfusion CT: an original method to perform ultra-low-dose CTA-enhanced perfusion CT. Neuroradiology. 2014;56(11):955–64.

156. Konstas AA, Goldmakher GV, Lee TY, Lev MH. Theoretic basis and technical implementations of CT perfusion in acute ischemic stroke, part 1: theoretic basis. AJNR Am J Neuroradiol. 2009;30(4):662–8.

157. Lin L, Bivard A, Parsons MW. Perfusion patterns of ischemic stroke on computed tomography perfusion. J Stroke. 2013;15(3):164–73.

158. Peretz S, Orion D, Last D, Mardor Y, Kimmel Y, Yehezkely S, et al. Incorporation of relative cerebral blood flow into CT perfusion maps reduces false 'at risk' penumbra. J Neurointerv Surg. 2018;10(7):657–62.

159. van der Hoeven EJ, Dankbaar JW, Algra A, Vos JA, Niesten JM, van Seeters T, et al. Additional diagnostic value of computed tomography perfusion for detection of acute ischemic stroke in the posterior circulation. Stroke. 2015;46(4):1113–5.

160. Sporns P, Schmidt R, Minnerup J, Dziewas R, Kemmling A, Dittrich R, et al. Computed tomography perfusion improves diagnostic accuracy in

acute posterior circulation stroke. Cerebrovasc Dis. 2016;41(5–6):242–7.

161. Shen J, Li X, Li Y, Wu B. Comparative accuracy of CT perfusion in diagnosing acute ischemic stroke: a systematic review of 27 trials. PLoS One. 2017;12(5):e0176622.

162. Pallesen LP, Lambrou D, Eskandari A, Barlinn J, Barlinn K, Reichmann H, et al. Perfusion computed tomography in posterior circulation stroke: predictors and prognostic implications of focal hypoperfusion. Eur J Neurol. 2018;25(5):725–31.

163. Nogueira RG, Jadhav AP, Haussen DC, Bonafe A, Budzik RF, Bhuva P, et al. Thrombectomy 6 to 24 hours after stroke with a mismatch between deficit and infarct. N Engl J Med. 2018;378(1):11–21.

164. Wintermark M, Reichhart M, Thiran JP, Maeder P, Chalaron M, Schnyder P, et al. Prognostic accuracy of cerebral blood flow measurement by perfusion computed tomography, at the time of emergency room admission, in acute stroke patients. Ann Neurol. 2002;51(4):417–32.

165. Albers GW, Marks MP, Kemp S, Christensen S, Tsai JP, Ortega-Gutierrez S, et al. Thrombectomy for stroke at 6 to 16 hours with selection by perfusion imaging. N Engl J Med. 2018;378(8):708–18.

166. Kidwell CS, Jahan R, Gornbein J, Alger JR, Nenov V, Ajani Z, et al. A trial of imaging selection and endovascular treatment for ischemic stroke. N Engl J Med. 2013;368(10):914–23.

167. Heit JJ, Zaharchuk G, Wintermark M. Advanced neuroimaging of acute ischemic stroke: penumbra and collateral assessment. Neuroimaging Clin N Am. 2018;28(4):585–97.

168. Bivard A, Krishnamurthy V, Stanwell P, Levi C, Spratt NJ, Davis S, et al. Arterial spin labeling versus bolus-tracking perfusion in hyperacute stroke. Stroke. 2014;45(1):127–33.

169. Zaharchuk G, El Mogy IS, Fischbein NJ, Albers GW. Comparison of arterial spin labeling and bolus perfusion-weighted imaging for detecting mismatch in acute stroke. Stroke. 2012;43(7):1843–8.

170. Grandin CB. Assessment of brain perfusion with MRI: methodology and application to acute stroke. Neuroradiology. 2003;45(11):755–66.

171. Wu L, Wu W, Tali ET, Yuh WT. Oligemia, penumbra, infarction: understanding Hypoperfusion with neuroimaging. Neuroimaging Clin N Am. 2018;28(4):599–609.

172. Kudo K, Terae S, Katoh C, Oka M, Shiga T, Tamaki N, et al. Quantitative cerebral blood flow measurement with dynamic perfusion CT using the vascular-pixel elimination method: comparison with H2(15) O positron emission tomography. AJNR Am J Neuroradiol. 2003;24(3):419–26.

173. Albers GW, Thijs VN, Wechsler L, Kemp S, Schlaug G, Skalabrin E, et al. Magnetic resonance imaging profiles predict clinical response to early reperfusion: the diffusion and perfusion imaging evaluation for understanding stroke evolution (DEFUSE) study. Ann Neurol. 2006;60(5):508–17.

174. Davis SM, Donnan GA, Parsons MW, Levi C, Butcher KS, Peeters A, et al. Effects of alteplase beyond 3 h after stroke in the echoplanar imaging thrombolytic evaluation trial (EPITHET): a placebo-controlled randomised trial. Lancet Neurol. 2008;7(4):299–309.

Medical Treatment

Kazunori Toyoda and Jong S. Kim

Introduction

Posterior circulation stroke (PCS) accounts for 20–40% of ischemic stroke [1–3] (see Chap. 3). In a single-center National Cerebral and Cardiovascular Center (NCVC) Stroke Registry from Japan [4], 22% of patients with ischemic stroke had posterior circulation stroke (PCS) (14.7% only in the posterior circulation and 7.7% both in the posterior and anterior circulations, Table 10.1, Fig. 10.1).

Although the basic pathophysiology of stroke appears to be the same, the optimal medical treatment strategy may be different considering that the stroke mechanisms and underlying characteristics of PCS are somewhat different from those of anterior circulation stroke (ACS), as discussed in Chap. 3. However, we were able to find very few appropriate articles on the treatment strategies specific for PCS. Most clinical trials were performed on patients with ACS and did not specifically include or exclude patients with PCS. Thus, scientific evidence for medical treatment has been principally established by using data on ACS, whereas specific treatment strategies for PCS have not been based on appropriately targeted clinical trials.

In this chapter, we first discuss the medical management based on the recommendations for overall stroke patients. We will then discuss the special points that should be addressed in the management of patients with PCS.

Critical Care in Acute Stroke

The first step of acute stroke care after recognition of stroke symptoms is a quick hospital visit using emergency medical services. Earlier arrival to stroke centers equipped for acute reperfusion therapy, i.e., intravenous thrombolysis and mechanical thrombectomy, increases the chance of receiving appropriate therapy with a shorter time delay; this, in turn, increases the chance to obtain better clinical outcomes. To facilitate quick hospital visits, public education regarding stroke warning signs is strongly recommended. "Act FAST" is a globally-known stroke awareness-raising campaign—sudden onset of face drooping, arm weakness, or speech difficulty are introduced as typical signs suggesting stroke [5]. These signs, mostly reflecting dysfunction of motor and speech systems, can undoubtedly appear in patients with PCS; however, these patients often present with other symptoms, such as vertigo, imbalance, double vision, and nausea. These are less often recognized as stroke symptoms by patients and even

K. Toyoda (✉)
Department of Cerebrovascular Medicine, National Cerebral and Cardiovascular Center, Osaka, Japan
e-mail: toyoda@ncvc.go.jp

J. S. Kim
Department of Neurology, Asan Medical Center, University of Ulsan, Seoul, South Korea
e-mail: jongskim@amc.seoul.kr

© Springer Nature Singapore Pte Ltd. 2021
J. S. Kim (ed.), *Posterior Circulation Stroke*, https://doi.org/10.1007/978-981-15-6739-1_10

Table 10.1 Baseline characteristics and stroke features in acute ischemic patients according to infarct distribution: National Cerebral and Cardiovascular Center (NCVC) Stroke Registry

	Posterior circulation stroke ($n = 662^a$)	Anterior circulation stroke ($n = 2301$)	P
Women	212 (32.0%)	958 (41.6%)	<0.001
Age, years	72.9 ± 12.5	74.5 ± 12.2	0.004
History of stroke	227 (34.3%)	703 (30.6%)	0.069
Ischemic heart disease	72 (10.9%)	263 (11.4%)	0.691
Atrial fibrillation	170 (25.7%)	869 (37.8%)	<0.001
Hypertension	541 (81.7%)	1756 (76.3%)	0.003
Dyslipidemia	350 (52.9%)	1153 (50.1%)	0.210
Diabetes mellitus	205 (31.0%)	531 (23.1%)	<0.001
Current smoking	121 (18.3%)	419 (18.2%)	0.968
Habitual drinking	272 (41.1%)	850 (36.9%)	0.053
Initial systolic blood pressure, mmHg	161.2 ± 28.9	159.8 ± 29.1	0.268
Initial diastolic blood pressure, mmHg	87.0 ± 17.7	87.8 ± 18.1	0.339
Initial NIH stroke scale score	3 [2–6]	5 [2–14]	<0.001
Stroke subtype by TOAST classification			<0.001
Cardioembolism	150 (22.7%)	881 (38.3%)	
Large-artery atherosclerosis	98 (14.8%)	328 (14.2%)	
Small vessel occlusion	137 (20.7%)	374 (16.3%)	
Other	277 (41.8%)	718 (31.2%)	
Receiving intravenous thrombolysis	39 (5.9%)	340 (14.8%)	<0.001
Receiving acute endovascular therapy	26 (3.9%)	122 (5.3%)	0.142

Number (%), mean ± standard deviation, or median [interquartile range]
Studied patients are the same as those in Ref. 4 ($n = 2965$), except for 2 patients whose infarct locations are unclear
Details of the NCVC Stroke Registry are introduced in Ref. 4
NIH: National Institutes of Health, TOAST: Trial of Org 10172 in Acute Stroke Treatment
[a]Including 435 patients with infarcts only in the posterior circulation and 227 patients with infarcts both in the posterior and anterior circulation

doctors, resulting in delaying a quick hospital visit. Indeed, prehospital and intrahospital time delays occur more often in patients with PCS than in those with ACS [6, 7].

The National Institutes of Health Stroke Scale (NIHSS) is an essential scoring system for quick assessment of neurological severity in stroke patients. The NIHSS is indispensable to stroke teams for judging a patient's eligibility for acute reperfusion therapy and other stroke care strategies. However, the scale is highly weighted toward neurological deficits caused by ACS. In 407 patients with PCS registered in the New England Medical Center posterior circulation registry, the most frequent symptoms were dizziness (47%), unilateral limb weakness (41%), dysarthria (31%), headache (28%), and nausea or vomiting (27%) [8]. Three of these five major

symptoms are not included in the components of the NIHSS. In a single-center comparison between 101 patients with PCS and 209 patients with ACS who did not undergo acute reperfusion therapy, the optimal cutoff baseline NIHSS scores for a modified Rankin Scale score of 0–2 at 3 months poststroke were ≤5 (sensitivity, 84%; specificity, 81%) and ≤8 (sensitivity, 80%; specificity, 82%), respectively [9]. In 7178 minor stroke patients (baseline NIHSS score of ≤4) registered in the Clinical Research Center for Stroke-5th division registry in South Korea, PCS with vertebrobasilar large vessel disease was independently associated with a modified Rankin Scale score of 2–6 at 3 months compared with ACS [10]. Thus, for patients with PCS, we should be careful about predicting chronic outcomes based on their NIHSS scores.

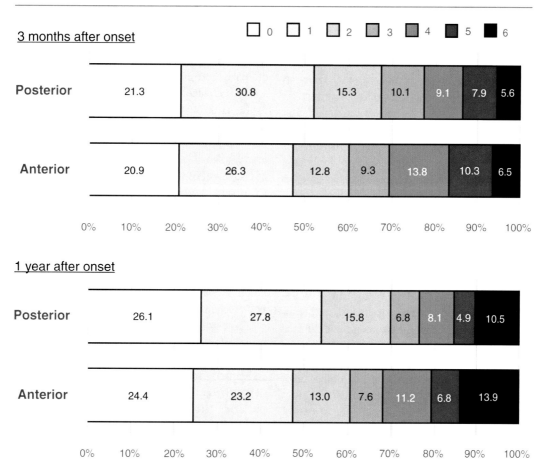

Fig. 10.1 Modified Rankin Scale scores at 3 months and 1 year after the onset of ischemic stroke according to infarct distribution: NCVC Stroke Registry. *NCVC* National Cerebral and Cardiovascular Center. (Newly analyzed using the dataset of Ref. 4)

Evidence for intravenous thrombolysis and mechanical thrombectomy was collected based on trials that mainly included patients with ACS. Therefore, mechanical thrombectomy for PCS remains understudied as compared to that for ACS. Nevertheless, most centers perform mechanical thrombectomy in appropriate PCA cases based on the trial results on ACS. These issues are described in Chap. 11. In an acute clinical setting for PCS, we should be extremely careful about sudden swelling and hemorrhagic transformation after cerebellar infarction, because they compress the brainstem and the fourth ventricle, subsequently resulting in hydrocephalus and brain-stem herniation (malignant cerebellar infarction) [3]. A large occipital infarction may also produce massive edema and hydrocephalus. A decreased level of consciousness is a reliable clinical symptom suggesting increased intracranial pressure with brain edema. Again, randomized trials for the efficacy of early decompressive craniectomy were performed in patients with ACS, but not in those with PCS. Nevertheless, decompressive craniectomy is being performed in patients with PCS and has been considered to be effective, especially for relatively young patients (e.g., <60 years in age) [11]. These surgical therapies are described in Chap. 13.

Antiplatelet Therapy

Antithrombotic therapy is an essential therapeutic strategy at every stage of stroke management, especially for secondary prevention. Antiplatelet therapy should be considered over anticoagulation for most patients with noncardioembolic stroke. Recent major trials on antiplatelet therapy for secondary stroke prevention seldom conducted subgroup analysis for posterior versus anterior circulation stroke. Nevertheless, it appears that therapeutic strategies involving antiplatelet agents are the same for patients with PCS and those with ACS.

There are differences in the recommendation of antiplatelet therapy between early after stroke and late after stroke. Globally, aspirin, a cyclooxygenase inhibitor, and clopidogrel, a thienopyridine derivative, are the two most-widely used oral antiplatelet agents. According to the guidelines set forth by American Heart Association/American Stroke Association, the combination of these two agents might be considered for initiation within 24 h of a minor ischemic stroke or transient ischemic attack (TIA) and continued for 21 days [12].

However, minor stroke can have diverse underlying mechanisms, and previous large-scale trials did not differentiate the detailed mechanisms. In patients with large-artery disease, especially with artery-to-artery embolism or in situ thrombotic occlusion, or in those who have systemic atherosclerosis (e.g., coronary heart disease, peripheral limb atherosclerosis), dual antiplatelets may be needed for a longer period of time, because these patients have a high risk of recurrent ischemic events. On the other hand, in patients with small-artery disease without evidence of atherosclerosis, dual antiplatelets may have to be used for a shorter period of time, because they are more susceptible to cerebral hemorrhages and at less risk for future ischemic stroke [13]. Thus, although the average period of dual antiplatelet use was 21 days in the recent CHANCE trial [14], the duration of administering dual antiplatelets may have to be adjusted based on the risk of recurrent ischemic stroke and hemorrhages in individual patients [15].

As compared to aspirin alone, cilostazol, a phosphodiesterase 3 inhibitor, in combination with aspirin attenuated the progression of intracranial atherosclerosis 6 months after ischemic stroke with stenosis of major intracranial arteries in the Trial of cilOstazol in Symptomatic intracranial arterial Stenosis (TOSS) [16]; of the 135 patients enrolled in the trial, 23 (17%) had basilar artery stenosis, and the others had stenosis in the M1 segment of the middle cerebral artery. In the Cilostazol Stroke Prevention Study for Antiplatelet Combination (CSPS.com) trial, the combination of cilostazol with aspirin or clopidogrel had a lower risk of ischemic stroke recurrence and a similar risk of severe or life-threatening bleeding compared to aspirin or clopidogrel alone in patients with high-risk noncardioembolic ischemic stroke [17]. Thus, the combination of cilostazol and aspirin or clopidogrel seems to be an effective and safe dual antiplatelet therapy that could be used even in the chronic stage of ischemic stroke. In the CSPS.com, 23% (430/1879) of participants had infarcts only in the posterior circulation. Subgroup analysis of the main outcomes according to the infarct location has not yet been performed.

Anticoagulation

Generally, the proportion of cardiac embolism is smaller in PCS than in ACS patients (see Chap. 3). Nevertheless, in the New England Medical Center Posterior Circulation registry, 40% of PCS patients had embolic stroke, and 24% of them were diagnosed with cardioembolism [18]. In South Korea, potential cardioembolic sources were found only in 11% of 591 consecutive patients with PCS in the Hallym Stroke Registry [19]. In the NCVC Stroke Registry, cardioembolism accounted for 23% of PCS and 38% of ACS (Table 10.1).

For patients with cardioembolic stroke, anticoagulation is the first-choice antithrombotic therapy, and anticoagulation therapeutic strategies used for PCS are not different from those for ACS. Vitamin K antagonists, typically warfarin, had been the sole oral anticoagulants for half a century until 2010; a direct thrombin inhibitor, dabigatran, and direct inhibitors of activated factor X, including rivaroxaban, apixaban, and edoxaban, were approved for clinical use in nonvalvular atrial fibrillation (NVAF) based on the evidence from randomized controlled trials comparing them with warfarin. The four newer anticoagulants are collectively named direct oral anticoagulants (DOACs) or nonvitamin K antagonist oral anticoagulants (NOACs). Meta-analyses of the randomized controlled trials showed that NOACs are at least as effective as warfarin for secondary stroke prevention in NVAF patients, with around half the risk of intracranial hemorrhage [20, 21]. The same trend was reported for NOACs versus warfarin on subsequent events after stroke in the real-world clinical setting, such as the Stroke Acute Management with Urgent Risk-factor Assessment and Improvement (SAMURAI)-NVAF study and a meta-analysis including the SAMURAI-NVAF [22, 23]. An interesting feature of the study and

meta-analysis was relatively early initiation of NOACs, with a median of 4 days after stroke onset in the SAMURAI-NVAF and 5 days in the meta-analysis [23, 24].

Of the 1192 participants in the SAMURAI-NVAF study, 175 had infarcts only in the posterior circulation. Kaplan–Meier curves for ischemic and hemorrhagic endpoints in these 175 patients are shown in Fig. 10.2. Contrary to the overall results described above, NOACs were significantly more effective than warfarin in reducing the risk of stroke or systemic embolism, but NOACs and warfarin were similar regarding the risk of intracranial hemorrhage. Note that the analyses used data from a small number of patients, and the results may have occurred by chance. For using anticoagulation as secondary prevention, there are no differences in guideline recommendations regarding the doses and timing of initiation between patients with PCS and those with ACS. However, as huge cerebellar or occipital infarcts can be fatal, especially when hemor-

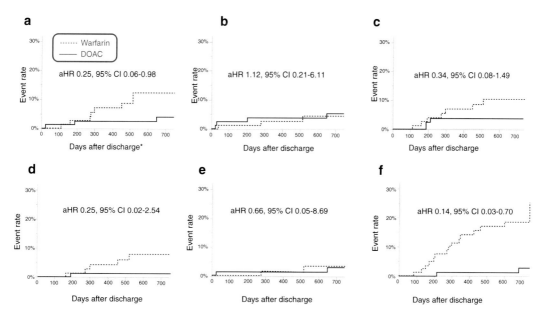

Fig. 10.2 Kaplan–Meier curves for clinical events in patients with posterior circulation stroke: SAMURAI-NVAF study. (**a**) Stroke/systemic embolism. (**b**) Major bleeding. (**c**) Ischemic events. (**d**) Ischemic stroke/TIA. (**e**) Intracranial hemorrhage. (**f**) Mortality. *Days after acute hospital discharge or 30 days after hospital admission, whichever occurred first. *aHR* adjusted hazard ratio (DOAC/warfarin) for sex, age, CHADS2 after the index stroke onset, admission National Institutes of Health Stroke Scale score, and serum creatinine, *DOAC* direct oral anticoagulant, *NVAF* nonvalvular atrial fibrillation, *SAMURAI* Stroke Acute Management with Urgent Risk-factor Assessment and Improvement (Newly analyzed using the dataset of Ref. 22)

rhagic transformation occurs, it would be better to delay the initiation of oral anticoagulants in these cases. Using a lower dose might be another strategy in the risk period.

Anticoagulation may also play a role in the prevention of ischemic stroke in patients without NVAF. As discussed in Chap. 3, patent foramen ovale (PFO)-related strokes appear to occur in the PCS more often than in the ACS. Randomized trials showed that PFO closure more effectively reduces future ischemic strokes than using antithrombotics alone in patients with high-risk PFO (large amount of shunt, large shunt size, presence of atrial septal aneurysm) [25–27]. However, antithrombotics are still needed in patients who do not undergo closure, e.g., those who are old, those who are unwilling to undergo the closure procedure, and those who have a low-risk PFO. A meta-analysis combining data from previous PFO closure studies showed that, in patients with cryptogenic stroke and PFO, anticoagulation (warfarin and NOACs combined) may be better for preventing recurrent ischemic stroke than aspirin (odds ratio, 0.48; 95% CI, 0.24–0.96; $P = 0.04$) [28]. Nevertheless, the current evidence is not strong enough to support the use of NOACs over aspirin in patients with PFO. Future trials are needed to determine the role of anticoagulants, especially NOACs or dual antiplatelets, in patients with PFO.

Finally, vertebral artery stump syndrome is an embolic stroke resulting from the occlusion of the stump of the vertebral artery origin. Kawano et al. [29] identified 12 (1.4%) patients with the syndrome in 865 acute PCS patients; of these, all three patients receiving antiplatelet therapy developed recurrent PCS during the acute phase. Therefore, anticoagulation may be needed in these patients.

Risk Factor Management

Risk factors for patients with PCS are described in Chap. 3. Patients with PCS should strictly control these risk factors for secondary stroke prevention. In this chapter, appropriate controls of blood pressure and lipid levels are described.

Blood Pressure Management

In the seventh report of the Joint National Committee on Prevention, Detection, Evaluation, and Treatment of High Blood Pressure (JNC7) guidelines, hypertension was defined as systolic blood pressure (BP) $\geq$140 mmHg or diastolic BP $\geq$90 mmHg, and antihypertensive pharmacotherapy was recommended for stroke survivors with BP $\geq$140/90 mmHg [30]. In contrast, newer guidelines by the American College of Cardiology/American Heart Association advocated changing the definition of hypertension to systolic BP $\geq$130 mmHg or diastolic BP $\geq$80 mmHg and described that a BP goal of <130/80 mmHg may be reasonable for stroke survivors [31] (Fig. 10.3). The results from the Secondary Prevention of Small Subcortical Strokes (SPS3) trial partly support the revised recommendations; in the trial, a systolic BP goal <130 mmHg tended to reduce the risk of any stroke recurrence and significantly reduced a risk of intracerebral hemorrhage in patients with recent lacunar stroke [32]. A meta-analysis of 4 randomized controlled trials, including the SPS3, Recurrent Stroke Prevention Clinical Outcome (RESPECT), and others, showed that intensive BP lowering to <130/80 mmHg significantly reduced a risk of any stroke recurrence (relative risk 0.78, 95% CI 0.64–0.96) and of hemorrhagic stroke (relative risk 0.25, 95% CI 0.07–0.90) [33]. As another supporting finding, the prospective, multicenter, observational Bleeding with Antithrombotic Therapy (BAT) Study, which involved 4009 patients taking oral antithrombotic agents for cardiovascular or cerebrovascular diseases, used receiver operating characteristic curve analysis over a median follow-up of 19 months to show that the optimal cutoff BP level for predicting the impending risk of intracranial hemorrhage was $\geq$130/81 mmHg [34].

There are no clear differences in recommendations on the timing for initiation of antihypertensive therapy, the target BP, and the choice of antihypertensive agents and other processes for BP lowering between PSC and ACS. Although hypertension is the leading risk factor for stroke in general, it was reported to be a more important

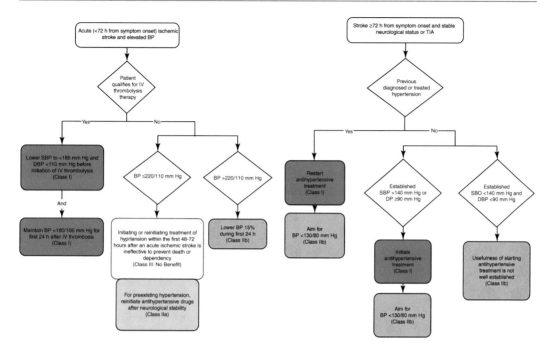

Fig. 10.3 Management of hypertension in patients with acute ischemic stroke (left) and those with a previous history of stroke (secondary stroke prevention, right). *BP* blood pressure, *DBP* diastolic blood pressure, *IV* intravenous, *SBP* systolic blood pressure, *TIA* transient ischemic attack. (Reprinted from Ref. 31)

risk factor in patients with PCS than those with ACS in previous studies (see Chap. 3) including NCVC Stroke Registry (82% vs. 76%, Table 10.1) and in a Korean study that enrolled only the patients with atherosclerotic stroke [35]. Therefore, hypertension control may have to be more strict in patients with PCS than in those with ACS.

One exception would be patients in the acute stage of stroke with elevated BP and an unstable neurological status. In particular, BP should be carefully managed in patients with hemodynamic failure associated with severe stenosis or occlusion of the vertebra-basilar arteries. These patients may show a fluctuating or gradually progressing neurological symptoms associated with decreased BP. In these cases, BP should be lowered cautiously until the neurological status becomes stable. Some patients show discontinuation of neurological progression or even improvement of symptoms with transient, pharmacologically induced hypertension [36]. Recent studies showed that this "induced pharmacological hypertension" is safe and feasible in patients with acute stroke, especially in patients with early neurological deterioration secondary to large-artery or small-artery disease [36, 37].

The potential benefit of induced hypertension has not been specifically examined in patients with PCS. However, given the fact that induced hypertension was done more frequently in patients with noncardioembolic stroke than in those with cardiogenic embolism [36], induced hypertension might be more useful in patients with PCS than in ACS patients. It has also been shown that excessive BP lowering may be hazardous even in the subacute–chronic stage if posterior fossa is hypoperfused due to severe atherosclerotic vertebrobasilar diseases. In this study, among patients with recent stroke or TIA associated with ≥50% stenosis of vertebral or basilar arteries, those with both low blood flow and BP <140/90 mm Hg had a significantly higher risk of subsequent stroke (hazard ratio of 4.5 [confidence interval 1.3–16.0], $P = 0.02$), compared with the other subgroups [38].

Lipid Management

Nowadays, it becomes easier to control low-density lipoprotein (LDL) cholesterol level, as pharmacotherapy has improved from classical statins to strong statins and proprotein convertase subtilisin/kexin type 9 (PCSK9) inhibitors. Recent guidelines and consensus statements on lipid control often use the terminology of atherosclerotic cardiovascular disease; the term usually includes two major conditions: coronary artery disease and ischemic stroke. Table 10.2 shows the risk categories of atherosclerotic cardiovascu-lar disease and the corresponding lipid-lowering goals [39]. The strict goal of an LDL cholesterol level of <70 mg/dL is recommended in the case of recent hospitalization for carotid vascular disease and that of <55 mg/dL is recommended in the case of progression of atherosclerotic cardiovascular disease after achieving an LDL cholesterol level of <70 mg/dL. However, such recommendations seem to be heavily influenced by evidence from studies on coronary artery disease. New guidelines on lipid control based purely on evidence from stroke research are required.

Table 10.2 Risk categories for atherosclerotic cardiovascular disease and corresponding lipid level reduction goals

		Treatment coals		
Risk category	Risk factors[a]/10-year risk[b]	LDL-C (mg/dL)	Non-HDL-C (mg/dL)	Apo B (mg/dL)
Extreme risk	– Progressive ASCVD including unstable angina in patients after achieving an LDL-C < 70 mg/dL	<55	<80	<70
	– Established clinical cardiovascular disease in patients with DM, CKD 3/4, or HeFH			
	– History of premature ASCVD (<55 male, <65 female)			
Very high risk	– Established or recent hospitalization for ACS, coronary, carotid or peripheral vascular disease, 10-year risk >20%	<70	<100	<80
	– Diabetes or CKD 3/4 with 1 or more risk factor(s)			
	– HeFH			
High risk	– ≥2 risk factors and 10-year risk 10–20%	<100	<130	<90
	– Diabetes or CKD 3/4 with no other risk factors			
Moderate risk	≤2 risk factors and 10-year risk <10%	<100	<130	<90
Low risk	0 risk factors	<130	<160	NR

Abbreviations: *ACS* acute coronary syndrome, *ASCVD* atherosclerotic cardiovascular disease, *CKD* chronic kidney disease, *DM* diabetes mellitus, *HDL-C* high-density lipoprotein cholesterol, *HeFH* heterozygous familial hypercholesterolemia, *LDL-C* low-density lipoprotein cholesterol, *MESA* Multi-Ethnic Study of Atherosclerosis, *NR* not recommended, *UKPDS* United Kingdom Prospective Diabetes Study

Reproduced with permission from Garber et al. *Endocr Pract.* 2017;23:207–238

Reprinted from Ref. 39

[a]Major independent risk factors are high LDL-C, polycystic ovary syndrome, cigarette smoking, hypertension (blood pressure ≥ 140/90 mm Hg or on hypertensive medication), low HDL-C (<40 mg/dL), family history of coronary artery disease (in male, first-degree relative younger than 55 years; in female, first-degree relative younger than 65 years), chronic renal disease (CKD) stage 3/4, evidence of coronary artery calcification and age (men ≥45; women ≥55 years), Subtract 1 risk factor if the person has high HDL-C

[b]Framingham risk scoring is applied to determine 10-year risk

In the recent multinational (French and Korean) comparison of 70 mg/dL and 100 mg/dL target LDL cholesterol levels after ischemic stroke (TST) trial, investigators enrolled patients who had a stroke in the previous 3 months or TIA within the previous 15 days with evidence of cerebrovascular or cardiac atherosclerosis. Patients were randomly assigned to target LDL cholesterol levels of less than 70 mg/dL or 100 ± 10 mg/dL. Statin with or without ezetimibe was used. The primary outcome was the composite of ischemic stroke, myocardial infarction, new symptoms requiring urgent coronary or carotid revascularization, and vascular death. A total of 2860 patients were enrolled, and follow-up was for a median of 3.5 years. The mean achieved LDL cholesterol levels were 65 and 96 mg/dL, respectively. The primary composite endpoint occurred in 121 (8.5%) and 156 (10.9%) patients, respectively (adjusted hazard ratio, 0.77 [95% CI, 0.61–0.98; $P = 0.035$]). The incidence of intracranial hemorrhages did not differ between the groups [40].

The result showed that LDL cholesterol <70 mg/dL, but not 100 mg/dL, should be the appropriate target for patients with atherosclerotic stroke. However, the difference was not evident when Korean patients were separately analyzed. Although this may be attributed to the smaller number of patients and shorter follow-up period for Korean (versus French) patients, the appropriate LDL target for Asian stroke patients still remains unclear. The LDL target for nonatherosclerotic (e.g., small vessel disease) also remains unknown. In the TST trial, the location of atherosclerosis was precisely analyzed for Korean patients, and it was found that there was no significant difference in the occurrence of primary outcome between patients with ACS and PCS (unpublished data).

Control for Other Risk Factors

In the previous studies (see Chap. 3), diabetes was found to be the more important risk factor in patients with PCS than in those with ACS (Table 10.1). In a study that enrolled only the patients with atherosclerotic stroke, diabetes mellitus (45% vs. 32%) and metabolic syndrome (34% vs. 28%) were more prevalent in patients with PCS than in those with ACS [35]. Therefore, PCS seems to be closely associated with metabolic derangement, and maintaining a healthy lifestyle such as a healthy diet, regular exercise, and weight control may be even more important in patients with PCS than in those with ACS. Cessation of smoking and heavy alcohol drinking should also be strongly recommended in patients with stroke regardless of the location of cerebral arterial diseases.

References

1. Merwick Á, Werring D. Posterior circulation ischaemic stroke. BMJ. 2014;348:g3175.
2. Nouh A, Remke J, Ruland S. Ischemic posterior circulation stroke: a review of anatomy, clinical presentations, diagnosis, and current management. Front Neurol. 2014;5:30.
3. Schulz UG, Fischer U. Posterior circulation cerebrovascular syndromes: diagnosis and management. J Neurol Neurosurg Psychiatry. 2017;88(1):45–53.
4. Toyoda K, Koga M, Yamagami H, Yokota C, Sato S, Inoue M, Tanaka T, Endo K, Fujinami J, Ihara M, Nagatsuka K, Minematsu K. Seasonal variations in neurological severity and outcomes of ischemic stroke: 5-year single-center observational study. Circ J. 2018;82(5):1443–50.
5. Kleindorfer DO, Miller R, Moomaw CJ, Alwell K, Broderick JP, Khoury J, Woo D, Flaherty ML, Zakaria T, Kissela BM. Designing a message for public education regarding stroke: does FAST capture enough stroke? Stroke. 2007;38(10):2864–8.
6. Sarraj A, Medrek S, Albright K, Martin-Schild S, Bibars W, Vahidy F, Grotta JC, Savitz SI. Posterior circulation stroke is associated with prolonged door-to-needle time. Int J Stroke. 2015;10(5):672–8.
7. Sommer P, Seyfang L, Posekany A, Ferrari J, Lang W, Fertl E, Serles W, Töll T, Kiechl S, Greisenegger S. Prehospital and intra-hospital time delays in posterior circulation stroke: results from the Austrian Stroke Unit Registry. J Neurol. 2017;264(1):131–8.
8. Searls DE, Pazdera L, Korbel E, Vysata O, Caplan LR. Symptoms and signs of posterior circulation ischemia in the New England Medical Center Posterior Circulation Registry. Arch Neurol. 2012;69(3):346–51.
9. Sato S, Toyoda K, Uehara T, Toratani N, Yokota C, Moriwaki H, Naritomi H, Minematsu K. Baseline NIH stroke scale score predicting outcome in anterior and posterior circulation strokes. Neurology. 2008;70(24 Pt 2):2371–7.

10. Kim JT, Park MS, Choi KH, Kim BJ, Han MK, Park TH, Park SS, Lee KB, Lee BC, Yu KH, Oh MS, Cha JK, Kim DH, Nah HW, Lee J, Lee SJ, Ko Y, Kim JG, Park JM, Kang K, Cho YJ, Hong KS, Choi JC, Kim DE, Ryu WS, Shin DI, Yeo MJ, Kim WJ, Lee J, Lee JS, Bae HJ, Saver JL, Cho KH. Clinical outcomes of posterior versus anterior circulation infarction with low National Institutes of Health stroke scale scores. Stroke. 2017;48(1):55–62.

11. Wijdicks EF, Sheth KN, Carter BS, Greer DM, Kasner SE, Kimberly WT, Schwab S, Smith EE, Tamargo RJ, Wintermark M, American Heart Association Stroke Council. Recommendations for the management of cerebral and cerebellar infarction with swelling: a statement for healthcare professionals from the American Heart Association/American Stroke Association. Stroke. 2014;45(4):1222–38.

12. Kernan WN, Ovbiagele B, Black HR, Bravata DM, Chimowitz MI, Ezekowitz MD, Fang MC, Fisher M, Furie KL, Heck DV, Johnston SC, Kasner SE, Kittner SJ, Mitchell PH, Rich MW, Richardson D, Schwamm LH, Wilson JA, American Heart Association Stroke Council, Council on Cardiovascular and Stroke Nursing, Council on Clinical Cardiology, Council on Peripheral Vascular Disease. Guidelines for the prevention of stroke in patients with stroke and transient ischemic attack: a guideline for healthcare professionals from the American Heart Association/American Stroke Association. Stroke. 2014;45(7):2160–236.

13. Benavente OR, Hart RG, McClure LA, Szychowski JM, Coffey CS, Pearce LA, SPS3 Investigators. Effects of clopidogrel added to aspirin in patients with recent lacunar stroke. N Engl J Med. 2012;367:817–25.

14. Wang Y, Wang Y, Zhao X, Liu L, Wang D, Wang C, Wang C, Li H, Meng X, Cui L, Jia J, Dong Q, Xu A, Zeng J, Li Y, Wang Z, Xia H, Johnston SC, CHANCE Investigators. Clopidogrel with aspirin in acute minor stroke or transient ischemic attack. N Engl J Med. 2013;369:11–9.

15. Wang Y, Johnston SC, Bath PM, Grotta JC, Pan Y, Amarenco P, Wang Y, Simon T, Kim JS, Jeng JS, Liu L, Lin Y, Wong KSL, Wang D, Li H. Acute dual antiplatelet therapy for minor ischaemic stroke or transient ischaemic attack. BMJ. 2019;364:l895.

16. Kwon SU, Cho YJ, Koo JS, Bae HJ, Lee YS, Hong KS, Lee JH, Kim JS. Cilostazol prevents the progression of the symptomatic intracranial arterial stenosis: the multicenter double-blind placebo-controlled trial of cilostazol in symptomatic intracranial arterial stenosis. Stroke. 2005;36(4):782–6.

17. Toyoda K, Uchiyama S, Yamaguchi T, Easton JD, Kimura K, Hoshino H, Sakai N, Okada Y, Tanaka K, Origasa H, Naritomi H, Houkin K, Yamaguchi K, Isobe M, Minematsu K, CSPS.com Trial Investigators. Dual antiplatelet therapy using cilostazol for secondary prevention in patients with high-risk ischaemic stroke in Japan: a multicentre, open-label, randomised controlled trial. Lancet Neurol. 2019;18(6):539–48.

18. Caplan LR, Wityk RJ, Glass TA, Tapia J, Pazdera L, Chang HM, Teal P, Dashe JF, Chaves CJ, Breen JC, Vemmos K, Amarenco P, Tettenborn B, Leary M, Estol C, Dewitt LD, Pessin MS. New England Medical Center Posterior Circulation registry. Ann Neurol. 2004;56(3):389–98.

19. Lee JH, Han SJ, Yun YH, Choi HC, Jung S, Cho SJ, Yu KH, Lee SM, Hwang SH, Song HK, Kwon KH, Lee BC. Posterior circulation ischemic stroke in Korean population. Eur J Neurol. 2006;13(7):742–8.

20. Salazar CA, del Aguila D, Cordova EG. Direct thrombin inhibitors versus vitamin K antagonists for preventing cerebral or systemic embolism in people with non-valvular atrial fibrillation. Cochrane Database Syst Rev. 2014;3:CD009893.

21. Bruins Slot KM, Berge E. Factor Xa inhibitors versus vitamin K antagonists for preventing cerebral or systemic embolism in patients with atrial fibrillation. Cochrane Database Syst Rev. 2018;3:CD008980.

22. Yoshimura S, Koga M, Sato S, Todo K, Yamagami H, Kumamoto M, Itabashi R, Terasaki T, Kimura K, Yagita Y, Shiokawa Y, Kamiyama K, Okuda S, Okada Y, Takizawa S, Hasegawa Y, Kameda T, Shibuya S, Nagakane Y, Ito Y, Matsuoka H, Takamatsu K, Nishiyama K, Fujita K, Kamimura T, Ando D, Ide T, Yoshimoto T, Shiozawa M, Matsubara S, Yamaguchi Y, Kinoshita N, Matsuki T, Takasugi J, Tokunaga K, Higashida K, Homma K, Kario K, Arihiro S, Toyoda K, SAMURAI Study Investigators. Two-year outcomes of anticoagulation for acute ischemic stroke with nonvalvular atrial fibrillation: SAMURAI-NVAF Study. Circ J. 2018;82(7):1935–42.

23. Seiffge DJ, Paciaroni M, Wilson D, Koga M, Macha K, Cappellari M, Schaedelin S, Shakeshaft C, Takagi M, Tsivgoulis G, Bonetti B, Kallmünzer B, Arihiro S, Alberti A, Polymeris AA, Ambler G, Yoshimura S, Venti M, Bonati LH, Muir KW, Yamagami H, Thilemann S, Altavilla R, Peters N, Inoue M, Bobinger T, Agnelli G, Brown MM, Sato S, Acciarresi M, Jager HR, Bovi P, Schwab S, Lyrer P, Caso V, Toyoda K, Werring DJ, Engelter ST, De Marchis GM, CROMIS-2, RAF, RAF-DOAC, SAMURAI, NOACISP LONGTERM, Erlangen and Verona registry collaborators. Direct oral anticoagulants versus vitamin K antagonists after recent ischemic stroke in patients with atrial fibrillation. Ann Neurol. 2019;85(6):823–34.

24. Toyoda K, Arihiro S, Todo K, Yamagami H, Kimura K, Furui E, Terasaki T, Shiokawa Y, Kamiyama K, Takizawa S, Okuda S, Okada Y, Kameda T, Nagakane Y, Hasegawa Y, Mochizuki H, Ito Y, Nakashima T, Takamatsu K, Nishiyama K, Kario K, Sato S, Koga M, SAMURAI Study Investigators. Trends in oral anticoagulant choice for acute stroke patients with nonvalvular atrial fibrillation in Japan: the SAMURAI-NVAF study. Int J Stroke. 2015;10(6):836–42.

25. Mas JL, Derumeaux G, Guillon B, Massardier E, Hosseini H, Mechtouff L, et al. Patent foramen ovale closure or anticoagulation vs. antiplatelets after stroke. N Engl J Med. 2017;377:1011–21.

26. Sondergaard L, Kasner SE, Rhodes JF, Andersen G, et al. Patent foramen ovale closure or antiplate-

let therapy for cryptogenic stroke. N Engl J Med. 2017;377:1033–42.

27. Lee PH, Song JK, Heo R, Lee S, Kim DH, et al. Cryptogenic stroke and high risk patent foramen ovale: the DEFEBSE-PFO trial. J Am Coll Cardiol. 2018;71:2335–42.

28. Kasner SE, Swaminathan B, Lavados P, Sharma M, Muir K, Veltkamp R, et al. Rivaroxaban or aspirin for patent foramen ovale and embolic stroke of undetermined source: a prespecified subgroup analysis from the NAVIGATE ESUS trial. Lancet Neurol. 2018;17:1053–60.

29. Kawano H, Inatomi Y, Hirano T, Yonehara T. Vertebral artery stump syndrome in acute ischemic stroke. J Neurol Sci. 2013;324(1–2):74–9.

30. Chobanian AV, Bakris GL, Black HR, Cushman WC, Green LA, Izzo JL Jr, Jones DW, Materson BJ, Oparil S, Wright JT Jr, Roccella EJ, Joint National Committee on Prevention, Detection, Evaluation, and Treatment of High Blood Pressure, National Heart, Lung, and Blood Institute, National High Blood Pressure Education Program Coordinating Committee. Seventh report of the joint national committee on prevention, detection, evaluation, and treatment of high blood pressure. Hypertension. 2003;42:1206–52.

31. Whelton PK, Carey RM, Aronow WS, Casey DE Jr, Collins KJ, Dennison Himmelfarb C, DePalma SM, Gidding S, Jamerson KA, Jones DW, MacLaughlin EJ, Muntner P, Ovbiagele B, Smith SC Jr, Spencer CC, Stafford RS, Taler SJ, Thomas RJ, Williams KA Sr, Williamson JD, Wright JT Jr. 2017 ACC/AHA/AAPA/ABC/ACPM/AGS/AphA/ASH/ASPC/NMA/PCNA guideline for the prevention, detection, evaluation, and management of high blood pressure in adults: a report of the American College of Cardiology/American Heart Association task force on clinical practice guidelines. Hypertension. 2018;71(6):e13–e115.

32. Benavente OR, Coffey CS, Conwit R, Hart RG, McClure LA, Pearce LA, Pergola PE, Szychowski JM, SPS3 Study Group. Blood-pressure targets in patients with recent lacunar stroke: the SPS3 randomised trial. Lancet. 2013;382(9891):507–15.

33. Kitagawa K, Yamamoto Y, Arima H, Maeda T, Sunami N, Kanzawa T, Eguchi K, Kamiyama K, Minematsu K, Ueda S, Rakugi H, Ohya Y, Kohro T, Yonemoto K, Okada Y, Higaki J, Tanahashi N, Kimura G, Umemura S, Matsumoto M, Shimamoto K, Ito S, Saruta T, Shimada K, Recurrent Stroke Prevention Clinical Outcome (RESPECT) Study Group. Effect of standard vs intensive blood pressure control on the risk of recurrent stroke: a randomized clinical trial and meta-analysis. JAMA Neurol. 2019;76(11):1309–18.

34. Toyoda K, Yasaka M, Uchiyama S, Nagao T, Gotoh J, Nagata K, Koretsune Y, Sakamoto T, Iwade K, Yamamoto M, Takahashi JC, Minematsu K, Bleeding with Antithrombotic Therapy (BAT) Study Group. Blood pressure levels and bleeding events during antithrombotic therapy: the bleeding with antithrombotic therapy (BAT) study. Stroke. 2010;41(7):1440–4.

35. Kim JS, Nah HW, Park SM, Kim SK, Cho KH, Lee J, Lee YS, Kim J, Ha SW, Kim EG, Kim DE, Kang DW, Kwon SU, Yu KH, Lee BC. Risk factors and stroke mechanisms in atherosclerotic stroke: intracranial compared with extracranial and anterior compared with posterior circulation disease. Stroke. 2012;43(12):3313–8.

36. Lee MH, Kim JG, Jeon SB, Kang DW, Kwon SU, Kim JS. Pharmacologically induced hypertension therapy for acute stroke patients. J Stroke. 2019;21(2):228–30.

37. Bang OY, Chung J-W, Kim S-K, Kim SJ, Lee MJ, Hwang J, Seo W-K, Ha YS, Sung SM, Kim EG, Sohn S-I, Han M-K. Therapeutic-induced hypertension in patients with noncardioembolic acute stroke. Neurology. 2019;93(21):e1955–63.

38. Amin-Hanjani S, Turan TN, Du X, Pandey DK, Rose-Finnell L, Richardson D, Elkind MS, Zipfel GJ, Liebeskind DS, Silver FL, Kasner SE, Gorelick PB, Charbel FT, Derdeyn CP. Higher stroke risk with lower blood pressure in hemodynamic vertebrobasilar disease: analysis from the VERiTAS study. J Stroke Cerebrovasc Dis. 2017;26(2):403–10.

39. Jellinger PS, Handelsman Y, Rosenblit PD, Bloomgarden ZT, Fonseca VA, Garber AJ, Grunberger G, Guerin CK, Bell DSH, Mechanick JI, Pessah-Pollack R, Wyne K, Smith D, Brinton EA, Fazio S, Davidson M. American Association of Clinical Endocrinologists and American College of Endocrinology guidelines for management of dyslipidemia and prevention of cardiovascular disease. Endocr Pract. 2017;23(Suppl 2):1–87.

40. Amarenco P, Kim JS, Labreuche J, Charles H, Abtan J, Béjot Y, Cabrejo L, Cha J-K, Ducrocq G, Giroud M, Guidoux C, Hobeanu C, Kim YJ, Lapergue B, Lavallée PC, Lee B-C, Lee KB, Leys D, Mahagne MH, Meseguer E, Nighoghossian N, Pico F, Samson Y, Sibon I, Steg PG, Sung SM, Touboul PJ, Touzé E, Varenne O, Vicaut É, Yelles N, Bruckert E, on behalf of the Treat Stroke to Target Investigators. A comparison of two LDL cholesterol targets after ischemic stroke. N Engl J Med. 2020;382(1):9. https://doi.org/10.1056/NEJMoa1910355.

Thrombolysis and Thrombectomy

11

Christine Hawkes, Kavit Shah, and Tudor G. Jovin

Summary

Posterior circulation stroke (PCS) comprises a minority of overall acute ischemic stroke (AIS) cases; however, it is associated with a disproportionally higher level of morbidity and mortality. Because its presenting symptoms may be ambiguous and insidious in onset, the diagnosis of PCS may require a stronger clinical acumen compared to that of anterior circulation stroke (ACS). However, like ACS, once recognized, acute reperfusion therapy such as thrombolytics or mechanical thrombectomy (MT) must be initiated immediately in eligible patients. Outcome data are relatively sparse for systemic thrombolysis or MT in PCS treatment compared to ACS; however, it is well established that in PCS due to basilar artery occlusion (BAO), the constellation of persistent vessel occlusion and moderate-to-severe clinical deficit at presentation is uniformly associated with death or severe disability. Multiple case series and reviews have demonstrated systemic and intra-arterial thrombolysis as promising recanalization methods for PCS. Furthermore, the advent of recent class I evidence of efficacy for MT in ACS, has established endovascular therapy (with or without IV thrombolysis depending on patient eligibility) as the standard of care for PCS due to BAO in many centers across the world. Just like in the case of ACS, where current guidelines recommend the recently expanded but still rigid time criteria for treatment selection, a growing body of literature suggests that time constraints should not limit treatment for select patients with BAO given that lack of treatment resulting in a uniformly poor outcome. While time is increasingly less considered, the primordial factor for patient selection in stroke populations, in each individual patient, the earlier reperfusion occurs, the higher the chance of a good outcome. Therefore, optimizing triage and transport to appropriate centers remains critical to achieving sustained growth in the number of eligible patients with better clinical outcomes. In addition, new-generation MT devices and adjunctive approaches to endovascular therapy, including neuroprotection, will be the next frontier in comprehensive acute PCS management.

C. Hawkes
McMaster University, Hamilton, ON, Canada
e-mail: christine.hawkes@medportal.ca

K. Shah
University of Pittsburgh Medical Center,
Pittsburgh, PA, USA
e-mail: shahkb2@upmc.edu

T. G. Jovin (✉)
Cooper Medical School of Rowan University,
Cooper University Hospital, Camden, NJ, USA
e-mail: Jovin-Tudor@CooperHealth.edu

Background

While posterior circulation stroke (PCS) accounts for only 20–30% of all acute ischemic stroke (AIS), it is associated with significant morbidity

© Springer Nature Singapore Pte Ltd. 2021
J. S. Kim (ed.), *Posterior Circulation Stroke*, https://doi.org/10.1007/978-981-15-6739-1_11

and mortality [1]. Stroke due to occlusion of proximal large vessels in the posterior circulation, involving the basilar artery (BA), both intracranial vertebral arteries (VAs), or one intracranial VA with atretic contralateral VA, carries a particularly poor prognosis. When all such untreated patients are considered, nearly 65% of patients can be left with severe deficits, and 40% will not survive [2]. Furthermore, in patients presenting with moderate-to-severe deficits, without reperfusion therapy, rates of good outcomes can be as low as 2% [3]. While the National Institute of Health Stroke Scale (NIHSS) is a less accurate measure of the severity of the neurological deficit in PCS compared to its ACS counterpart, an NIHSS ≥10 is highly associated with death or severe disability without reperfusion therapy [4].

Clinical Symptomatology and Clot Location

Similar to ACS, prompt recognition and institution of treatment aimed to reperfuse the ischemic brain is essential. Recognition of PCS symptoms, however, may be more difficult given the more complex nuances of patient's presenting symptoms, particularly as the NIHSS is not as reliable for these strokes [5–7]. Unlike an ACS that may present with specific symptoms suggestive of impairment of certain brain regions, such as hemiparesis, hemisensory loss, hemifield cut, aphasia, or neglect, the symptoms of a PCS can be nonspecific with dizziness, headache, or slight incoordination. These relatively ambiguous symptoms may present as recurrent transient ischemic attacks (TIAs), which represent the prodromal symptoms of a full-blown BA occlusion (BAO) syndrome in 25–60% of cases, when untreated [8, 9].

The mode of symptom presentation may indicate the pathophysiologic mechanism of BAO. Typically, the prodromal, stuttering symptoms occur in patients with proximal BA occlusions, which are more likely to be related with atherothrombosis whereas the abrupt, sudden symptoms associated with mid/distal BA occlusion are more frequently associated with embolic

mechanisms [10–12]. These distal embolic occlusions have higher recanalization rates compared to their proximal, atherosclerotic counterparts [3, 13–15].

Thrombolytic Therapy

Historical Context

The potential benefit of thrombolytic therapy in acute PCS was recognized as early as 1958. In their series of 3 patients treated with intravenous (IV) fibrinolysin, Sussman and Fitch made several important observations. They understood that time to treatment was essential, based on the finding that angiographic proof of recanalization within 6 hours correlated with a favorable prognosis. They also reported that while a surgical approach can satisfactorily recanalize an occluded vessel, by the time this is achieved, the tissue at risk will likely be irreversibly damaged [16].

Despite numerous early case reports of successful IV thrombolytic therapy for AIS, this treatment became standard of care only after 1995 landmark National Institute of Neurological Disorders and Stroke (NINDS) IV tissue plasminogen activator (t-PA) trial, which established the benefit of t-PA in acute AIS when treated within 3 h of last seen well (LSW) [17]. Later, the use of IV t-PA was established out to 4.5 h from LSW [18].

While IV thrombolysis remains the standard of care for AIS, its utilization in BAO is low. It has been reported that among all patients who receive thrombolysis, only 5% have BAO [19]. Furthermore, the aforementioned pivotal t-PA trials either had a low proportion of PCS (5% in NINDS) or did not delineate how many PCS were included (ECASS III). More recently, single-arm studies have investigated outcomes in PCS treated with IV t-PA. A retrospective study of 116 patients treated with IV t-PA over 13 years reported rates of recanalization of 65% with trends toward favorable outcomes [15]. Another retrospective study reported 53% recanalization rates associated with 22% favorable outcomes and 50% mortality [3]. Lastly, the prospective

Basilar Artery International Cooperation Study (BASICS) group captured data on 121 patients treated with IV t-PA who achieved nearly 70% recanalization rates with 16% mortality; however, it is worth noting that a third of these patients received rescue intra-arterial (IA) thrombolysis [4]. Rates of symptomatic intracerebral hemorrhage (sICH) in these groups ranged from 6% to 16%, which is higher than that observed with IV t-PA treatment in ACS. However, two studies reported lower rates of sICH in PCS compared to ACS [20, 21]. When comparing outcomes with IV thrombolysis in PCS with ACS, a large single-center study found a higher rate of favorable outcomes in the former than in the latter [21]. Overall, despite the lack of evidence from randomized control trials (RCTs) of IV thrombolysis in stroke due to BAO, studies suggest that IV t-PA is relatively safe and likely to be efficacious for this subgroup of patients.

Intra-Arterial Thrombolysis

In addition to systemic thrombolysis, local IA thrombolysis has been used to treat AIS with thrombolytics such as streptokinase, urokinase, or prourokinase. The first RCTs assessing the feasibility of IA thrombolytic treatment were Prolyse in Acute Cerebral Thromboembolism (PROACT) and PROACT II. The latter included patients with AIS due to occlusion of the M1 or M2 MCA segment who could be treated within 6 hours of LSW. Investigators compared clinical outcomes in patients treated with IA prourokinase administered within the thrombus to standard medical therapy [22, 23]. Despite the increased risk of sICH, PROACT II found a significant benefit in favor of IA therapy [23]. The primary clinical outcome at 90 days (modified Rankin Scale [mRS] score $\leq$ 2) was achieved in 40% of the treatment group and 25% of the controls, $p = 0.043$ [23]. The positive results of PROACT II in the context of the particularly dismal natural history of stroke due to BAO have led to cessation of equipoise such that there have been virtually no RCTs examining the benefit of IA lytics for this type of stroke. One RCT of IA

streptokinase conducted in Australia enrolled only 16 patients before being stopped due to slow enrollment and lack of funding [24]. In this study, 4 of the 8 patients in the IA streptokinase group achieved a favorable outcome (mRS 0–3), while only one favorable outcome was observed in the 8 control patients. Since Zeumer et al. firstly described IA streptokinase therapy for BAO in a young woman in 1982 [25], several papers published have attested to the feasibility, relative safety, and higher than expected outcomes of this approach compared to historical controls [3, 4, 26–31].

Mechanical (Nonpharmacological) Endovascular Treatment

Evolution of Endovascular Treatment

Narrow time windows and the risk of hemorrhage associated with thrombolytic agents prompted the design and application of mechanical thrombectomy (MT) devices. Endovascular clot retrieval provides the potential for rapid flow restoration, with a decreased incidence of clot fragmentation and distal embolism [32]. Catheter-based, retrieval/aspiration systems began to be used in AIS patients who were either ineligible for or had failed IV t-PA administration; initially, they were largely used in conjunction with thrombolytic infusion.

MERCI Device

The first device to receive U.S. Food and Drug Administration (FDA) approval for clot retrieval was the MERCI device [33]. Results from the single-arm Mechanical Embolus Removal in Cerebral Ischemia (MERCI) trial demonstrated the efficacy of the MERCI system in restoring the patency of occluded intracranial vessels within 8 hours of AIS [34]; 48% of occluded vessels were recanalized, a rate significantly higher than that of the control arm in the PROACT II trial (18%) [23, 32]. After adjuvant therapy (IA t-PA, angioplasty, snare), the rate of recanalization reached to 60.3%. Furthermore, successful revascularization was found to be an independent predictor of decreased mortality and favorable neurological outcome at 90 days [34]. Similar results were noted in the Multi MERCI trial, which included patients treated with IV t-PA prior to MT and used a modified version of the original MERCI device [35]. These trials are mainly of historical importance as the MERCI device is no longer used in clinical practice.

Penumbra Aspiration System

The Penumbra System (Penumbra Inc., Alameda, CA) is an aspiration device through which the thrombus can be retrieved from the occluded vessel. The aspiration device is advanced coaxially to the level of the thrombus through a guide catheter, and an aspiration pump or aspiration syringe is connected to the reperfusion catheter. Based on the results of the Penumbra Pivotal trial demonstrating a recanalization rate of thrombolysis in myocardial infarction (TIMI) 2–3 of 81.6% and rates of mRS 0–2 of 20%, coupled with a rate of sICH of 11.2%, the Penumbra device received FDA approval in 2008 [36]. Ever since, newer-generation reperfusion catheters with an increasingly larger diameter and improved navigability have been designed, which have substantially improved procedural results with this device [37].

Stentrievers

Retrievable stent thrombectomy devices (stentrievers) are self-expanding stent-like structures attached to a microwire that are designed to capture the thrombus. These devices emerged as favorable methods for MT in stroke after the first two such devices (Solitaire and Trevo) showed overwhelmingly superior rates of recanalization and better clinical outcomes in a head-to-head comparison against the MERCI device [38, 39].

Another technique, manual aspiration thrombectomy, has also been used in the treatment of

large vessel occlusion. This technique was initially described for use in the extracranial posterior circulation and later in the BA [40–42]. Single-arm studies supported the use of manual aspiration as part of a multimodality recanalization strategy [43].

Early Evidence for Endovascular Treatment

Many of the early trials on MT excluded PCS [22, 23, 44–47]. MERCI and Multi MERCI enrolled a total of 26 patients with BAO and 1 patient with VA plus bilateral posterior cerebral artery occlusions [34, 35]. While lacking a control group, a consistent finding of all the early MT trials was that favorable outcomes were seen in significantly higher proportions in patients who achieved recanalization compared to those without [48]. The first large randomized endovascular stroke trial, the Endovascular Therapy after Intravenous t-PA versus t-PA Alone for Stroke (IMS III) trial, included only 4 patients with BAO. This trial was stopped prior to completing enrollment of the planned sample size due to futility [49]. In the Penumbra Pivotal trial, only 11 patients with vertebrobasilar occlusion were included [36]. As such, limited conclusions can be drawn regarding the efficacy of MT with early-generation devices from these small numbers of patients. A summary of various endovascular trials including patients with posterior circulation stroke is shown in Table 11.1.

BASICS represents an international, multicenter prospective registry that enrolled patients presenting with BAO confirmed by CTA or MRA. Patients were treated with best medical management, including IV t-PA (within 4.5 h of the estimated time of BAO) or antithrombotics, or best medical management plus IA therapy [4]. IA therapy had to be initiated within 6 h, and the strategy used was at the discretion of the treating neurointerventionalist, including IA thrombolysis (with urokinase) or IA stenting. Analysis of the BASICS registry data revealed no statistically significant difference in poor outcome (defined

Table 11.1 Summary of trials including patients with posterior circulation large vessel occlusion

Trial	Patients treated	Time window	Recanalization	Mortality at 90 days
MERCI Multi MERCI	27	<8 h	21 (78%) TIMI II or more	12 (44%)
Penumbra pivotal	11	<8 h	Unknown	Unknown
SWIFT	2 (roll in) 1 (SOLITAIRE) 1 (MERCI0	<8 h	Unknown	Unknown
TREVO 2	7 (TREVO) 5 (MERCI)	<8 h	Unknown	Unknown
IMS III	4	Procedure start <5 h, end <7 h	Unknown	Unknown
BASICS	288	No limit	207 (72%) TIMI II or more	Unknown
ENDOSTROKE registry	148	No limit	111 (79%) TICI 2b-3	43 (35%)
BEST	66	<8 h	47 (71.4%) TICI 2b-3	22 (33.3%)

as mRS 4–6 at 1 month) between patients treated with IV thrombolysis or antithrombotics alone compared to intra-arterial therapy (55% of patients) [4]. A portion of patients (10%) included in the registry had no treatment, either because symptoms were mild while already on antithrombotics or because further treatment was considered futile. Overall, 68% of patients had a poor outcome, with a mortality rate of 36%. However, successful recanalization with IA therapy was associated with higher likelihood of favorable outcomes. In this nonrandomized study, there was also a suspected bias toward more aggressive treatment in patients with a more severe presentation, which is a confounder of worse outcome [4]. Another limitation of this registry is that modern stentrievers were not available at the time of the study.

Modern Endovascular Trials

In 2015, five prospective RCTs showed overwhelming benefit for MT performed largely with stentrievers in patients with AIS due to LVO presenting in the early time window [50–54]. Another positive trial was published in 2016 [55]. However, none of these studies included patients with BAO. Subsequent trials showing arguably stronger benefit of MT than that observed in the early time window trials were seen in patients presenting from 6 to 24 h with evidence of substantial areas of salvageable brain on neuroimaging. However, these trials also did not include BAO [56, 57].

Observational data from the Endovascular Stroke Treatment Registry (ENDOSTROKE), an international registry of patients aged 18 or older who underwent attempted MT, showed that only 34% of patients with BAO and attempted MT had a good clinical outcome at 3 months, despite 79% recanalization rate of thrombolysis in cerebral infarction (TICI) 2b-3 [58]. This confirms previously held beliefs that, at comparable recanalization rates, clinical outcomes with MT for BAO are poorer than those seen in ACS. Factors predictive of favorable outcomes included young age and low NIHSS at presentation [58]. This suggests that acute stroke due to BAO continues to remain a formidable challenge requiring a multifaceted approach as recanalization alone may be insufficient in achieving a good outcome.

There is limited randomized controlled data on BAO treatment with MT (Table 11.1). Acute Basilar Artery Occlusion: Endovascular Interventions versus Standard Medical Treatment (BEST) was a RCT evaluating endovascular treatment of BAO compared to standard care (including IV t-PA in eligible patients) within 8 h of estimated occlusion time [59]. The trial was stopped early due to excessive crossovers and a progressive drop in recruitment, underscoring again the ethical challenges associated with conducting BAO trials. The trial aimed to demonstrate that MT for BAO (when performed within 8 h of estimated occlusion time) yields a higher rate of favorable clinical outcomes expressed as an mRS score of 0–3 compared to standard medical therapy. The study enrolled 131 patients, 66 allocated to intervention and 65 allocated to control, including patients treated with IV t-PA (30%) as part of standard medical therapy. The intention-to-treat analysis of BEST failed to show a statistically significant benefit in favor of MT (rates of mRS 0–3 in MT were 42.4% vs 32.3 in controls, $p = 0.232$, which was attributed to the high number (21.5%) of crossovers from medical therapy to MT in the medical group). When analyzed "per protocol," a significant difference in the primary outcome between MT and control patients was found (44.4% vs 25.5%, respectively, $p = 0.036$). A nonstatistically significant increase in sICH was noted in the MT group compared to the control group (7.9% compared to 0%, $p = 0.064$). Despite lack of class I evidence, due to the very poor likelihood of favorable clinical outcomes in patients with BAO without recanalization, MT is currently offered at most endovascular centers as a part of routine care protocols.

Selection Criteria for Endovascular Treatment

Selection based on imaging played an important role in the success of the landmark MT trials, especially in those patients enrolled in the extended time window. Just like with the ACS, key questions that imaging aims to answer in PCS are: is it an ischemic or hemorrhagic stroke? is there a large vessel occlusion? what is the extent of infarcted tissue? and what is the extent of "at-risk" (penumbral) tissue? With regard to MT for ACS, our understanding of imaging's role as a patient selection tool for MT has been continuously evolving. It has long been believed that patients with large baseline infarcts should not be treated because of futility or even harm in the form of reperfusion injury, resulting in sICH or malignant edema. However, data from a large pooled analysis of nearly 1800 patients directly contradicts this concept by showing that in the early time window, even patients with large baseline infarcts still stand to benefit from MT [60]. Furthermore, baseline infarct size, regardless of imaging modalities through which it is being measured, while a strong prognostic factor, is not capable of identifying which patients benefit and which patients do not benefit from MT. Whether the same findings apply to BAO stroke remains to be established.

Similar to the ACS, CTA is a reliable method for identifying vascular occlusions in the PCS [61]. However, detection of early ischemic changes based on noncontrast CT is more difficult in the PCS compared to ACS. Using areas of hypoattenuation on CTA source images improves the accuracy of infarct size estimation [62]. The posterior circulation Acute Stroke Prognosis Early CT Score (pc-ASPECTs) allots 10 points to the normal posterior circulation and deducts one point for early region with early ischemic changes on CTA source images [63]. One point is subtracted for early ischemic changes in the right or left thalamus, cerebellar hemispheres, or posterior cerebral artery territory. Two points are deducted for early ischemic changes in the midbrain or pons. Just like its anterior equivalent, pc-ASPECTS appears to be a powerful prognostic factor. In a case series of patients treated with endovascular therapy for BAO, of patients with recanalization of the BA, 70% of those with a pc-ASPECTS score of ≥ 8 had a favorable outcome, compared to those with scores <8 having 9% favorable outcomes (RR 12.1; 95% CI 1.7 to 84.9) [63]. Because of the low rates of favorable outcomes noted in patients with low pc-ASPECTS, this score has been proposed as a way to improve selection of patients for future trials. However, the absence of a control group in the case series describing the association of pre-intervention pc-ASPECTS with clinical outcomes does not rule out the possibility that clinical benefit may still exist in patients with low pc-ASPECTS scores who undergo MT compared to those who do not.

Another method of quantifying early ischemic changes in the PCS is the Pons Midbrain Index [64]. This system involves scoring each side of the pons and midbrain from 0 to 2 on the CTA source images; 0, no hypoattenuation; 1, equal or less than 50% hypoattenuation; or 2, more than 50% hypoattenuation. A study conducted on patients from the BASICS registry revealed that those with a Pons Midbrain Index of <3 were less likely to die and more likely to have a favorable outcome compared to those patients with a comparatively higher index [65].

Multiple scoring systems for brainstem DWI lesions on MRI have also been proposed to quantify infarct burden in patients with BAO, including using pc-ASPECTS with MRI [66, 67]. Regardless of the scoring system used, the absence of extensive infarct on MRI is associated with a favorable outcome with mechanical MT [68]. In addition to infarct volume, infarct topography is of crucial importance with regard to prognosis in these patients. Based on a retrospective review of patients treated with MT for BAO who underwent a postprocedure MRI, one group reported that the only significant predictors of favorable outcome (mRS 0–2) were age (OR 0.84, 95% CI 0.74–0.91, $p = 0,018$) and infarct volume in the brainstem (OR 0.25, 95% CI 0.11–0.61, $p = 0,002$) [69]. Time to treatment and infarct volume were not associated with clinical outcomes for strokes outside of the brainstem. Another study also demonstrated a lack of association between time to treatment and clinical outcomes, specifically in patients with BAO who underwent MT for BAO [70]. Identical to the rates of favorable (33%) outcomes seen in a similarly large case series of patients treated in earlier time window (median time to treatment 300 min), rates of favorable outcomes in the study conducted by Starr et al. were 33% and time to treatment was not associated with the likelihood of a favorable outcome [71]. Rangaraju et al. described the Pittsburgh Outcomes in Thrombectomy for anterior circulation stroke (POST) score as a prognostic tool that aims to inform physicians and family members of the likelihood of a favorable outcome after MT for BAO and thus aid in the post-MT care decision-making process [72]. However, this score has been validated for patients with ACS only.

Using strict time criteria as selection criteria for treatment of BAO has been called into question by multiple authors. The presentation of BAO can be insidious and protean, making an accurate determination of symptom onset timing very challenging [8]. Studies have shown that patients with BAO treated more than 24 h from LSW can have clinical outcomes and rates of sICH that are comparable to those seen in patients treated early [70, 71]. The highly developed collateral arterial network in the posterior circulation, reverse filling of the BA, and a layer of plasma flow between the clot and artery wall have been proposed to maintain brainstem viability for longer time after BAO compared to occlusions in the anterior circulation [73]. On the contrary, Grevik et al. analyzed a cohort of 619 patients with BAO from BASICS and found that time to treatment is an independent predictor of outcome, along with age, baseline NIHSS, hyperlipidemia, and minor prodromal stroke symptoms. Although the therapeutic time window may be longer in BAO patients than in ACS patients, the importance of prompt and active therapy to save the penumbra area should also be emphasized in BAO treatment.

Technical Considerations

The anatomy of the vertebrobasilar circulation can pose technical challenges in MT. The caliber of the vessels in the posterior circulation is generally smaller than that of large arteries in the anterior circulation, requiring careful consideration when selecting catheters and devices [74]. There are also a number of anatomical variations in the posterior circulation, such as VA termination at the posterior inferior cerebellar artery [75]. Some anatomical characteristics may represent an advantage. For example, the lesser tortuosity of the VA compared to the internal carotid artery makes direct thromboaspiration feasible in the

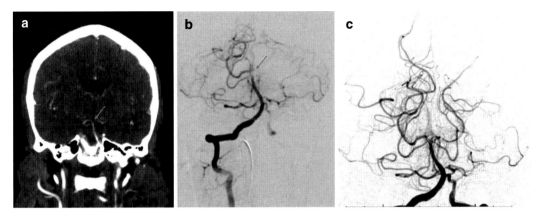

Fig. 11.1 A middle-aged woman with a history of atrial fibrillation on anticoagulation was admitted to the hospital for workup of new-onset, recurrent seizures. During her hospitalization, she was found to be unresponsive during a routine nursing check, which prompted a stroke code activation. NIHSS performed by the Stroke team was cal-culated at 29. STAT CTA demonstrated a basilar tip occlu-sion (**a**, arrow). She went for emergent endovascular thrombectomy, where the first base catheter run demon-strated the basilar tip occlusion (**b**, arrow). She underwent thromboaspiration and achieved TICI 2B recanalization (**c**)

vertebrobasilar system [41–43]. An example is demonstrated in Fig. 11.1.

A subgroup of patients with PCS has tandem BAO and VA occlusions (intracranially or extra-cranially), making access to the BAO more challenging, especially when the contralateral VA is hypoplastic or occluded. Access can be through the patent VA, or the occluded VA, which depending on the location and etiology of the occlusion (e.g., atherosclerotic) may require stenting or angioplasty. The choice of the approach should be tailored to the individual ana-tomic and clinical considerations [76, 77]. Some studies suggest that once base catheter access is achieved in the VA and the BA is accessed via microcatheter, contralateral VA low flow, from either an occlusion or hypoplasia, is associated with better recanalization and lower risk of distal embolization [75]. This may be due to the lack of flow reversal when the contralateral VA is patent during aspiration. When standard access is not possible, for instance, if the VA ostium is occluded and thus not visible, alternative approaches to access the BA have been employed. These approaches include obtaining retrograde access through the posterior communicating artery, using thyrocervical collaterals in a chroni-cally occluded VA, or using a hypoplastic contra-lateral VA access to pass a microwire retrograde

through the occluded VA ostium to delineate its location [78–80].

Treatment of VA ostium high-grade stenosis or occlusion is also a consideration when the occluded VA represents the only access site to the BAO. Since occlusion of the VA results in a low flow state, and because of the high propensity for re-occlusion with angioplasty alone, stenting should be the preferred choice. There are gener-ally two approaches, consisting either of stenting the vessel prior to accessing the distal lesion or more commonly of placing a stent at the end of the procedure after the distal reperfusion is com-plete [76]. The former approach has the main advantage of allowing intracranial access and is required when access cannot be established oth-erwise. It may also allow placement of larger bore guide catheters that may not be able to be navigated through a severe ostial stenosis [81]. The latter approach more rapidly restores flow to the ischemic tissue, avoids the risk of dislodge-ment of the stent with passage of a large sheath through the stent, and can be done after the intra-cranial work is complete [80]. Both approaches require the use of dual antiplatelet therapy (peri-procedurally, this can be in the form of IV GP IIb/IIIa inhibitors), which can be of concern, especially in patients with large cerebellar infarcts who may require open surgical decompressive surgery. Thus, if the likelihood of posterior fossa decompression is deemed to be high, VA angioplasty may be the best alternative. Because of the relatively high incidence of atherosclerotic lesions underlying the occlusion compared to anterior circulation occlusions, especially in the proximal segment of the BA, consideration should be given to acute angioplasty or (preferably) stenting, especially when MT yields either no recanalization or recanalization with residual high-grade stenosis. This can be accomplished with self-expanding stents, balloon-mounted stents, or detachable stentrievers (Solitaire AB) [82, 83]. This angioplasty with or without stenting is often performed in Asian countries where intracranial atherosclerotic occlusion is relatively common [84]. An example is demonstrated in Fig. 11.2.

Treatment for LVOs with balloon-mounted stents as a second-line approach after MT in patients with presumed intracranial atherosclerosis has been shown to have reperfusion rates and clinical outcomes comparable to MT [82].

However, the rates of sICH and mortality were higher than those seen with traditional MT devices in this cohort of high-risk patients, a significant proportion of whom had BAO. While the advent of modern intermediate catheters has made delivery of balloon-mounted stents in the BA feasible with high reliability, the need for immediate antiplatelet agent administration to prevent stent thrombosis, with their ensuing hemorrhagic risk, especially in those patients who receive IV t-PA, is potential limitation of this technology. Larger randomized studies are needed to assess the safety and efficacy of this treatment modality.

Future Directions

Ongoing clinical trials, including the Basilar Artery Occlusion Chinese Endovascular Trial (BAOCHE) and BASIC, hope to address some of the gaps in evidence for endovascular treatment of BAO [85, 86]. Trials examining neuro-

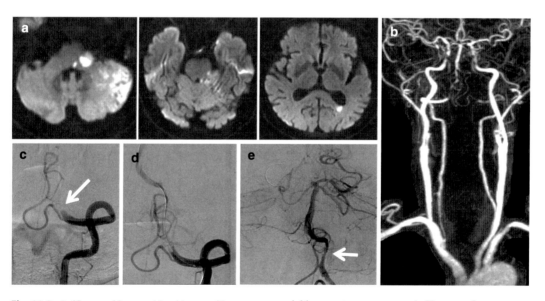

Fig. 11.2 A 65-year-old man with a history of hypertension and diabetes mellitus developed recurrent episodes of dizziness for a few days, followed by sudden vertigo, dysarthria, and gait ataxia. Diffusion-weighted MRI showed acute infarcts in the right pons, cerebellar peduncle, cerebellum, and occipital area (**a**). MR angiogram showed bilateral steno-occlusion in the distal vertebral arteries (VAs) (**b**). Initially, he was alert, but he became drowsy and his symptoms progressed. He went for emergent endovascular thrombectomy. Catheter angiogram showed occlusion of the right distal VA (**c**, arrow). Thrombectomy was performed with a stentriever, and residual stenosis was managed with angioplasty and intracranial stent application (**d**) to maintain patency of the dominant left vertebral artery (**e**). He became alert and was discharged with mild dysarthria only

protectants, which include the Field Randomization of NA-1 Therapy in Early Responders and No-NO, are also underway [87]. It is hoped that neuroprotectant drugs may result in prolongation of the therapeutic time window by transforming "fast progressors" into "slow progressors." Other potentially beneficial effects of neuroprotectant agents include mitigation of reperfusion injury and apoptosis and inflammation [88, 89]. Technological solutions are being proposed to address the challenges of endovascular treatment for PCS. For example, stentrievers are being developed with the ability to detach should the lesion require stenting. This could be particularly useful for the PCS where there is a higher likelihood of underlying intracranial atherosclerotic disease [90]. Transporting patients to the appropriate medical center is necessary to facilitate timely treatment, particularly with PCS where there is a higher rate of misdiagnosis [91]. Finally, improvement in systems of care is needed to increase access to timely endovascular treatment for patients with large vessel occlusion including those with BAO.

References

1. Gulli G, Marquardt L, Rothwell P, Markus H. Stroke risk after posterior circulation stroke/transient ischemic attack and its relationship to site of vertebrobasilar stenosis. Stroke. 2013;44(3):598–604.
2. Schonewille W. Outcome in patients with basilar artery occlusion treated conventionally. J Neurol Neurosurg Psychiatry. 2005;76(9):1238–41.
3. Lindsberg P, Mattle H. Therapy of basilar artery occlusion. Stroke. 2006;37(3):922–8.
4. Schonewille W, Wijman C, Michel P, Rueckert C, Weimar C, Mattle H, et al. Treatment and outcomes of acute basilar artery occlusion in the Basilar Artery International Cooperation Study (BASICS): a prospective registry study. Lancet Neurol. 2009;8(8):724–30.
5. Kim J, Park M, Choi K, Kim B, Han M, Park T, et al. Clinical outcomes of posterior versus anterior circulation infarction with low National Institutes of Health stroke scale scores. Stroke. 2017;48(1):55–62.
6. Inoa V, Aron A, Staff I, Fortunato G, Sansing L. Lower NIH stroke scale scores are required to accurately predict a good prognosis in posterior circulation stroke. Cerebrovasc Dis. 2014;37(4):251–5.
7. Heldner M, Zubler C, Mattle H, Schroth G, Weck A, Mono M, et al. National Institutes of Health stroke scale score and vessel occlusion in 2152 patients with acute ischemic stroke. Stroke. 2013;44(4):1153–7.
8. Ferbert A, Brückmann H, Drummen R. Clinical features of proven basilar artery occlusion. Stroke. 1990;21(8):1135–42.
9. Caplan L, Wityk R, Glass T, Tapia J, Pazdera L, Chang H, et al. New England medical center posterior circulation registry. Ann Neurol. 2004;56(3):389–98.
10. Mattle H, Arnold M, Lindsberg P, Schonewille W, Schroth G. Basilar artery occlusion. Lancet Neurol. 2011;10(11):1002–14.
11. Nouh A, Remke J, Ruland S. Ischemic posterior circulation stroke: a review of anatomy, clinical presentations, diagnosis, and current management. Front Neurol. 2014;5:30.
12. Markus H, van der Worp H, Rothwell P. Posterior circulation ischaemic stroke and transient ischaemic attack: diagnosis, investigation, and secondary prevention. Lancet Neurol. 2013;12(10):989–98.
13. Caplan L. "Top of the basilar" syndrome. Neurology. 1980;30(1):72.
14. Eckert B, Kucinski T, Pfeiffer G, Groden C, Zeumer H. Endovascular therapy of acute vertebrobasilar occlusion: early treatment onset as the Most important factor. Cerebrovasc Dis. 2002;14(1):42–50.
15. Sairanen T, Strbian D, Soinne L, Silvennoinen H, Salonen O, Artto V, et al. Intravenous thrombolysis of basilar artery occlusion. Stroke. 2011;42(8):2175–9.
16. Sussman B, Fitch T. Thrombolysis with fibrinolysin in cerebral arterial occlusion. J Am Med Assoc. 1958;167(14):1705.
17. National Institute of Neurological Disorders and Stroke rt-PA Stroke Study Group. Tissue Plasminogen Activator for Acute Ischemic Stroke. N Eng J Med. 1995;333(24):1581–8.
18. Hacke W, Kaste M, Bluhmki E, Brozman M, Dávalos A, Guidetti D, et al. Thrombolysis with alteplase 3 to 4.5 hours after acute ischemic stroke. N Engl J Med. 2008;359(13):1317–29.
19. Weimar C, Goertler M, Harms L, Diener H. Distribution and outcome of symptomatic stenoses and occlusions in patients with acute cerebral ischemia. Arch Neurol. 2006;63(9):1287.
20. Pagola J, Ribo M, Alvarez-Sabin J, Rubiera M, Santamarina E, Maisterra O, et al. Thrombolysis in anterior versus posterior circulation strokes: timing of recanalization, ischemic tolerance, and other differences. J Neuroimaging. 2011;21(2):108–12.
21. Sarikaya H, Arnold M, Engelter S, Lyrer P, Mattle H, Georgiadis D, et al. Outcomes of intravenous thrombolysis in posterior versus anterior circulation stroke. Stroke. 2011;42(9):2498–502.
22. del Zoppo G, Higashida R, Furlan A, Pessin M, Rowley H, Gent M. PROACT: a phase II randomized trial of recombinant pro-urokinase by direct arterial delivery in acute middle cerebral artery stroke. Stroke. 1998;29(1):4–11.
23. Furlan A, Higashida R, Wechsler L, Gent M, Rowley H, Kase C, et al. Intra-arterial prourokinase for acute ischemic stroke. JAMA. 1999;282(21):2003.

24. Donnan G, Davis S, Chambers B, Gates P, Hankey G, McNeil J, et al. Streptokinase for acute ischemic stroke with relationship to time of administration: Australian streptokinase (ASK) trial group. JAMA. 1996;276(12):961–6.
25. Zeumer H, Hacke W, Kolmann H, Poeck K. Lokale Fibrinolysetherapie bei Basilaris-Thrombose. Dtsch Med Wochenschr. 2008;107(19):728–31.
26. Berg-Dammer E, Felber S, Henkes H, Nahser H, Kühne D. Long-term outcome after local intra-arterial fibrinolysis of basilar artery thrombosis. Cerebrovasc Dis. 2000;10(3):183–8.
27. Renard D, Landragin N, Robinson A, Brunel H, Bonafe A, Heroum C, et al. MRI-based score for acute basilar artery thrombosis. Cerebrovasc Dis. 2008;25(6):511–6.
28. Chandra R, Law C, Yan B, Dowling R, Mitchell P. Glasgow coma scale does not predict outcome post-intra-arterial treatment for basilar artery thrombosis. Am J Neuroradiol. 2011;32(3):576–80.
29. Kashiwagi J, Kiyosue H, Hori Y, Okahara M, Tanoue S, Sagara Y, et al. Endovascular recanalization of acute intracranial vertebrobasilar artery occlusion using local fibrinolysis and additional balloon angioplasty. Neuroradiology. 2010;52(5):361–70.
30. Yu Y, Niu L, Gao L, Zhao Z, Deng J, Qu Y, et al. Intraarterial thrombolysis and stent placement for acute basilar artery occlusion. J Vasc Interv Radiol. 2010;21(9):1359–63.
31. Hacke W, Zeumer H, Ferbert A, Brückmann H, del Zoppo G. Intra-arterial thrombolytic therapy improves outcome in patients with acute vertebrobasilar occlusive disease. Stroke. 1988;19(10):1216–22.
32. Nogueira R, Liebeskind D, Sung G, Duckwiler G, Smith W. Predictors of good clinical outcomes, mortality, and successful revascularization in patients with acute ischemic stroke undergoing thrombectomy: pooled analysis of the mechanical embolus removal in cerebral ischemia (MERCI) and multi MERCI trials. Stroke. 2009;40(12):3777–37783.
33. Pierre Gobin Y, Starkman S, Duckwiler G, Grobelny T, Kidwell C, Jahan R, et al. MERCI 1. Stroke. 2004;35(12):2848–54.
34. Smith W, Sung G, Starkman S, Saver J, Kidwell C, Gobin Y, et al. Safety and efficacy of mechanical embolectomy in acute ischemic stroke: results of the MERCI trial. Stroke. 2005;36(7):1432–8.
35. Smith W, Sung G, Saver J, Budzik R, Duckwiler G, Liebeskind D, et al. Mechanical thrombectomy for acute ischemic stroke. Stroke. 2008;39(4):1205–12.
36. Penumbra Pivotal Stroke Trial Investigators. The Penumbra Pivotal Stroke Trial. Stroke. 2009;40(8):2761–8.
37. Turk A, Siddiqui A, Fifi J, De Leacy R, Fiorella D, Gu E, et al. Aspiration thrombectomy versus stent retriever thrombectomy as first-line approach for large vessel occlusion (COMPASS): a multicentre, randomised, open label, blinded outcome, non-inferiority trial. Lancet. 2019;393(10175):998–1008.
38. Saver J, Jahan R, Levy E, Jovin T, Baxter B, Nogueira R, et al. Solitaire flow restoration device versus the Merci retriever in patients with acute ischaemic stroke (SWIFT): a randomised, parallel-group, non-inferiority trial. Lancet. 2012;380(9849):1241–9.
39. Nogueira R, Lutsep H, Gupta R, Jovin T, Albers G, Walker G, et al. Trevo versus Merci retrievers for thrombectomy revascularisation of large vessel occlusions in acute ischaemic stroke (TREVO 2): a randomised trial. Lancet. 2012;380(9849):1231–40.
40. Nedeltchev K, Remonda L, Do D, Brekenfeld C, Ozdoba C, Arnold M, et al. Acute stenting and thromboaspiration in basilar artery occlusions due to embolism from the dominating vertebral artery. Neuroradiology. 2004;46(8):686–91.
41. Chapot R, Houdart E, Mounayer C, Saint-Maurice J, Merland J. Thromboaspiration in the basilar artery: report of two cases. Am J Neuroradiol. 2002;23:282–4.
42. Jankowitz B, Aleu A, Lin R, Jumaa M, Kanaan H, Kostov D, et al. Endovascular treatment of basilar artery occlusion by manual aspiration thrombectomy. J Neurointerv Surg. 2010;2(2):110–4.
43. Jankowitz B, Aghaebrahim A, Zirra A, Spataru O, Zaidi S, Jumaa M, et al. Manual aspiration thrombectomy. Stroke. 2012;43(5):1408–11.
44. Ogawa A, Mori E, Minematsu K, Taki W, Takahashi A, Nemoto S, et al. Randomized trial of intraarterial infusion of urokinase within 6 hours of middle cerebral artery stroke. Stroke. 2007;38(10):2633–9.
45. Ciccone A, Valvassori L, Nichelatti M, Sgoifo A, Ponzio M, Sterzi R, et al. Endovascular treatment for acute ischemic stroke. N Engl J Med. 2013;368(10):904–13.
46. Kidwell C, Jahan R, Gornbein J, Alger J, Nenov V, Ajani Z, et al. A trial of imaging selection and endovascular treatment for ischemic stroke. N Engl J Med. 2013;368(10):914–23.
47. Lansberg M, Straka M, Kemp S, Mlynash M, Wechsler L, Jovin T, et al. MRI profile and response to endovascular reperfusion after stroke (DEFUSE 2): a prospective cohort study. Lancet Neurol. 2012;11(10):860–7.
48. Lutsep H, Rymer M, Nesbit G. Vertebrobasilar revascularization rates and outcomes in the MERCI and multi-MERCI trials. J Stroke Cerebrovasc Dis. 2008;17(2):55–7.
49. Broderick J, Palesch Y, Demchuk A, Yeatts S, Khatri P, Hill M, et al. Endovascular therapy after intravenous t-PA versus t-PA alone for stroke. N Engl J Med. 2013;368(10):893–903.
50. Berkhemer O, Fransen P, Beumer D, van den Berg L, Lingsma H, Yoo A, et al. A randomized trial of intra-arterial treatment for acute ischemic stroke. N Engl J Med. 2015;372(1):11–20.
51. Goyal M, Demchuk A, Menon B, Eesa M, Rempel J, Thornton J, et al. Randomized assessment of rapid endovascular treatment of ischemic stroke. N Engl J Med. 2015;372(11):1019–30.
52. Jovin T, Chamorro A, Cobo E, de Miquel M, Molina C, Rovira A, et al. Thrombectomy within 8 hours after

symptom onset in ischemic stroke. N Engl J Med. 2015;372(24):2296–306.

53. Campbell B, Mitchell P, Kleinig T, Dewey H, Churilov L, Yassi N, et al. Endovascular therapy for ischemic stroke with perfusion-imaging selection. N Engl J Med. 2015;372(11):1009–18.

54. Saver J, Goyal M, Bonafe A, Diener H, Levy E, Pereira V, et al. Stent-retriever thrombectomy after intravenous t-PA vs. t-PA alone in stroke. N Engl J Med. 2015;372(24):2285–95.

55. Bracard S, Ducrocq X, Mas J, Soudant M, Oppenheim C, Moulin T, et al. Mechanical thrombectomy after intravenous alteplase versus alteplase alone after stroke (THRACE): a randomised controlled trial. Lancet Neurol. 2016;15(11):1138–47.

56. Nogueira R, Jadhav A, Haussen D, Bonafe A, Budzik R, Bhuva P, et al. Thrombectomy 6 to 24 hours after stroke with a mismatch between deficit and infarct. N Engl J Med. 2018;378(1):11–21.

57. Albers G, Marks M, Kemp S, Christensen S, Tsai J, Ortega-Gutierrez S, et al. Thrombectomy for stroke at 6 to 16 hours with selection by perfusion imaging. N Engl J Med. 2018;378(8):708–18.

58. Singer O, Berkefeld J, Nolte C, Bohner G, Haring H, Trenkler J, et al. Mechanical recanalization in basilar artery occlusion: the ENDOSTROKE study. Ann Neurol. 2015;77(3):415–24.

59. Liu X, Dai Q, Ye R, Zi W, Liu Y, Wang H et al. Basilar artery occlusion endovascular intervention versus standard medical treatment (BEST) trial. Presentation presented at World Stroke Organization; 2018.

60. Roman L, Menon B, Blasco J, Hernández-Pérez M, Dávalos A, Majoie C, et al. Imaging features and safety and efficacy of endovascular stroke treatment: a meta-analysis of individual patient level data. Lancet Neurol. 2018;17(10):895–904.

61. Graf J, Skutta B, Kuhn F, Ferbert A. Computed tomographic angiography findings in 103 patients following vascular events in the posterior circulation; potential and clinical relevance. J Neurol. 2000;247(10):760–6.

62. Coutts S, Lev M, Eliasziw M, Roccatagliata L, Hill M, Schwamm L, et al. ASPECTS on CTA source images versus unenhanced CT. Stroke. 2004;35(11):2472–6.

63. Puetz V, Sylaja P, Coutts S, Hill M, Dzialowski I, Mueller P, et al. Extent of Hypoattenuation on CT angiography source images predicts functional outcome in patients with basilar artery occlusion. Stroke. 2008;39(9):2485–90.

64. Schaefer P, Yoo A, Bell D, Barak E, Romero J, Nogueira R, et al. CT angiography-source image hypoattenuation predicts clinical outcome in posterior circulation strokes treated with intra-arterial therapy. Stroke. 2008;39(11):3107–9.

65. Pallesen L, Khomenko A, Dzialowski I, Barlinn J, Barlinn K, Zerna C, et al. CT-angiography source images indicate less fatal outcome despite coma of patients in the basilar artery international cooperation study. Int J Stroke. 2016;12(2):145–51.

66. Cho T, Nighoghossian N, Tahon F, Némoz C, Hermier M, Salkine F, et al. Brain stem diffusion-weighted imaging lesion score: a potential marker of outcome in acute basilar artery occlusion. Am J Neuroradiol. 2008;30(1):194–8.

67. Karameshev A, Arnold M, Schroth G, Kappeler L, Stein P, Gralla J, et al. Diffusion-weighted MRI helps predict outcome in basilar artery occlusion patients treated with intra-arterial thrombolysis. Cerebrovasc Dis. 2011;32(4):393–400.

68. Nagel S, Herweh C, Köhrmann M, Huttner H, Poli S, Hartmann M, et al. MRI in patients with acute basilar artery occlusion – DWI lesion scoring is an independent predictor of outcome. Int J Stroke. 2011;7(4):282–8.

69. Jadhav A, Nanduri S, Starr M, Aghaebrahim A, Zaidi S, Jumaa M et al. Infarct location and volumes as predictors of outcome after endovascular recanalization of basilar artery occlusion. Presentation presented at international stroke conference; 2013.

70. Bouslama M, Haussen D, Aghaebrahim A, Grossberg J, Walker G, Rangaraju S, et al. Predictors of good outcome after endovascular therapy for vertebrobasilar occlusion stroke. Stroke. 2017;48(12):3252–7.

71. Starr MT, Jadhav AP, Zaidi SF, Jumaa MA, Reddy VK, Hammer MD, Jankowitz BT, Wechsler LR, Jovin TG. Treatment of basilar artery occlusion without time constraints: clinical outcomes, safety and predictors of favorable results [unpublished manuscript]. Pittsburgh: University of Pittsburgh Medical Center; 2016.

72. Rangaraju S, Liggins J, Aghaebrahim A, Streib C, Sun C, Gupta R, et al. Pittsburgh outcomes after stroke MT score predicts outcomes after endovascular therapy for anterior circulation large vessel occlusions. Stroke. 2014;45(8):2298–304.

73. Lindsberg P, Pekkola J, Strbian D, Sairanen T, Mattle H, Schroth G. Time window for recanalization in basilar artery occlusion. Neurology. 2015;85(20):1806–15.

74. Ring B, Waddington M. Intraluminal diameters of the intracranial arteries. Vasc Surg. 1967;1(3):137–51.

75. Boeckh-Behrens T, Pree D, Lummel N, Friedrich B, Maegerlein C, Kreiser K, et al. Vertebral artery patency and thrombectomy in basilar artery occlusions. Stroke. 2019;50(2):389–95.

76. Cohen J, Leker R, Gomori J, Eichel R, Rajz G, Moscovici S, et al. Emergent revascularization of acute tandem vertebrobasilar occlusions: endovascular approaches and technical considerations—confirming the role of vertebral artery ostium stenosis as a cause of vertebrobasilar stroke. J Clin Neurosci. 2016;34:70–6.

77. Siebert E, Bohner G, Zweynert S, Maus V, Mpotsaris A, Liebig T, et al. Revascularization techniques for acute basilar artery occlusion. Clin Neuroradiol. 2019;29(3):435–43.

78. Liu W, Kung D, Mahaney K, Rossen J, Jabbour P, Hasan D. Anterior-to-posterior circulation approach for mechanical thrombectomy of an acutely occluded basilar artery using the penumbra aspiration system. World Neurosurg. 2012;77(2):398.e17–20.

79. Morales A, Parry P, Jadhav A, Jovin T. A novel route of revascularization in basilar artery occlusion and review of the literature. Case Rep. 2015;2015:bcr2015011723.

80. Gross B, Jadhav A, Jankowitz B, Jovin T. Recanalization of tandem vertebrobasilar occlusions with contralateral vertebral occlusion or hypoplasia via either direct passage or the SHERPA technique. Interv Neurol. 2018;8:13–9.

81. Puri A, Kühn A, Kwon H, Khan M, Hou S, Lin E, et al. Endovascular treatment of tandem vascular occlusions in acute ischemic stroke. J Neurointerv Surg. 2014;7(3):158–63.

82. Gross B, Desai S, Walker G, Jankowitz B, Jadhav A, Jovin T. Balloon-mounted stents for acute intracranial large vessel occlusion secondary to presumed atherosclerotic disease: evolution in an era of supple intermediate catheters. J Neurointerv Surg. 2019;11(10):975–8.

83. Zhao Y, Jin M, Liu Q, Liu D, Chen D, Du B. A long-term follow-up results of Enterprise stent in treatment of severe symptomatic basilar artery atherosclerotic stenosis. Zhonghua Nei Ke Za Zhi. 2016;55(5):372–6.

84. Lee JS, Hong JM, Kim JS. Diagnostic and therapeutic strategies for acute intracranial atherosclerosis-related occlusions. J Stroke. 2017;19(2):143–51.

85. Basilar Artery Occlusion Chinese Endovascular Trial - ClinicalTrials.gov [Internet]. Clinicaltrials.gov. 2019 [cited 21 April 2019]. Available from: https://clinicaltrials.gov/ct2/show/NCT02737189?term=Basilar+Artery+Occlusion+Chinese+Endovascular+Trial&rank=1

86. Basilar Artery International Cooperation Study - ClinicalTrials.gov [Internet]. Clinicaltrials.gov. 2019 [cited 21 April 2019]. Available from: https://clinicaltrials.gov/ct2/results?cond=&term=Basilar+Artery+International+Cooperation+Study+&cntry=&state=&city=&dist=

87. Field Randomization of NA-1 Therapy in Early Responders - ClinicalTrials.gov [Internet]. Clinicaltrials.gov. 2019 [cited 23 April 2019]. Available from: https://clinicaltrials.gov/ct2/show/NCT02315443

88. Kim JS, Lee KB, Park JH, Sung SM, Oh K, Kim EG, Chang DI, Hwang YH, Lee EJ, Kim WK, Ju C, Ryu JM. Safety and efficacy of otaplimastat in patients with acute ischemic stroke receiving rtPA (SAFE-TPA): a multicenter, randomised, double-blind, placebo-controlled phase II study. Ann Neurol. 2020;87(2):233–45.

89. Kim JS. tPA helpers in the treatment of acute ischemic stroke: are they ready for clinical use? J Stroke. 2019;21(2):160–74.

90. Lee J, Hong J, Lee K, Suh H, Demchuk A, Hwang Y, et al. Endovascular therapy of cerebral arterial occlusions: intracranial atherosclerosis versus embolism. J Stroke Cerebrovasc Dis. 2015;24(9):2074–80.

91. Arch A, Weisman D, Coca S, Nystrom K, Wira C, Schindler J. Missed ischemic stroke diagnosis in the emergency department by emergency medicine and neurology services. Stroke. 2016;47(3):668–73.

Angioplasty and Stenting for Posterior Circulation Stroke

12

Hugh S. Markus

Approximately 20–40% of all ischaemic strokes occur in the posterior circulation, and about a quarter of these are caused by either vertebral or basilar artery stenosis [1]. Despite its frequency, the optimal management for vertebrobasilar stenosis is not clear. This is in marked contrast to carotid stenosis for which large randomised controlled trials have provided robust evidence showing that removal of the stenosis by carotid endarterectomy improves outcome [2].

Prospective natural history studies have shown that symptomatic vertebrobasilar stenosis is associated with a high risk of early recurrent stroke, particularly in the first few weeks, and that the temporal pattern of recurrence is very similar to that seen for carotid artery disease [3, 4]. The risk is particularly high for intracranial disease for which it was reported to be 33% in the first 90 days of follow-up, compared to 16% for extracranial disease, in a pooled individual patient analysis of two prospective follow-up studies in patients presenting with posterior circulation TIA or stroke who all had CTA or MRA to identify stenosis [5]. This high early recurrent stroke risk raises a question as to whether vertebral and basilar stenosis should be treated with revascularisation in a similar fashion to carotid endarterectomy for carotid stenosis.

The vertebral artery is much less accessible than the carotid artery, and therefore, although surgical endarterectomy approaches have been used, these have not been widely adopted [1]. In contrast, angioplasty and stenting have been widely used to treat vertebrobasilar stenoses.

Vertebral stenting has been shown to be technically feasible in many studies, largely small case series. Systematic reviews data have reported very low complication rates for extracranial vertebral stenosis (as low as 1% or less for origin stenosis), but higher rates of 5–10% for intracranial vertebral stenosis [6, 7]. However, such case series are open to selection and publication bias and therefore do not provide robust data. This can only be provided by randomised control trials. Recently, a number of randomised control trials have evaluated stenting in patients with symptomatic vertebral artery stenosis, the largest of which, the Vertebral Artery Ischaemia Trial (VIST), was published in 2017 [8]. Data from a number of these have been pooled in a recent individual patient analysis [9]. In this review, the results of these trials and the pooled analysis are presented.

There is less data on stenting basilar artery stenosis, but data from the Stenting and Aggressive Management for the Prevention of Recurrent stroke in Intracranial Stenosis (SAMMPRIS) trial [10] and from individual case reports have shown a much higher complication rate. This is consistent with our experience, with complications including both basilar artery

H. S. Markus (✉)
Stroke Research Group, Neurology Unit, Department of Clinical Neurosciences, University of Cambridge, Cambridge, UK
e-mail: hsm32@medschl.cam.ac.uk

© Springer Nature Singapore Pte Ltd. 2021
J. S. Kim (ed.), *Posterior Circulation Stroke*, https://doi.org/10.1007/978-981-15-6739-1_12

rupture and stroke secondary to occlusion of perforating arteries arising from the basilar artery. These results had led to much less enthusiasm for basilar artery stenosis, and this was not included in the recent trials, which were limited to vertebral stenosis.

Randomised Clinical Trials

Five randomised trials have assessed the effectiveness of angioplasty and stenting in symptomatic vertebral artery stenosis. Two of these, SAMMPRIS [10] and Vitesse Intracranial Stent Study for Ischaemic Therapy (VISSIT), were confined to intracranial stenosis [11]. They included patients with intracranial vessel stenosis in multiple arterial locations, and vertebral artery stenosis made up a minority of the participants. Two other recent trials, VIST [8] and Vertebral Artery Stenting on Trial (VAST) [12], included both intracranial and extracranial stenosis. One trial (Carotid and Vertebral Artery Transluminal Angioplasty Study (CAVATAS)), which was conducted in the 1990s, recruited almost exclusively patients with extracranial disease [13].

The natural history data showing a higher recurrent stroke risk for intracranial, compared with extracranial, vertebral stenosis [5] combined with the reported higher peri-operative risk for intracranial stenosis [7] suggest that the risk–benefit ratio may differ for intra- and extracranial stenosis. Therefore, it is important to not only analyse the results of these trials for all vertebral stenosis but also to determine whether there may be specific treatment benefits for intracranial and extracranial stenosis.

CAVATAS recruited 16 patients with symptomatic vertebral stenosis (15 were extracranial all of the origin of the vertebral artery and 1 intracranial), of which 8 were randomised to angioplasty/stenting [13]. Because it was performed in the 1990s, older equipment was used and most patients randomised to endovascular therapy received angioplasty alone (6 cases) rather than with stenting (2 cases). The mean time between symptoms and randomisation was long at 92 days (range 5–376 days), and in those randomised to

angioplasty, there was a mean additional time from randomisation to the procedure of 45 days (range 7–148 days). This means that many patients were treated after the acute period during which there is a high risk of recurrent stroke. Patients were followed for a mean of 4.5 years in the endovascular group and 4.9 years in the medical group. There were no recurrent strokes in the vertebrobasilar territory in either treatment arm during the follow-up. There was 1 non-fatal and 1 fatal carotid territory stroke in the endovascular treatment arm.

There were no further trials that included patients with extracranial vertebral stenosis until VAST and VIST, which were published in 2015 and 2017, respectively. VAST aimed for a sample size of 180 but only recruited 115 of which 83% had extracranial stenosis [12]; 57 patients were assigned to stenting and 58 to medical treatment alone with a median interval between most recent symptoms and randomisation of 25 days. During a median follow-up of 3 years, there were 7 strokes in the medical treatment group and 8 strokes in the stenting group. More early recurrent strokes (defined as within 30 days) occurred in the stenting arm (3 versus 1) while more strokes during longer-term follow-up occurred in the medical arm (7 versus 4). Of the 3 early strokes that occurred in the stenting arm, 2 occurred in 9 patients with intracranial stenosis (22%) while only 1 occurred in the 48 patients with extracranial stenosis (2%). The results of VAST were underpowered to detect any treatment difference between the two arms, and it provided a neutral result. Nevertheless, it did suggest that the early stroke risk of stenting in patients with intracranial stenosis was high, while the risk for patients with extracranial stenosis was low.

VIST aimed to recruit 540 patients with 50% or greater symptomatic vertebral stenosis [8]. However, recruitment was closed by the funder NIHR HTA after 181 patients were enrolled due to recruitment being slower than expected. In retrospect, this was an unfortunate decision. It is of note that the carotid endarterectomy trials ECST and NASCET, which transformed the management of symptomatic carotid stenosis, took much longer to reach their sample size than expected, and without funding being continued beyond the original planned deadline would not have had their transformational effect on management of carotid artery disease [14, 15]. Three patients in VIST did not contribute follow-up data, which left 88 patients in the medical group and 91 in the intervention group. Mean follow-up was 3.5 years. As in VAST, stenosis was predominantly extracranial (78.7% versus 21.3%). Similar to VAST, the peri-procedural stroke rate was very low in extracranial stenosis (no complications), while it was much higher in intracranial stenosis (2 strokes in 13 patients). The primary endpoint of fatal or non-fatal stroke occurred in 5 patients in the stent group versus 12 patients in the medical group (hazard ratio 0.40:95% CI 0.14–1.13, $P = 0.08$). The absolute risk reduction was 25 strokes per 1000 person-years. Therefore, although there was an approximately 60% reduction in the rate of recurrent stroke in patients in the stenting arm, this difference was not significant. However, post hoc analyses did show a suggestion of benefit. When the time from randomisation was controlled (this was shorter in the stenting arm), the hazard ratio for the primary endpoint was 0.34 (95% CI 0.12–0.98 $P = 0.046$). A second post hoc analysis also trying to take into account this difference in baseline risk due to the stented arm being recruited sooner after symptoms looked at patients who had been randomised within 2 weeks after the last symptoms. This revealed a hazard ratio for the primary endpoint of 0.30 (95% CI 0.09–0.99, $P = 0.048$).

Therefore, although the results of VIST were suggestive of a possible treatment effect, the primary endpoint was not significant. They do, however, suggest that if funding had been continued to allow the planned sample size to be reached, VIST may well have produced a definitive result. Strengths of VIST were that no patients were lost to follow-up. However, there are a number of limitations. First, the planned sample size was not reached. Second, a number of patients randomised to stenting did not have greater than 50% stenosis at angiogram when the procedure was due to be performed and therefore were treated conservatively. This emphasises the need

for careful assessment of non-invasive imaging (which in VIST was CT and MR angiography) in any such trials. A further potential criticism is that patients in the stenting arm were more likely to receive dual antiplatelet therapy with aspirin and clopidogrel than those in the medical treatment alone arm. Some data suggest that this dual antiplatelet therapy may be associated with less recurrent stroke risk in patients with symptomatic large artery stenosis.

SAMMPRIS and VISSIT randomised only patients with intracranial stenosis. In SAMMPRIS, 451 patients with a variety of large vessel intracranial stenosis were randomised, of which 60 (13%) had intracranial stenosis [10]. Another difference in SAMMPRIS was that all patients in the medical arm were treated with a very intensive management protocol, which comprised dual antiplatelet therapy with aspirin and clopidogrel for the first 90 days, intensive management of risk factors including blood pressure and cholesterol, and a focus on lifestyle modification with advice on smoking cessation, weight loss, and exercise. It is of note that the recurrent stroke rate in the medical arm in SAMMPRIS was much lower than had been expected, and this may be a reflection of this intensive management programme.

A criticism that has been labelled against SAMMPRIS is the use of the Wingspan self-extending stent. Since the study, it has been suggested that this stent is associated with an increased risk of peri-procedural complications. However, a similar overall result was reported in VISSIT, which used a different stent, a balloon-expandable stent, and there was a similar high risk of early complications. VISSIT randomised 112 patients with symptomatic intracranial stenosis in a variety of intracerebral arteries with a median time to randomisation of 15 days in the medical arm and 9 in the stenting arm [11]. There was a similar overall outcome to SAMMPRIS with 1-year stroke rates of 9.4% in the medical arm and 34.5% in the stenting arm. Most strokes in the stenting arm occurred in the peri-operative period. A breakdown for those patients with vertebrobasilar stenosis is not presented in the paper, and it has not been possible to obtain further information from the corresponding authors. Nevertheless, the overall results in VISSIT were similar to those seen in SAMMPRIS.

What Do the Results of Randomised Trials Tell Us?

Meta-analyses of the published data, including SAMMPRIS, VAST, and VIST (similar analyses could not be done with the VISSIT data due to the inability to obtain vertebral artery specific data), found no evidence of any treatment benefit for intracranial stenosis [8]. Results were largely neutral without any clear benefit for medical therapy. Although results for extracranial stenosis were not significant, they suggested a possible benefit with a hazard ratio of 0.66 (95% CI 0.25–1.72) [8]. A more recent analysis used individual patient data from the three trials [9]. This approach allows a more detailed assessment of treatment efficacy and also enables effects in specific subgroups to be studied. The pooled analysis included a total of 168 subjects randomised to medical treatment (46 intracranial and 122 extracranial) and 186 randomised to stenting (64 intracranial and 122 extracranial). In those randomised to stenting, the peri-procedural stroke or death rate was higher for intracranial stenosis than for extracranial stenosis (15.6% versus 0.8%, $P = 0.00005$). There was a total of 1036 years of follow-up, and in the overall population, the hazard ratio for any stroke in the stenting arm compared with the medical arm was 0.81 (95% CI 0.45–1.44). For extracranial stenosis alone, it was 0.63 (0.27–1.46), and for intracranial stenosis alone, it was 1.06 (0.46–2.42).

Therefore, there was no benefit for stenting in vertebral stenosis as a whole. The results in intracranial stenosis confirmed a high peri-procedural risk of stroke and also showed no evidence of any long-term benefit with a hazard ratio at almost unity. The hazard ratio of 0.63 for extracranial stenosis would be consistent with a benefit but could also be consistent with no benefit for stenting. The conclusion was that further trials are warranted for extracranial stenosis. In contrast,

trials would only be indicated for intracranial stenosis if the peri-operative risk associated with intracranial stenosis could be reduced [9].

How Should Current Data Influence Clinical Practice?

The most definitive data come from the individual patient pooled analysis [9]. This does not provide a definitive answer as to whether stenting is better than medical treatment but does provide useful pointers to guide practice until more clinical trial data are available.

For intracranial stenosis, the data suggest that medical therapy is the treatment of choice, and only if this fails, should stenting be considered. For extracranial stenosis, because the peri-procedural risk has been confirmed to be very low, both best medical therapy and stenting do represent reasonable treatment choices.

The trials have recruited patients with reasonably symptomatic stenosis, most of whom have had a single TIA or minor stroke. It has been suggested that there may be specific subgroups of patients who may specifically benefit from vertebral stenting. This includes patients with recurrent events despite the best medical therapy and patients in whom the stenosis results in haemodynamic compromise: for example, those who have a tight stenosis with an atretic or absent contralateral vertebral stenosis [16]. Whether these subgroups do particularly benefit from vertebral revascularisation can only definitively be answered with clinical trials.

Whether stenting or best medical treatment is chosen, it is important that the best medical treatment is intensive. The SAMMPRIS trial was consistent with a marked benefit from intensive secondary preventative therapy, and this fits with recent data showing the benefits of intensive treatment of cardiovascular risk factors. Increasing evidence suggests that dual antiplatelet therapy with aspirin and clopidogrel is more effective than aspirin alone in preventing stroke in patients with recent symptomatic large artery stenosis, both extracranial and intracranial, particularly in the first few weeks after symptoms when the risk of recurrent stroke is highest. This was initially suggested by a greater reduction of asymptomatic emboli detected on transcranial Doppler ultrasound in randomised trials in both extracranial [17] and intracranial carotid stenosis [18]. Recent trials randomising patients within the first 24 hours after minor stroke or TIA (CHANCE and POINT) have shown that aspirin and clopidogrel dual therapy, compared with aspirin alone, reduces early recurrent stroke risk by about one third [19, 20]. Interestingly, in CHANCE, the benefit seemed to be greatest in patients with large artery stenosis [21], while another trial SOCRATES showed no benefit for a new antiplatelet agent ticagrelor against aspirin when given to all patients with recent stroke and TIA, but a subgroup analysis suggested that there was a benefit in patients presenting with large artery stenosis [22]. Therefore, our practice is to treat all patients with large artery stenosis, including those with both intra- and extracranial vertebral stenosis, with aspirin and clopidogrel for the first 1–3 months after symptom onset after which we switch them to clopidogrel alone. We would also treat them with intensive statin therapy and aim to reduce blood pressure to 130 mmHg systolic. SAMMPRIS also emphasised the importance of lifestyle medications such as smoking cessation, a healthy diet, and exercise.

Does the Type of Stent Matter?

Both VIST and VAST used a variety of different stents, the choice being left with the operator. SAMMPRIS was criticised for using the Wingspan stent because of its potentially higher peri-operative risk [23]. As yet, it is uncertain whether different stents may be safer. Because the peri-operative stroke risk is very low for extracranial stenosis with current stents, the need for safer options is not pressing. However, stents or other technical advances, which could reduce the high peri-procedural stroke rate reported for intracranial stenosis, might alter the risk–benefit ratio for treating this disease.

Restenosis has been reported following stenting, particularly for vertebral artery origin steno-

sis [24]. Data do suggest that drug-eluting stents may be associated with a reduced risk [25]. A meta-analysis of available data, largely from non-randomised case series, reported a restenosis rate of 33.6% with bare-metal stents and 15.5% with drug-eluting stents [26]. Whether this translates into clinical benefit remains uncertain. Most restenoses remain asymptomatic and in VIST, in which almost stents were non-drug eluting, the long-term recurrent stroke rate in those receiving stenting was low [8]. More trials are required in this area.

It has been suggested that distal embolic protection devices might reduce the risk of peri-procedural embolisation. In a randomised trial, 61 patients were randomised to a self-expanding stent with an embolic protection device and 66 to bare-metal stents without embolic protection. Diffusion-weighted lesions on MRI were less frequent after the procedure in those receiving embolic protection (3.3 v 18.6%) [27]. However, the devices can themselves be associated with increased risk as they have to be advanced through the stenosis and can cause damage, and further trials would be required to demonstrate improved clinical outcome before their widespread use could be recommended, particularly for extracranial stenosis in which the perioperative risk is very low without the use of such devices.

VIST also highlighted diagnostic challenges that need to be incorporated into any future trials. It relied on CT angiography and contrast-enhanced MRA to screen for vertebral stenoses. Although previous studies had shown good sensitivity for both techniques in the detection of vertebral stenosis compared with intra-arterial digital subtraction angiography [28], in VIST 23 of the 91 patients randomised to stenting were found not to have stenosis of more than 50% on digital subtraction angiography performed at the time of stenting [8]. Subsequent central review of all pre-randomisation CTA and MRA imaging revealed that in approximately half of these cases, expert neuroradiological review would not have confirmed stenoses on the non-invasive imaging, while in the other half of the cases, central review found entry imaging to be of insufficient quality to confirm stenosis. These data emphasise the importance of non-invasive imaging being reviewed by expert neuroradiologists before any decision is made on stenting. It also emphasises the need for careful ongoing quality control in any future studies with ongoing review of non-invasive entry imaging, possibly with confirmation of stenosis on central review prior to randomisation.

References

1. Markus HS, van der Worp HB, Rothwell PM. Posterior circulation ischaemic stroke and transient ischaemic attack: diagnosis, investigation, and secondary prevention. Lancet Neurol. 2013;12:989–98.
2. Rothwell PM, Eliasziw M, Gutnikov SA, Fox AJ, Taylor DW, Mayberg MR, et al. Analysis of pooled data from the randomized controlled trials of endarterectomy for symptomatic carotid stenosis. Lancet. 2003;361:107–16.
3. Gulli G, Khan S, Markus HS. Vertebrobasilar stenosis predicts high early recurrent stroke risk in posterior circulation stroke and TIA. Stroke. 2009;40:2732–7.
4. Flossmann E, Rothwell PM. Prognosis of vertebrobasilar transient ischaemic attack and minor stroke. Brain. 2003;126:1940–54.
5. Gulli G, Marquardt L, Rothwell PM, Markus HS. Stroke risk after posterior circulation stroke/transient ischemic attack and its relationship to site of vertebrobasilar stenosis: pooled data analysis from prospective studies. Stroke. 2013;44:598–604.
6. Stayman AN, Nogueira RG, Gupta R. A systematic review of stenting and angioplasty of symptomatic extracranial vertebral artery stenosis. Stroke. 2011;42:2212–6.
7. Eberhardt O, Naegele T, Raygrotzki S, Weller M, Ernemann U. Stenting of vertebrobasilar arteries in symptomatic atherosclerotic disease and acute occlusion: case series and review of the literature. J Vasc Surg. 2006;43:1145–54.
8. Markus HS, Larsson SC, Kuker W, Schulz UG, Ford I, Rothwell PM, Clifton A, Investigators VIST. Stenting for symptomatic vertebral artery stenosis: the vertebral artery Ischaemia stenting trial. Neurology. 2017;89:1229–36.
9. Markus HS, Harshfield EL, Compter A, Kuker W, Kappelle LJ, Clifton A, et al.; Vertebral Stenosis Trialists' Collaboration. Stenting for symptomatic vertebral artery stenosis: a preplanned pooled individual patient data analysis. Lancet Neurol. 2019;18:666–73.
10. Chimowitz MI, Lynn MJ, Derdeyn CP, Turan TN, Fiorella D, Lane BF, et al. Stenting versus aggressive medical therapy for intracranial arterial stenosis. N Engl J Med. 2011;365:993–1003.
11. Zaidat OO, Fitzsimmons BF, Woodward BK, Wang Z, Killer-Oberpfalzer M, Wakhloo A, et al. Effect of a balloon-expandable intracranial stent vs medical therapy on risk of stroke in patients with symptomatic intracranial stenosis: the VISSIT randomized clinical trial. JAMA. 2015;313:1240–8.
12. Compter A, van der Worp HB, Schonewille WJ, Vos JA, Boiten J, Nederkoorn PJ, et al. Stenting versus medical treatment in patients with symptomatic vertebral artery stenosis: a randomised open-label phase 2 trial. Lancet Neurol. 2015;14:606–14.
13. Coward LJ, McCabe DJ, Ederle J, Featherstone RL, Clifton A, Brown MM. Long term outcome after angioplasty and stenting for symptomatic vertebral artery stenosis compared with medical treatment in the carotid and vertebral artery transluminal angioplasty study (CAVATAS): a randomized trial. Stroke. 2007;38:1526–30.
14. Randomised trial of endarterectomy for recently symptomatic carotid stenosis: final results of the MRC European Carotid Surgery Trial (ECST). Lancet. 1998;351(9113):1379–87.
15. North American Symptomatic Carotid Endarterectomy Trial Collaborators, HJM B, Taylor DW, Haynes RB, Sackett DL, Peerless SJ, Ferguson GG, et al. Beneficial effect of carotid endarterectomy in symptomatic patients with high-grade carotid stenosis. N Engl J Med. 1991;325:445–53.
16. Wang ZL, Gao BL, Li TX, Cai DY, Zhu LF, Bai WX, et al. Symptomatic intracranial vertebral artery atherosclerotic stenosis ($\geq$70%) with concurrent contralateral vertebral atherosclerotic diseases in 88 patients treated with the intracranial stenting. Eur J Radiol. 2015;84:1801–4.
17. Markus HS, Droste DW, Kaps M, Larrue V, Lees KR, Siebler M, et al. Dual antiplatelet therapy with clopidogrel and aspirin in symptomatic carotid stenosis evaluated using doppler embolic signal detection: the clopidogrel and aspirin for reduction of emboli in symptomatic carotid stenosis (CARESS) trial. Circulation. 2005;111:2233–40.
18. Wong KS, Chen C, Fu J, Chang HM, Suwanwela NC, Huang YN, et al.; CLAIR study investigators. Clopidogrel plus aspirin versus aspirin alone for reducing embolisation in patients with acute symptomatic cerebral or carotid artery stenosis (CLAIR study): a randomised, open-label, blinded-endpoint trial. Lancet Neurol. 2010;9:489–97.
19. Wang Y, Wang Y, Zhao X, Liu L, Wang D, Wang C, et al.; CHANCE Investigators. Clopidogrel with aspirin in acute minor stroke or transient ischemic attack. N Engl J Med. 2013;369:11–9.
20. Johnston SC, Easton JD, Farrant M, Barsan W, Conwit RA, Elm JJ, Featherstone RL, Clifton A, Brown MM, the POINT Investigators. Clopidogrel and aspirin in acute ischemic stroke and high-risk TIA. N Engl J Med. 2018;379:215–25.
21. Liu L, Wong KS, Leng X, Pu Y, Wang Y, Jing J, et al.; CHANCE Investigators. Dualantiplatelet

therapy in stroke and ICAS: subgroup analysis of CHANCE. Neurology. 2015;85:1154–62.

22. Amarenco P, Albers GW, Denison H, Easton JD, Evans SR, Held P, et al.; SOCRATES Steering Committee and Investigators. Efficacy and safety of ticagrelor versus aspirin in acute stroke or transient ischaemic attack of atherosclerotic origin: a subgroup analysis of SOCRATES, a randomised,double-blind, controlled trial. Lancet Neurol. 2017;16:301–10.

23. Farooq MU, Al-Ali F, Min J, Gorelick PB. Reviving intracranial angioplasty and stenting "SAMMPRIS and beyond". Front Neurol. 2014;5:101.

24. Chen W, Huang F, Li M, Jiang Y, He J, Li H, et al. Incidence and predictors of the in-stent restenosis after vertebral artery ostium stenting. J Stroke Cerebrovasc Dis. 2018;27:3030–5.

25. Tank VH, Ghosh R, Gupta V, Sheth N, Gordon S, He W, et al. Drug eluting stents versus bare metal stents for the treatment of extracranial vertebral artery disease: a meta-analysis. J Neurointerv Surg. 2016;8:770–4.

26. Langwieser N, Buyer D, Schuster T, Haller B, Laugwitz KL, Ibrahim T. Bare metal vs. drug-eluting stents for extracranial vertebral artery disease: a meta-analysis of nonrandomized comparative studies. J Endovasc Ther. 2014;21:683–92.

27. Geng X, Hussain M, Du H, Zhao L, Chen J, Su W, et al. Comparison of self-expanding stents with distal embolic protection to balloon-expandable stents without a protection device in the treatment of symptomatic vertebral artery origin stenosis: a prospective randomized trial. J Endovasc Ther. 2015;22:436–44.

28. Khan S, Rich P, Clifton A, Markus HS. Noninvasive detection of vertebral artery stenosis: a comparison of contrast-enhanced MR angiography, CT angiography, and ultrasound. Stroke. 2009;40:3499–503.

Surgical Therapy

13

Christopher J. Stapleton
and Sepideh Amin-Hanjani

Introduction

Acute stroke in the posterior circulation, either ischemic or hemorrhagic, can require urgent surgical therapy for management of life-threatening brainstem compression. Underlying atherosclerotic or occlusive vertebrobasilar disease resulting in posterior circulation ischemic events can also occasionally benefit from surgical revascularization. This chapter will review the surgical options for these situations.

Surgical Revascularization

A variety of extracranial and intracranial surgical options can be utilized for revascularization of the posterior fossa. Advances in endovascular technology and technique, such as submaximal angioplasty [1, 2], have reduced the need for surgical approaches to neurovascular diseases affecting the posterior circulation; nevertheless, strategies for surgical interventions remain an important tool in patient management.

Patients presenting with refractory vertebrobasilar insufficiency (VBI) despite maximal medical therapy [3] are potential candidates for posterior circulation revascularization. Bypass

for revascularization in the setting of posterior fossa ischemia has been less studied than anterior circulation ischemia [4, 5]. This is likely due to the relative prevalence of the conditions [6, 7], the availability and evolution of endovascular techniques for treatment of vertebrobasilar stenosis [1–3], and the relatively higher morbidity and technical complexity of posterior circulation bypass. However, various extracranial–intracranial (EC-IC) bypass options to the posterior circulation are feasible, including occipital artery (OA) to posterior inferior cerebellar artery (PICA) (Fig. 13.1) and superficial temporal artery (STA) to superior cerebellar artery (SCA) or posterior cerebral artery (PCA) bypasses (Fig. 13.2) [8, 9]. Additionally, a variety of surgical options for revascularization of the extracranial vertebral artery are also available [10, 11].

Patient Evaluation and Selection

Athero-Occlusive Vertebrobasilar Disease

As with other stroke syndromes, standard evaluation for patients presenting with VBI includes parenchymal brain imaging and vascular imaging, typically performed initially with a combination of magnetic resonance imaging (MRI) and magnetic resonance angiography (MRA). If vertebrobasilar occlusive disease is evident, imaging and clinical presentation can ascertain the etiology as atherosclerotic (versus dissection or

C. J. Stapleton · S. Amin-Hanjani (✉)
Department of Neurosurgery, University of Illinois at Chicago, Chicago, IL, USA
e-mail: cstapleton@mgh.harvard.edu;
hanjani@uic.edu

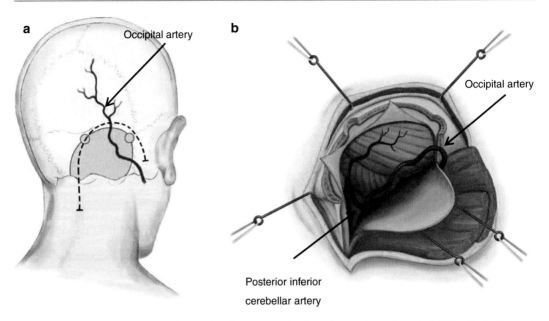

Fig. 13.1 Illustrations demonstrating occipital artery (OA) to posterior inferior cerebellar artery (PICA) bypass. (**a**) A hockey-stick-shaped incision is placed extending from the mastoid to the midline and a retrosigmoid or far lateral craniotomy is performed. (**b**) The OA is dissected and anastomosed to the tonsillomedullary loop of the PICA

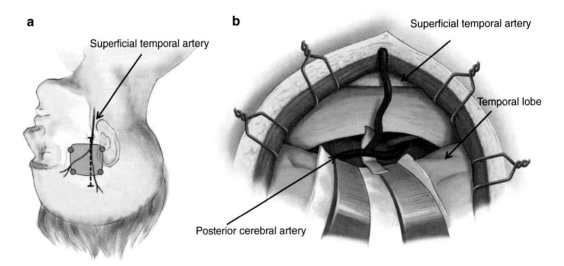

Fig. 13.2 Illustrations demonstrating superficial temporal artery (STA) to posterior cerebral artery (PCA) bypass. (**a**) An incision is placed overlying the STA, the STA dissected, and a subtemporal craniotomy is performed. (**b**) The PCA is exposed in the ambient cistern adjacent to the oculomotor nerve and superior cerebellar artery (SCA) and a STA-PCA bypass is created

extrinsic compression). Flow compromise within the vertebrobasilar system and distal arterial tree is difficult to evaluate as imaging methods standardly used in evaluation of anterior circulation ischemia are less useful in assessment of the posterior circulation due to the more compact brain territory and skull base artifacts. An alternative method for assessing posterior circulation blood flow relies on large vessel flow measurement performed using quantitative magnetic resonance angiography (QMRA), a technique utilizing phase-contrast MR to measure vessel-specific volumetric flow rates. QMRA thus provides a technique to directly measure posterior circulation vessel flow [12]. The observational Vertebrobasilar Flow Evaluation and Risk of Transient Ischemic Attack and Stroke (VERiTAS) study demonstrated that patients with vertebrobasilar occlusive disease with evidence of flow compromise, as determined by QMRA, are at higher risk of recurrent stroke [13, 14]. In VERiTAS, patients with VBI from steno-occlusive vertebrobasilar disease with normal flow in their distal intracranial vasculature had a recurrent stroke-free survival rate of 96% and 87% at 12 and 24 months, respectively, while those patients with low distal flow had stroke-free survival rates of only 78% and 70%, respectively [14]. Flow assessment with QMRA, therefore, may be used to identify the subset of patients with VBI who are most likely to benefit from revascularization.

Presently, however, the indications for surgical revascularization are limited as no prospective or randomized studies have been performed to assess the efficacy of surgical intervention, and the procedures carry the risk of morbidity. Overall, surgical revascularization of the posterior circulation carries a higher risk and lower patency rates than that seen with anterior circulation bypass. Patency rates for OA-PICA bypass range from 88% to 100%, with mortality rates averaging 4% [15]. For STA-PCA and STA-SCA bypass, a review of 86 bypasses compiled from several series revealed patency rates in the 78–90% range, with mortality averaging 12% [15, 16] and serious morbidity of 20%. Though these series reported improvement in symptoms in a subset of patients, the morbidity and mortality associated with such revascularization procedures have introduced caution when entertaining surgical bypass options, particularly for patients with poor neurological condition or medical comorbidities. Nonetheless, more recent advances in microsurgical and neuroanesthetic techniques, as well as improvements in perioperative neuro-

intensive care management, do allow posterior circulation revascularization to be successfully undertaken in selected patients with no other options for management.

Prior to surgical revascularization, the first approach is to optimize all medical therapeutic options, including maximizing antithrombotic regimens, judicious blood pressure control, aggressive lipid lowering with statins, glycemic control, and smoking cessation. Anticoagulation with warfarin has not shown benefit over antiplatelet therapy and higher risk of complications in patients with intracranial atherosclerotic intracranial disease [17]. If the patient has recurrent ischemia despite these measures, and the disease is not amenable to endovascular therapy, then bypass options will be considered, but only if comorbid cardiac or medical conditions are not prohibitive for undergoing general anesthesia and surgery with acceptable risk. Particular caution should be used in considering bypass distal to a high-grade vessel stenosis, for example, in the case of distal bypass for severe basilar stenosis. Distal bypass can create competing flow at the location of disease, which has the potential to promote thrombosis at the site of stenosis [18] and causes perforator occlusion and local infarction with devastating consequence.

Vertebrobasilar Dissection

It is important to recognize the etiology of VBI. Posterior circulation stroke due to vertebral artery dissection is typically managed differently from atherosclerotic disease, with surgical revascularization considered only in cases of chronic dissection or occlusion with associated hypoperfusion. For acute dissections, while the evidence is incomplete, anticoagulation with heparin followed by oral anticoagulation therapy for 3–6 months remains popular in many centers [19]. This practice is supported by several small case series demonstrating good outcome with low complication rates in patients receiving anticoagulation [20, 21]. There are centers that prefer dual antiplatelets to anticoagulation. There are no randomized clinical trials that have directly compared antiplatelet therapy to anticoagulation [22]. Certain features, such as severe

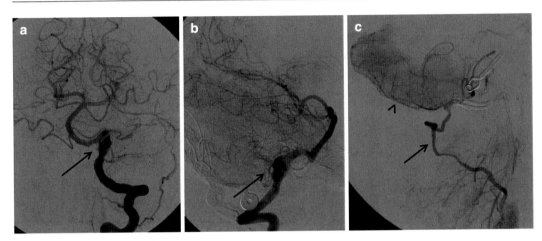

Fig. 13.3 (**a**) Anteroposterior and (**b**) lateral left vertebral artery angiograms demonstrating a dissecting vertebral artery aneurysm (arrow) in a patient presenting with subarachnoid hemorrhage. (**c**) The patient underwent occipital artery (OA—arrow) to posterior inferior cerebellar artery (PICA—arrowhead) bypass with trapping of the aneurysmal segment

stenosis or intraluminal thrombus in association with the dissection, tend to favor anticoagulation, whereas a large associated infarction would favor antiplatelets. Imaging is repeated after 3 months, and anticoagulation or antiplatelets are continued if the pathology persists. Long-term antiplatelets can be considered, especially in the setting of persistent vessel abnormality or risk factors such as a history of connective tissue diseases or recurrent dissections. Oral anticoagulation is contraindicated in intracranial dissections as these are prone to subarachnoid hemorrhage and in the presence of a large infarct with associated mass effect or intracranial extension of the dissection [21].

In rare patients with ischemic symptoms refractory to medical management and in those with expanding or ruptured dissecting aneurysms, endovascular therapy may be indicated. Endovascular therapy is the initial therapy of choice when medical therapy fails or is contraindicated [23, 24]. Procedures include balloon angioplasty followed by placement of one or more balloon-expandable or self-expanding stents. Associated dissecting aneurysms may require coil embolization or the deployment of a covered stent [25]. Surgery remains an option of final resort if medical therapy fails and endovascular options are not feasible. Refractory isch-

emic symptoms related to hypoperfusion can be addressed using bypass for flow augmentation, while dissecting aneurysms typically require vessel sacrifice and revascularization to obliterate the aneurysm while preserving distal flow (Fig. 13.3).

Preoperative Assessment

Patients who are considered for posterior circulation bypass should undergo angiography to delineate the intracranial vasculature with selective external carotid injections to evaluate the caliber and course of donor branches, such as the STA or OA when needed. If there is concern regarding the adequacy of the in situ donors, alternative bypass strategies using interposition grafts (saphenous vein or radial artery) can be entertained. In patients with VBI, where atherosclerosis is the primary etiology for the vertebrobasilar disease encountered in such patients, systemic atherosclerotic disease is also often present. Therefore, preoperative cardiac and medical clearance, including echocardiography and stress testing, for cardiac risk stratification is an important element of preoperative assessment.

If interposition grafts are anticipated, saphenous vein can be harvested in the calf or thigh following preoperative ultrasound mapping to determine the suitability (size and length) of the vein. For radial artery, the vessel is generally harvested from the nondominant arm after ensuring adequate ulnar artery collaterals to the hand with Allen's test.

Perioperative and Anesthetic Considerations

Patients should be placed on full dose (325 mg) aspirin, ideally beginning a week prior to surgery or at least the morning of surgery. Other antiplatelet agents, such as clopidogrel, are generally avoided due to bleeding risk, particularly in cases involving intracranial surgery. For patients requiring dual antiplatelets due to high thrombotic risk, the second agent can be discontinued a week prior to surgery and replaced with enoxaparin or equivalent until the day prior to surgery. Patients who are on warfarin anticoagulation are converted to intravenous heparin, which is withheld 6 h prior to surgery as antiplatelets are administered.

Arterial line and central venous access is routinely obtained for surgery. Antibiotic prophylaxis is administered prior to skin incision and maintained for 48 h postoperatively. Throughout the surgery, normovolemia, normocapnia, and normotension (based upon the patient's baseline blood pressure) are maintained. For tenuous patients with VBI who are blood pressure dependent, even extreme hypertension is maintained throughout until the bypass has been completed. Somatosensory evoked potential (SSEP) and motor evoked potential (MEP) can also be used for physiologic monitoring during the surgery and can be useful in alerting the operative team to inadequate blood pressure maintenance during the case. Scalp electrodes for electroencephalographic (EEG) monitoring are placed outside the surgical field, which are used to monitor induction of metabolic burst suppression during temporary vessel occlusion for bypass. Inhalational agents are preferentially used for burst suppression as they increase cerebral blood flow in comparison to barbiturates; intravenous anesthetics for burst suppression may be required if SSEP and MEP are also monitored, as evoked potentials can also be suppressed otherwise.

For intracranial bypass operations, lumbar drain for cerebrospinal fluid (CSF) drainage is used preferentially for brain relaxation to avoid the need for intravenous diuretics (furosemide), hyperosmolar agents (mannitol), or hyperventilation. Prior to cross-clamping of major vessels, intravenous heparin is administered. For entirely extracranial operations, full dosing with weight-appropriate heparin (routine dose 5000 U) is performed 5 min prior to initial vessel occlusion. For intracranial operations, smaller doses (generally 2000 U) are administered prior to temporary vessel occlusion. The heparin is not reversed postoperatively but rather allowed to wear off on its own.

Postoperative Management

Patients are continued on aspirin 325 mg daily, starting immediately postoperatively. Patients are observed in the intensive care unit postoperatively and are kept well hydrated, with avoidance of hypotension. Pressure over the location of the bypass graft (by nasal oxygen cannula or glasses) is avoided to prevent direct mechanical occlusion. In patients with bypass for ischemia, it is especially important to avoid hypertension given the potential risk for hyperperfusion hemorrhage, although this appears to occur less commonly in the posterior circulation, and with STA or OA grafts, than larger higher flow interposition grafts. Potential postoperative complications include epidural hematoma or wound infection and postoperative graft occlusion. Patients are discharged on daily aspirin.

Extracranial Surgical Options

Extracranial revascularization procedures focus on vertebral artery disease. The pathologies involved are primarily occlusive diseases, such as atherosclerotic stenosis or occlusion of the vertebral artery, or direct external compression by bony cer-

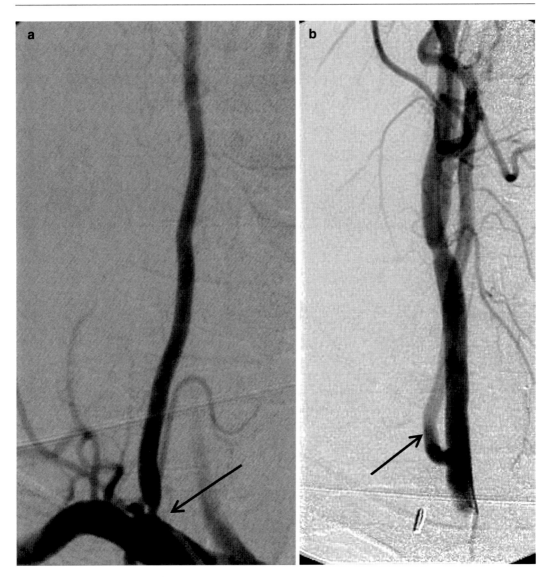

Fig. 13.4 (a) Right subclavian artery anteroposterior angiogram demonstrating severe right vertebral origin stenosis (arrow). (b) Following vertebral-carotid transposition, there is filling of the vertebral artery (arrow) via injection of the common carotid artery

vical osteophytes. The most commonly utilized surgical options for treatment are vertebral-carotid transposition, carotid-to-vertebral bypass, and osteophyte foraminal decompression.

Vertebral-Carotid Transposition

Vertebral-carotid transposition (VCT) is performed for treatment of vertebral artery origin stenosis (Fig. 13.4). Although direct vertebral origin endarterectomy [10] through a subclavian approach is also an option, it is seldom used as VCT offers a more simple and effective method of revascularization. The potential limitation of VCT is the requirement for simultaneous occlusion of both carotid and vertebral arteries; however, given the proximal location of temporary occlusion on the common carotid and proximal vertebral, cervical, and muscular collaterals distally invariably prevent cerebral ischemia. If the carotid artery is stenotic or otherwise compromised, transposition to another location of the subclavian artery can be used. Similarly, if transposition is not feasible because of the inadequate length of the proximal vertebral artery, an interposition vein or prosthetic graft bypass can be performed from the subclavian with end-to-end anastomosis to the vertebral artery [26, 27]. Although this procedure does not interrupt carotid blood flow, it requires two anastomoses and is time consuming. The proximal vertebral artery can also be transposed from the subclavian artery to the thyrocervical trunk [11, 27]. Occasionally, obstruction at the vertebral origin is extrinsic, caused by compression due to bands from the tendon of the anterior scalene or the longus colli muscle [10, 28]. These ligaments, muscles, and bands overlying the artery can be excised. In some cases, the sympathetic ganglia or nerve fibers constrict the artery. If the ganglia are divided, a mild Horner's syndrome will develop. Segmental resection and end-to-end anastomosis of the vessel can be used when obstruction is caused by entrapment, but the vertebral artery must be long and its diameter adequate.

Extracranial Carotid-to-Vertebral Bypass

Vein grafts can be used to bypass disease at a more proximal aspect of the vertebral artery by connecting the distal vertebral to the carotid (Fig. 13.5) [28, 29]. The V2 segment of the vertebral is partially encased in a bony channel as it travels through the transverse foramina of the C1 through C6 cervical segments. Anatomically, however, the vertebral has more redundancy and is more easily accessible at the distal V2 segment (between C1 and C2), where anastomosis is favorable [28]. The graft can be attached to the external carotid, or the external carotid itself can be transposed onto the vertebral [29]. The advantage of the external carotid as the donor supply is that the proximal anastomosis does not interfere with the cerebral circulation. Although vein grafts to the mid-V2 segment can be performed successfully [30] using an anterior approach to expose both the vertebral artery and the carotid artery, the C1-C2 vertebral artery segment, accessed via the anterolateral approach, is particularly amenable to bypass. In the C1-C2 interspace, a 2-cm segment of the vessel can be

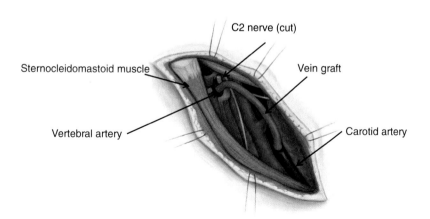

Fig. 13.5 Illustration demonstrating the extracranial carotid-to-vertebral bypass. An incision is placed along the medial border of the sternocleidomastoid and extended posteriorly toward the mastoid; initial exposure through the platysma, medial to the sternocleidomastoid reveals the contents of the carotid sheath. The contents of the carotid sheath are retracted medially to palpate the transverse processes of C1 and C2; the overlying levator scapulae muscle is divided, revealing the anterior ramus of the C2 nerve, which is cut and retracted to expose the underlying VA. A vein graft is placed with anastomosis onto the vertebral artery and the common carotid artery

exposed without the need for bony removal and unroofing of the vertebral canal necessary in the mid-V2 segment.

Osteophyte Decompression

Endovascular treatment is typically the first choice of treatment for intrinsic stenotic lesions affecting the posterior circulation, but extrinsic compression with osteoarthritic spurs in the cervical region is associated with good results from surgical decompression [31].

Various forms of local, nonforaminal vertebral artery compression have been described. If a diagnosis of static or rotational vertebral artery compression is established by dynamic vertebral imaging, surgical treatment is recommended. Conservative medical therapy consists of anticoagulation or neck immobilization, either by instructing the patient to refrain from head turning or by the use of a collar. However, conservative measures alone can be associated with a stroke rate of approximately 50% [32]. Severe local obstruction of the distal vertebral artery caused by compression from arterial branches or neighboring nerves can be treated by using the posterolateral approach with division of the obstruction. Bow hunter's syndrome due to constriction of the distal segment of the vertebral artery, with occlusion following lateral head rotation, can also occur [33]. Traditionally, these patients have been fused between the occiput, C1, and C2 to limit head rotation and vertebral artery compression. In younger patients, however, it is best to explore the anatomy and remove the compressive pathology.

Intracranial Surgical Options

The primary EC-IC bypass options for the posterior fossa include the STA to PCA or SCA bypass and the OA to PICA or anterior inferior cerebellar artery (AICA) bypass [8, 9]. Other described variants include the use of vein interposition grafts to the SCA or PCA [34–36].

STA-PCA (or SCA) Bypass

A subtemporal approach is used to gain access to the PCA or SCA (Fig. 13.2). The bypass is typically performed on the right side if possible so that manipulation of the temporal lobe is on the nondominant side. A Doppler is utilized to map the STA starting at the level of the zygoma. The skin incision is placed to overlie the STA trunk just anterior to the tragus in the region of the zygoma and extend along the course of the vessel. The goal is to dissect at least 8–10 cm of STA in order to have enough length to reach subtemporally to the PCA or SCA. A temporal craniotomy is performed. The zygomatic arch and prominent elevations of the middle fossa floor are drilled to create a flat plane of approach. The dura is opened as a semicircular flap, which is retracted inferiorly.

The microscope is utilized for all intradural aspects of the procedure. The temporal lobe is elevated, with coagulation of any small anterior bridging veins as needed. Typically, the SCA will come into view first at the edge of the tentorium, although it is often necessary to cut the tentorium to better visualize the lateral course of the vessel. Further elevation of the temporal lobe will bring the P2 segment of the PCA into view. The PCA provides a substantially larger recipient vessel than the SCA, which can therefore accommodate a higher flow bypass; in cases when the STA is inadequate and a radial artery or saphenous vein interposition graft is necessary, donor–recipient size mismatch precludes use of the SCA. When using the PCA, however, greater temporal lobe retraction is needed, and it can be more difficult to identify a perforator-free zone along the P2 segment than along the lateral SCA. Perforators in this region must be preserved, and if absolutely necessary, should be occluded with temporary clips during anastomosis rather than sacrificed. Once the STA has been prepared, it is useful to check the "cut flow" of the vessel to determine its flow capacity and adequacy for the bypass [37].

The STA-PCA or SCA anastomosis is performed in an end-to-side fashion. The STA is cut at a slight bevel and can be fish-mouthed to enlarge the opening. If an interposition vein or artery graft is used, it should be cut at a right angle; otherwise, the opening will be too long. After completion of the bypass, blood flow measurement provides confirmation of the patency and function of the bypass. The dura is loosely tacked with a slit created for passage of the STA. The bone is replaced, but the inferior opening is enlarged to accommodate the graft avoiding any kinking or pressure on the vessel. The muscle is re-approximated loosely and left open inferiorly to avoid pressure on the graft, and the skin is closed with care.

OA-PICA (or AICA) Bypass

The OA-PICA bypass is traditionally performed through a lateral suboccipital approach (Fig. 13.1). The skin incision is planned as a hockey-stick flap based over midline and toward the side of interest, ending over the region of the mastoid process. The occipital artery is identified in the midpoint of the horizontal portion of the incision, where it is transected, dissected, and occluded with a temporary clip on the proximal end after the suboccipital muscles have been elevated. The skin and muscle flap are retracted laterally and inferiorly. A lateral suboccipital craniotomy is performed, and the dura is opened in a hockey-stick fashion near the midline.

The microscope is utilized for all intradural aspects of the procedure. The ipsilateral cerebellar tonsil is elevated, bringing the tonsillomedullary segment of the PICA into view. This is the preferred location of anastomoses as a lengthy perforator-free portion can be readily obtained, and the loop of the vessel can be mobilized and elevated to reduce the depth of the anastomosis. If revascularization distal to the PICA is needed, the AICA can also be used as a recipient, although the PICA is much more easily accessible. Once the PICA or AICA recipient has been prepared, the "cut flow" of the donor OA vessel can be checked to evaluate its flow capacity.

An end-to-side anastomosis of the OA-PICA or AICA is performed. The OA is beveled and fish-mouthed. Following completion of the anastomosis, the flow in the OA graft is measured.

The dura is tacked loosely, and the dural opening is covered. The superior portion of the bone can be replaced, but with care to avoid pressure on the graft. The lateral suboccipital musculature sometimes needs to be trimmed to prevent pressure on the exit point of the OA, and the midline muscle closure is performed with care to avoid kinking of the graft.

Stroke Decompression

Background and Indications

Cerebellar Infarction
Unlike for cerebral infarctions with malignant edema, there are no large-scale and long-term prospective studies evaluating the efficacy of posterior fossa decompression after stroke. However, the utility of suboccipital craniectomy (SOC) with or without cerebellar resection or ventricular drainage was first described in 1956 [38–40], and numerous single- and multi-institutional reports indicate that SOC can reduce mortality and improve long-term outcomes in patients with space-occupying cerebellar infarcts [41].

For patients with posterior fossa stroke, several studies have identified a progressive decline in consciousness as the primary indication for surgical intervention [42–47]. Tsitsopoulos et al. noted that long-term functional outcomes after SOC were correlated with a patient's immediate preoperative level of consciousness and advocated for decompression before or early in the course of a patient's decline. Important causes of a reduced level of consciousness include brainstem compression and hydrocephalus. While the treatment for brainstem compression from an edematous cerebellum is decompression, some authors advocate for ventriculostomy alone in the setting of hydrocephalus without obvious brainstem compression [43]. In a study of 44 patients, Raco et al. found that 88% of patients with acute hydrocephalus requiring ventriculostomy made a good recovery without SOC. However, Chen et al. noted that ventricular drainage alone without decompression increased the risk of upward transtentorial herniation [48]. Even when a ventricular drain is placed, several authors have noted that early SOC allows for earlier removal of the drain (often within 72 h) by restoring cerebrospinal fluid (CSF) pathways, which reduces the risk of infection and need for permanent CSF diversion [48, 49]. Cranial nerve involvement is an early sign of brainstem involvement and increased infratentorial pressure, and suboccipital decompression should be undertaken in patients with these signs. In series by Jüttler et al. and Pfefferkorn et al., 68% and >82%, respectively, of patients who required SOC developed cranial nerve palsies prior to intervention [44, 45]. While radiographic criteria have been developed to guide the neurosurgeon's decision-making process [42], it is generally agreed that the patient's clinical condition is the most important factor in the management algorithm.

The timing of suboccipital decompression is controversial, as no prospective, randomized studies have been performed. Of the 84 patients in a study by Jauss et al., 18% were awake/drowsy, 35% were somnolent/stuporous, and 47% were comatose at the time of surgery. Whereas 86% of the awake/drowsy patients experienced a good functional outcome, only 76% and 47% of the somnolent/stuporous and comatose patients, respectively, had a good outcome [42]. In a similar fashion, Tsitsopoulos et al. noted that patients with a better preoperative neurological status did better than those with neurological compromise [46]. While these data indicate that a patient's preoperative neurological status is an important indicator of postoperative outcome, these studies generally do not provide a medical management cohort for comparative purposes.

Cerebellar Hemorrhage

Multiple studies have attempted to evaluate the indications for surgery in the setting of spontaneous cerebellar hemorrhage. A number of variables are relevant to surgical decision making. There is general consensus that cerebellar hemorrhage patients who are comatose or deteriorate neurologically warrant surgical hematoma evacuation; typically, such patients present with large hematomas. In patients who present with Glasgow Coma Score (GCS) ≥ 13, indications for surgery have been less well defined but have included various thresholds for hematoma sizes ranging from >3 cm to >5 cm or presence of marked effacement of the fourth ventricle. Surgical indications for patients in very poor neurological status at presentation are also controversial. Some authors have recommended conservative measures in the setting of deep coma and acute hydrocephalus that does not resolve with CSF diversion, absent brain stem reflexes or tetraplegia, deep coma in combination with >5 cm hemorrhage, and deep coma of more than 2 h duration [50]. However, even deeply comatose patients with minimal brainstem reflexes have been reported to benefit from rapid surgical evacuation of hematoma, favoring an aggressive surgical approach.

Other variables in addition to the absolute hematoma size and GCS have also been reported to be relevant to decision making about surgical intervention. A lower size threshold has been proposed for vermian than cerebellar hemisphere hemorrhage based on the anatomically closer location of vermian hemorrhages to the brain stem and the CSF pathways [51, 52]. The presence of a 'tight' posterior fossa, defined as effaced posterior fossa basal cisterns and fourth ventricle as well as enlarged third and lateral ventricles, has also been proposed as an important factor, with the notion that hematoma size thresholds for surgery should be reduced by 1 cm in such a context [52].

Recent guidelines for the management of spontaneous intracerebral hemorrhage recommend that cerebellar hemorrhages in patients who are deteriorating clinically or who have evidence of brainstem compression and/or hydrocephalus warrant surgical evacuation [53]. With hemorrhages smaller than 3 cm with no brainstem compression or hydrocephalus, patients can be treated medically with favorable outcomes; hematomas >3 cm are generally at high risk for subsequent deterioration and warrant evacuation (Fig. 13.6).

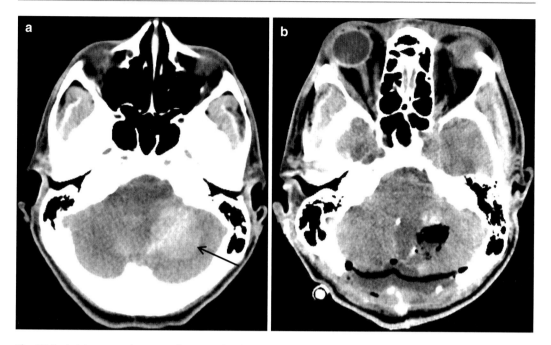

Fig. 13.6 Axial computed tomography scans showing (**a**) a large hemorrhage (arrow) in the left cerebellar hemisphere before and (**b**) after suboccipital decompression and hematoma evacuation

Suboccipital Decompression and Ventriculostomy

In the setting of infarction, the principal goal of suboccipital craniectomy is to provide space for the infarcted cerebellum to swell in order to relieve pressure on the fourth ventricle and brainstem (Fig. 13.7). In general, a wide craniectomy, at least 6 cm in width, is performed from the transverse sinuses superiorly to the foramen magnum inferiorly. The underlying dura is opened widely, and while some authors advocate for resection of the infarcted cerebellums [46, 47, 54], more recent evidence suggests that the area of restricted diffusion on MRI may be reversible [55]. Therefore, over-aggressive resection may in fact hinder recovery and impair long-term functional outcomes. The posterior arch of C1 may also be removed to achieve further decompression. Duraplasty is performed to allow maximal decompression. For cerebellar hemorrhage, the goal is for hematoma evacuation. Typically, suboccipital craniotomy (with replacement of the bone flap) rather than craniectomy can be per-formed, if the posterior fossa contacts are well decompressed with removal of the hematoma.

The role of ventriculostomy alone in acute cerebellar infarction and hemorrhage is an issue of debate. Some neurosurgeons advocate for ventriculostomy alone in patients with cerebellar infarctions who decline due to the development of hydrocephalus [43]. In a series by Jauss et al., however, 41% of somnolent/stuporous and 50% of comatose patients experienced a good outcome after SOC compared with only 27% and 33%, respectively, after ventricular drainage alone. Ventriculostomy alone carries the risk of upward transtentorial herniation. Studied in the setting of cerebellar hemorrhage, van Loon et al. noted this in 2 of 30 patients with space-occupying cerebellar hemorrhages. Some authors endorse CSF drainage only in the presence of small hematomas, or alternatively draining judiciously (either intermittently only for high intracranial pressure, or continuously, but at a higher level such as 15–20 cmH₂O), to reduce risk of upward herniation. Ultimately, while some

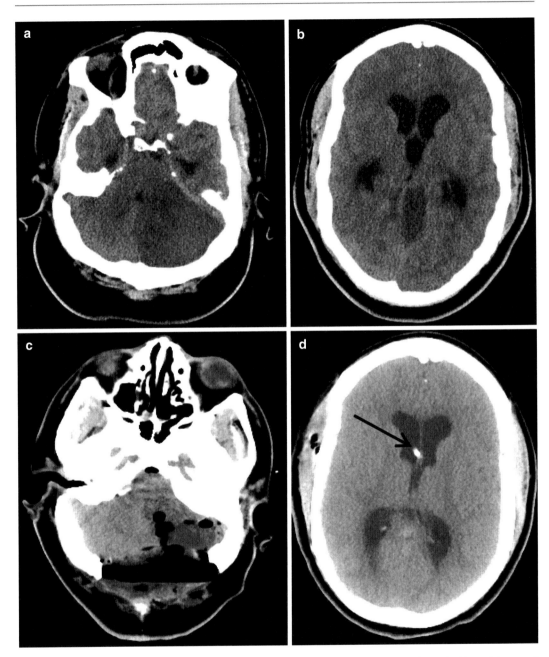

Fig. 13.7 Axial computed tomography scans showing (**a**) a large left posterior inferior cerebellar artery territory infarction (arrow) with (**b**) hydrocephalus. (**c**) A suboc- cipital decompression was performed with partial removal of the infarcted cerebellum, and (**d**) an external ventricu- lar drain (arrow) was placed for the hydrocephalus

patients with malignant cerebellar edema from stroke or cerebellar hemorrhage may improve with ventricular drainage alone, suboccipital decompression remains the most definitive method of reducing posterior fossa intracranial pressure. Therefore, although ventricular drainage can be necessary to relieve hydro- cephalus, ventriculostomy alone without plans for concomitant surgical evacuation is not gen- erally recommended [53].

References

1. Dumont TM, Kan P, Snyder KV, Hopkins LN, Siddiqui AH, Levy EI. Revisiting angioplasty without stenting for symptomatic intracranial atherosclerotic stenosis after the stenting and aggressive medical management for preventing recurrent stroke in intracranial stenosis (SAMMPRIS) study. Neurosurgery. 2012;71(6):1103–10.
2. Dumont TM, Sonig A, Mokin M, Eller JL, Sorkin GC, Snyder KV, et al. Submaximal angioplasty for symptomatic intracranial atherosclerosis: a prospective phase I study. J Neurosurg. 2016;125(4):964–71.
3. Chimowitz MI, Lynn MJ, Derdeyn CP, Turan TN, Fiorella D, Lane BF, et al. Stenting versus aggressive medical therapy for intracranial arterial stenosis. N Engl J Med. 2011;365(11):993–1003.
4. Group EIBS. Failure of extracranial-intracranial arterial bypass to reduce the risk of ischemic stroke. Results of an international randomized trial. N Engl J Med. 1985;313(19):1191–200.
5. Powers WJ, Clarke WR, Grubb RL, Videen TO, Adams HP, Derdeyn CP, et al. Extracranial-intracranial bypass surgery for stroke prevention in hemodynamic cerebral ischemia: the carotid occlusion surgery study randomized trial. JAMA. 2011;306(18):1983–92.
6. Chimowitz MI, Kokkinos J, Strong J, Brown MB, Levine SR, Silliman S, et al. The warfarin-aspirin symptomatic intracranial disease study. Neurology. 1995;45(8):1488–93.
7. Sacco RL, Kargman DE, Gu Q, Zamanillo MC. Race-ethnicity and determinants of intracranial atherosclerotic cerebral infarction. The Northern Manhattan Stroke Study. Stroke. 1995;26(1):14–20.
8. Ausman JI, Diaz FG, Dujovny M. Posterior circulation revascularization. Clin Neurosurg. 1986;33:331–43.
9. Hopkins LN, Martin NA, Hadley MN, Spetzler RF, Budny J, Carter LP. Vertebrobasilar insufficiency. Part 2. Microsurgical treatment of intracranial vertebrobasilar disease. J Neurosurg. 1987;66(5):662–74.
10. Spetzler RF, Hadley MN, Martin NA, Hopkins LN, Carter LP, Budny J. Vertebrobasilar insufficiency. Part 1: Microsurgical treatment of extracranial vertebrobasilar disease. J Neurosurg. 1987;66(5):648–61.
11. Berguer R, Flynn LM, Kline RA, Caplan L. Surgical reconstruction of the extracranial vertebral artery: management and outcome. J Vasc Surg. 2000;31(1 Pt 1):9–18.
12. Amin-Hanjani S, Du X, Zhao M, Walsh K, Malisch TW, Charbel FT. Use of quantitative magnetic resonance angiography to stratify stroke risk in symptomatic vertebrobasilar disease. Stroke. 2005;36(6):1140–5.
13. Amin-Hanjani S, Du X, Rose-Finnell L, Pandey DK, Richardson D, Thulborn KR, et al. Hemodynamic features of symptomatic Vertebrobasilar disease. Stroke. 2015;46(7):1850–6.
14. Amin-Hanjani S, Pandey DK, Rose-Finnell L, Du X, Richardson D, Thulborn KR, et al. Effect of hemodynamics on stroke risk in symptomatic atherosclerotic Vertebrobasilar occlusive disease. JAMA Neurol. 2016;73(2):178–85.
15. Hopkins LN, Budny JL. Complications of intracranial bypass for vertebrobasilar insufficiency. J Neurosurg. 1989;70(2):207–11.
16. Ausman JI, Diaz FG, Vacca DF, Sadasivan B. Superficial temporal and occipital artery bypass pedicles to superior, anterior inferior, and posterior inferior cerebellar arteries for vertebrobasilar insufficiency. J Neurosurg. 1990;72(4):554–8.
17. Chimowitz MI, Lynn MJ, Howlett-Smith H, Stern BJ, Hertzberg VS, Frankel MR, et al. Comparison of warfarin and aspirin for symptomatic intracranial arterial stenosis. N Engl J Med. 2005;352(13):1305–16.
18. Massimo C, Orazio A, Felice F. Bypass surgery in patients with intracranial stenotic lesions. Postoperative morbidity and angiographic findings. J Neurosurg. 1985;62(4):532–8.
19. Engelter ST, Brandt T, Debette S, Caso V, Lichy C, Pezzini A, et al. Antiplatelets versus anticoagulation in cervical artery dissection. Stroke. 2007;38(9):2605–11.
20. Lucas C, Moulin T, Deplanque D, Tatu L, Chavot D. Stroke patterns of internal carotid artery dissection in 40 patients. Stroke. 1998;29(12):2646–8.
21. Schievink WI. The treatment of spontaneous carotid and vertebral artery dissections. Curr Opin Cardiol. 2000;15(5):316–21.
22. Lyrer P, Engelter S. Antithrombotic drugs for carotid artery dissection. Stroke. 2004;35(2):613–4.
23. DeOcampo J, Brillman J, Levy DI. Stenting: a new approach to carotid dissection. J Neuroimaging. 1997;7(3):187–90.
24. Phatouros CC, Higashida RT, Malek AM, Meyers PM, Lefler JE, Dowd CF, et al. Endovascular treatment of noncarotid extracranial cerebrovascular disease. Neurosurg Clin N Am. 2000;11(2):331–50.
25. Biggs KL, Chiou AC, Hagino RT, Klucznik RP. Endovascular repair of a spontaneous carotid artery dissection with carotid stent and coils. J Vasc Surg. 2004;40(1):170–3.
26. Berguer R, Feldman AJ. Surgical reconstruction of the vertebral artery. Surgery. 1983;93(5):670–5.
27. Diaz FG, Ausman JI, de los Reyes RA, Pearce J, Shrontz C, Pak H, et al. Surgical reconstruction of the proximal vertebral artery. J Neurosurg. 1984;61(5):874–81.
28. Carney AL. In: Robicsek F, editor. Vertebral artery surgery: pathology, hemodynamics, and technique. New York: Macmillan; 1986.
29. Berguer R, Morasch MD, Kline RA. A review of 100 consecutive reconstructions of the distal vertebral artery for embolic and hemodynamic disease. J Vasc Surg. 1998;27(5):852–9.
30. Kakino S, Ogasawara K, Kubo Y, Kobayashi M, Kashimura H, Ogawa A. Symptomatic occlusion at the origin of the vertebral artery treated using external carotid artery-cervical vertebral artery bypass with interposed saphenous vein graft. Surg Neurol. 2008;69(2):164–8; discussion 8

31. Venteicher AS, Quddusi A, Coumans JV. Anterolateral approach for a cervical nerve root compression syndrome due to an ectatic vertebral artery. Oper Neurosurg (Hagerstown). 2019;17(1):E29–32.

32. Kuether TA, Nesbit GM, Clark WM, Barnwell SL. Rotational vertebral artery occlusion: a mechanism of vertebrobasilar insufficiency. Neurosurgery. 1997;41(2):427–32; discussion 32-3

33. Sorensen BF. Bow hunter's stroke. Neurosurgery. 1978;2(3):259–61.

34. Hopkins LN, Budny JL, Spetzler RF. Revascularization of the rostral brain stem. Neurosurgery. 1982;10(3):364–9.

35. Sundt TM, Piepgras DG, Houser OW, Campbell JK. Interposition saphenous vein grafts for advanced occlusive disease and large aneurysms in the posterior circulation. J Neurosurg. 1982;56(2):205–15.

36. Russell SM, Post N, Jafar JJ. Revascularizing the upper basilar circulation with saphenous vein grafts: operative technique and lessons learned. Surg Neurol. 2006;66(3):285–97.

37. Amin-Hanjani S, Du X, Mlinarevich N, Meglio G, Zhao M, Charbel FT. The cut flow index: an intra-operative predictor of the success of extracranial-intracranial bypass for occlusive cerebrovascular disease. Neurosurgery. 2005;56(1 Suppl):75–85; discussion 75–85

38. Fairburn B, Oliver LC. Cerebellar softening; a surgical emergency. Br Med J. 1956;1(4979):1335–6.

39. Lindgren SO. Infarctions simulating brain tumours in the posterior fossa. J Neurosurg. 1956;13(6):575–81.

40. Lehrich JR, Winkler GF, Ojemann RG. Cerebellar infarction with brain stem compression. Diagnosis and surgical treatment. Arch Neurol. 1970;22(6):490–8.

41. Agarwalla PK, Stapleton CJ, Ogilvy CS. Craniectomy in acute ischemic stroke. Neurosurgery. 2014;74(Suppl 1):S151–62.

42. Jauss M, Krieger D, Hornig C, Schramm J, Busse O. Surgical and medical management of patients with massive cerebellar infarctions: results of the German-Austrian cerebellar infarction study. J Neurol. 1999;246(4):257–64.

43. Raco A, Caroli E, Isidori A, Salvati M. Management of acute cerebellar infarction: one institution's experience. Neurosurgery. 2003;53(5):1061–5; discussion 5–6

44. Jüttler E, Schweickert S, Ringleb PA, Huttner HB, Köhrmann M, Aschoff A. Long-term outcome after surgical treatment for space-occupying cerebellar infarction: experience in 56 patients. Stroke. 2009;40(9):3060–6.

45. Pfefferkorn T, Eppinger U, Linn J, Birnbaum T, Herzog J, Straube A, et al. Long-term outcome after suboccipital decompressive craniectomy for malignant cerebellar infarction. Stroke. 2009;40(9):3045–50.

46. Tsitsopoulos PP, Tobieson L, Enblad P, Marklund N. Clinical outcome following surgical treatment for bilateral cerebellar infarction. Acta Neurol Scand. 2011;123(5):345–51.

47. Tsitsopoulos PP, Tobieson L, Enblad P, Marklund N. Surgical treatment of patients with unilateral cerebellar infarcts: clinical outcome and prognostic factors. Acta Neurochir. 2011;153(10):2075–83.

48. Chen HJ, Lee TC, Wei CP. Treatment of cerebellar infarction by decompressive suboccipital craniectomy. Stroke. 1992;23(7):957–61.

49. Mathew P, Teasdale G, Bannan A, Oluoch-Olunya D. Neurosurgical management of cerebellar haematoma and infarct. J Neurol Neurosurg Psychiatry. 1995;59(3):287–92.

50. Dammann P, Asgari S, Bassiouni H, Gasser T, Panagiotopoulos V, Gizewski ER, et al. Spontaneous cerebellar hemorrhage--experience with 57 surgically treated patients and review of the literature. Neurosurg Rev. 2011;34(1):77–86.

51. Kirollos RW, Tyagi AK, Ross SA, van Hille PT, Marks PV. Management of spontaneous cerebellar hematomas: a prospective treatment protocol. Neurosurgery. 2001;49(6):1378–86; discussion 86–7

52. Salvati M, Cervoni L, Raco A, Delfini R. Spontaneous cerebellar hemorrhage: clinical remarks on 50 cases. Surg Neurol. 2001;55(3):156–61; discussion 61

53. Morgenstern LB, Hemphill JC, Anderson C, Becker K, Broderick JP, Connolly ES, et al. Guidelines for the management of spontaneous intracerebral hemorrhage: a guideline for healthcare professionals from the American Heart Association/American Stroke Association. Stroke. 2010;41(9):2108–29.

54. Hornig CR, Rust DS, Busse O, Jauss M, Laun A. Space-occupying cerebellar infarction. Clinical course and prognosis. Stroke. 1994;25(2):372–4.

55. Kidwell CS, Alger JR, Saver JL. Beyond mismatch: evolving paradigms in imaging the ischemic penumbra with multimodal magnetic resonance imaging. Stroke. 2003;34(11):2729–35.

Non-atherosclerotic, Uncommon Diseases

14

Jong S. Kim

Dissection

General Remark

Cervicocerebral artery dissections account for 1–2% of all ischemic strokes [1–3] and 10–25% of ischemic strokes in young and middle-aged patients [4, 5]. According to population-based studies, the incidence of spontaneous arterial dissections was 1.7–3.0/100,000 in the internal carotid arteries (ICAs) and 1.0–1.5/100,000 in the vertebral arteries (VAs) [1, 6, 7]. The prevalence is higher in man than in woman [8, 9], and females are younger and more often have migraine and multiple dissections [8].

Cervicocerebral artery dissections can result from either primary intimal tear with secondary dissection into the media layer or primary intramedial hemorrhage. An intimal tear will let circulating blood to enter the wall of the arteries and to form an intramural hematoma (false lumen). The intramural hematoma is located within the medial layer or near the intimal or adventitial layer. A subintimal dissection leads to luminal stenosis and obstruction, resulting in an ischemic event. A subadventitial dissection may cause aneurysmal formation (dissecting aneurysm) and subarachnoid hemorrhage (SAH) when it ruptures.

Dissection can be etiologically categorized as traumatic and spontaneous (nontraumatic). However, the definition of "traumatic" is difficult to make because physicians may not be sure of the causality when very minor trauma or neck rotation was described by the patient. Inherent conditions predisposing spontaneous arterial dissections include fibromuscular dysplasia, cystic medial necrosis, $\alpha 1$ antitrypsin deficiency, Ehlers–Danlos syndrome type IV, Marfan's syndrome, autosomal dominant polycystic kidney disease, tuberous sclerosis, migraine, and hyperhomocysteinemia [3, 10]. However, dissection usually occurs in isolation without definite evidence of connective tissue diseases. Nevertheless, ultrastructural morphological aberrations of dermal connective tissue were found in more than half of patients with spontaneous cervical artery dissections [11]. It has also been shown that patients with dissection have increased vascular tortuosity than age/sex-matched normal controls [12].

It has traditionally been recognized that intracranial dissection is less frequent than extracranial dissection [3]. However, the frequency of intracranial dissections may have been underestimated because the diagnosis of intracranial dissection is more difficult to make than that of the extracranial counterpart. Extensive workup, such as repeated angiogram studies [13], or additional utilization of high-resolution vessel wall MRI [14, 15], will increase the diagnostic rate of intracranial dissection [16] (Fig. 14.1) (see also Chap. 9).

J. S. Kim (✉)
Department of Neurology, Asan Medical Center, University of Ulsan, Seoul, South Korea
e-mail: jongskim@amc.seoul.kr

© Springer Nature Singapore Pte Ltd. 2021
J. S. Kim (ed.), *Posterior Circulation Stroke*, https://doi.org/10.1007/978-981-15-6739-1_14

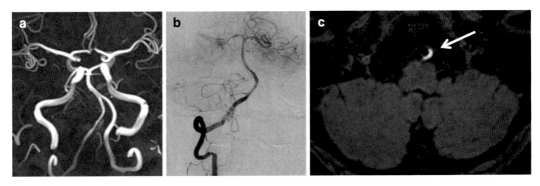

Fig. 14.1 A 47-year-old, previously healthy man suddenly developed severe right occipito-nuchal headache. MRI findings were normal. MRA (**a**) and conventional angiogram (**b**) showed suspicious narrowing of the right distal vertebral artery (VA). Precontrast T1 weighted high-resolution vessel wall MRI showed a high signal intensity (**c**, arrow) consistent with wall hematoma associated with VA dissection

With advanced imaging, a recent study on dissections causing ischemic stroke or transient ischemic attack (TIA) [16] reported that intracranial arterial dissection is two times more common than extracranial arterial dissection. The most frequent site was the distal VA.

In contrast to the extracranial cervical arteries, the intracranial arteries lack external elastic lamina and have only a thin adventitial layer. Therefore, intracranial dissections more easily lead to the development of dissecting aneurysm and subsequent SAH [17, 18]. Pathological studies have shown that subadventitial dissections are more frequent in the VA than in the middle cerebral artery (MCA) [19, 20]. This could explain the relatively low frequency of SAH in patients with MCA dissection. Trauma, either serious or minor one, seems to be more closely associated with extracranial dissections than intracranial dissections [3, 16, 18]. As in atherothrombotic infarction, arterial dissections produce stroke or TIA by way of artery-to-artery embolism, in situ occlusion, branch occlusion, or hypoperfusion [21].

Clinical Manifestations

Dissection in Anterior Circulation

In the anterior circulation, dissections most often occur in the ICA followed by the proximal MCA. Distal ICA dissection occasionally extends to the MCA. Both ICA and MCA dissections often produce cerebral infarction or TIA, while SAH is uncommon [22]. Most patients show vascular luminal stenosis, and a small number of patients have aneurysmal dilatation or double lumen. Symptoms are those with MCA ischemia such as hemiparesis, aphasia, hemineglect, and visual field defect. Rotational neck vessel injury is a probable cause of ICA dissection while the exact mechanism of MCA dissection is not clear. Some suggested that the impact of the MCA against the sphenoid ridge may cause an intimal tear and dissection [23]. Congenital vessel wall defects are often found in patients with anterior circulation dissection [22]. In one study, RNF gene polymorphism, a genetic variation associated with moyamoya disease, is found in about one-third of patients with anterior circulation dissection [24]. Dissection may account for the fusiform aneurysms arising from the MCA [19]. Dissections occurring in the anterior cerebral artery (ACA) is uncommon, but nowadays being more easily detected by high-resolution vessel wall imaging. In a study of 18 patients with nontraumatic ACA dissections, 9 had ischemia, 5 had SAH, and 4 patients had both [25].

Dissection in Posterior Circulation

In the posterior circulation, dissection most commonly develops in the VA. Although extracranial VA dissection has been traditionally emphasized [26, 27], recent reports from Asia showed that intracranial VA dissection is a more common cause of ischemic stroke [28]. The VA dissection is often associated with trauma associated with rotating neck motion such as chiropractic procedures or other neck manipulations [29]. Some arise from very minor trauma that include heavy coughing, falling on the back, and turning the head back to a car. Many others, however, do not have such a history [29–33]. The most common symptom of VA dissection is pain in the posterior head, posterior neck, or both. The posterior neck pain may radiate to the shoulder. Headache and neck pain may be the only complaint (Fig. 14.1). Ischemic symptoms and signs may develop at the same time as the pain or after a delay of hours to a few days.

Extracranial VA dissection often results in artery-to-artery embolism and produces ischemic strokes or TIA in the posterior fossa. When the dissection extends to the intracranial VA, it may produce ischemic stroke in the medulla and cerebellum by way of branch occlusion. Intracranial VA dissections most frequently involve the VA near the origin of the posterior inferior cerebellar artery (PICA). The dissection occasionally extends into the basilar artery (BA). Intracranial VA dissection often produces ischemic stroke in the medulla (usually lateral medulla) and the cerebellum by way of occlusion of the VA perforators or PICA (branch occlusion) (Fig. 14.2). Dissection may rupture and produce SAH (Fig. 8.4 in Chap. 8). The dissection may act as a mass lesion compressing the brainstem, cranial nerves, or vessels [34]. In a study on 31 cases with intracranial VA dissections, 55% had headache, 48% had infarction involving the brainstem or cerebellum, and 10% presented with SAH [35].

BA dissections are uncommon and usually carry a more grave prognosis than VA dissections. They often produce extensive, bilateral pontine infarction clinically manifested as sudden altered consciousness and quadriparesis [36]. In a review of 38 cases with BA dissections, there were brainstem ischemia in 27, SAH in 5, and both in 6 patients. Thirty patients (79%) died

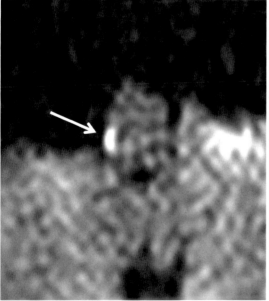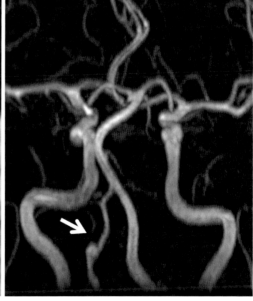

Fig. 14.2 A 35-year-old woman suddenly developed dizziness, gait instability, and sensory deficits in the left lower limb preceded by posterior neck pain for 3 days. Diffusion-weighted MRI showed a right caudal lateral medullary infarction (arrow, left image). MRA showed distal vertebral artery (VA) dissecting aneurysm (arrow, right image). The infarction was probably caused by perforator occlusion associated with VA dissection

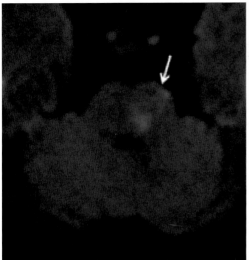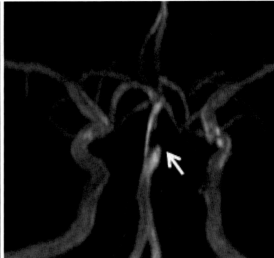

Fig. 14.3 An 81-year-old woman presented with dysarthria and right hemiparesis. Diffusion-weighted MRI shows left pontine infarction (arrow, left images). MRA shows dissecting aneurysm in the basilar artery (arrow, right image). (Modified from Kwon et al. Intracranial and extracranial arterial dissection presenting with ischemic stroke: Lesion location and stroke mechanism. Journal of the Neurological Sciences 358 (2015) 371–376)

[37]. However, a more recent study showed that unilateral pontine infarction with a favorable outcome is actually more common [38] (Fig. 14.3).

Dissections occurring in the posterior cerebral artery (PCA) are rare [39] and are often difficult to diagnose unless high-resolution vessel wall MRI is used (Fig. 14.4). In a review of 40 patients with PCA dissections, 15 had ischemia, 15 had SAH, and 6 had an aneurismal mass effect. Precipitating factors were found in nearly half of cases, including trauma, migraine, substance abuse, migraine, and the postpartum status [40]. The symptoms of ischemic stroke include visual field defect and hemisensory change.

Isolated dissections of the posterior inferior cerebellar artery (PICA) without involvement of the VA may present with cerebellar infarction, medullary infarction, or SAH [41, 42]. One report suggested that dissections occurring in the proximal PICA tend to produce ischemic symptoms, while those in the distal portion tend to cause SAH [43]. PICA dissection presenting with ischemic symptoms may have been underdiagnosed, partly because cerebral angiography is often omitted, and partly because it is difficult to assess the PICA with MRA. A study [13] reported that of 167 patients with isolated PICA territory

infarction, PICA dissection was the cause of stroke in 10 patients (6%). In 6 of these 10 patients, PICA dissections had not been suspected on initial MRA and were confirmed by follow-up MRA or digital subtraction angiography. Utilizing high-resolution vessel wall MRI will definitely increase the diagnostic sensitivity (Fig. 14.5). Thus, extensive workups are needed to diagnose PICA dissection in suspected cases. Dissections occurring in the anterior inferior cerebellar artery (AICA) and SCA are rare and may produce infarction or SAH [44] (Fig. 14.6).

Studies involving a large number of patients with posterior circulation dissection are rare. In a study from South Korea, among 159 symptomatic dissections, there were dissections in the VA in 77 (intracranial 39, extracranial 38), BA in 12, PICA in 8, and PCA in 4. In a study on 286 patients with posterior circulation stroke from Taipei [45], 74 patients were determined to be caused by dissection. The location of dissection was initiated in the VA (66.2%), BA (27.0%), PICA (5.4%), and PCA (1.4%). In this study, intracranial VA dissection was twice as common as extracranial VA dissection. There were 10% mortalities, and 30% of the patients had poor functional outcomes (modified Rankin

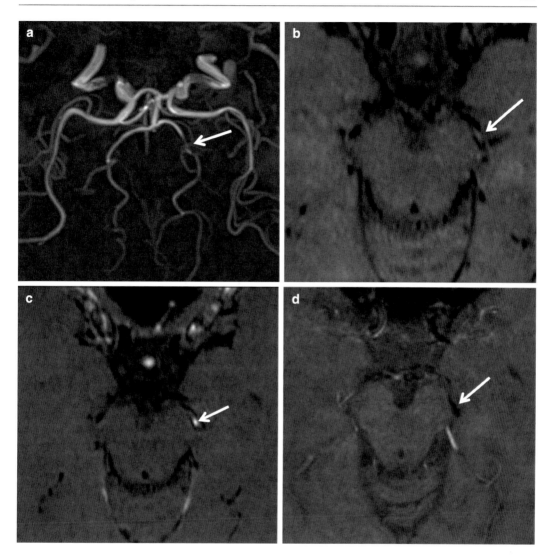

Fig. 14.4 A 65-year-old woman had head injury after falling down. She had headache and dizziness and 5 days later developed transient tingling sensation in the right face and limb. Neurological examination was normal, and brain MRI did not show any abnormality. MRA showed a focal stenosis in the P2 portion of the left posterior cerebral artery (PCA) (arrow, **a**). High-resolution vessel wall MRI showed iso-intense signal on precontrast T1-weighted image (arrow, **b**), strong enhancement on contrast T1 image (arrow, **b**), and dark signal on susceptibility-weighted image (arrow, **d**) on the wall of the PCA, consistent with intramural hematoma. The patient had transient ischemic attack, probably due to PCA dissection caused by head trauma

Scale ≥ 4) at 3-month follow-up. NIHSS scores >8 were independently associated with poor functional outcome. Another study from South Korea assessed 191 patients with symptomatic unruptured intracranial vertebrobasilar dissection [46]. Clinical manifestations were ischemic symptoms with headache ($n = 97$) or without headache ($n = 13$) and headache without ischemic symptoms ($n = 81$). During the follow-up period (mean, 46 months), none developed hemorrhages, and all patients without ischemic presentation had favorable outcomes (modified Rankin Scale, 0–1). Of the 102 patients with ischemic presentation, outcomes were favorable in 92 and unfavorable in 10 patients. Four patients died, and only one died as a result of BA dissection. Old age and BA involvement were independent predictors of unfavorable

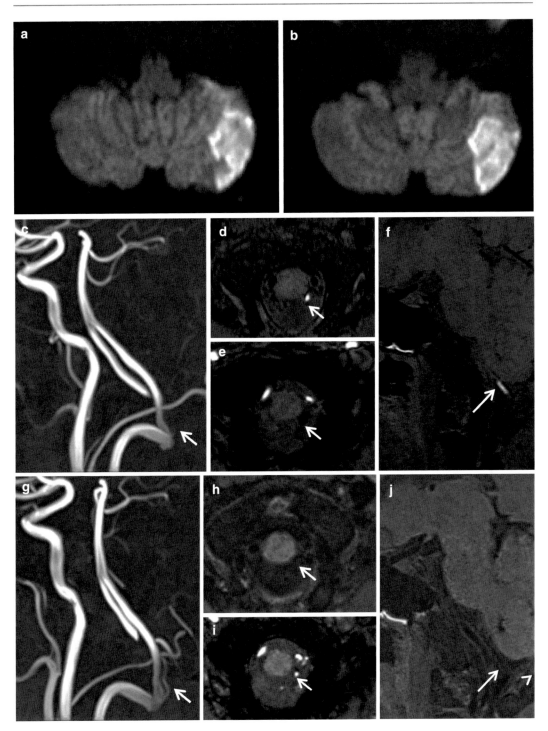

Fig. 14.5 A 46-year-old man without vascular risk factors suddenly developed vertigo, nausea, and gait instability. Examination showed mild dysarthria and right limb ataxia. Diffusion-weighted MRI showed left posterior inferior cerebellar artery (PICA) territory infarction (**a**, **b**). TOF-MRA shows left PICA occlusion (**c**). Axial precontrast T1-weighted image (high signal, **d**) and susceptibility-weighted image (dark signal, **e**) and sagittal contrast T1-weighted image (enhancement, **f**) show intramural hematoma in left PICA. One month later, TOF-MRA shows normalization of left PICA (**g**). Axial precontrast T1-weighted image (**h**) and susceptibility-weighted image (**i**) and sagittal contrast T1-weighted image (**j**) show complete normalization of the previous left PICA dissection

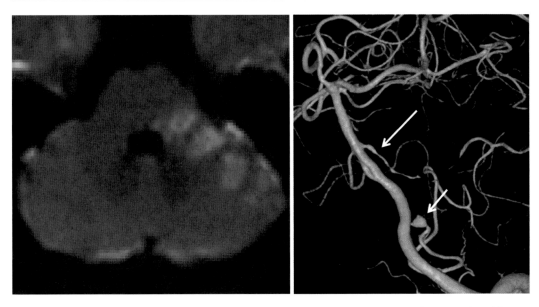

Fig. 14.6 A 63-year-old man developed dizziness and gait instability. Examination showed left facial palsy, hearing difficulty, dysarthria, and left limb ataxia. Diffusion-weighted MRI showed an infarction in the left anterior inferior cerebellar artery (AICA) territory (left image). Angiogram showed luminal narrowing with proximal dilataion and distal occlusion of AICA, consistent with dissection (long arrow, right image). An aneurysmal dilatation in the proximal portion of the PICA was also observed (short arrow, right image)

outcomes in these patients. These results suggest that clinical outcomes for nonhemorrhagic posterior circulation dissection are generally favorable, but old age, BA involvement, and initial severe neurological deficits may predict poor outcome.

Fusiform (Dolichoectatic) Dilatation

With the advent of imaging techniques, fusiform, tortuous, elongated, ectatic arteries (dolichoectasia) are increasingly recognized. They are most often observed in the BA [47]. The intracranial VA may also be affected. Occurrence in the distal ICA and MCA is rare. In some, the arterial abnormalities are widespread and affect other vessels such as the abdominal aorta [47, 48]. The etiologies of fusiform arterial dilatation remain unclear but may involve degenerative processes under genetic influences that lead to structural arterial defects characterized by fibrous dysplasia, internal elastic lamina degeneration, and fibrous and collagen replacement of the media [49]. In adults, atherosclerotic changes in the vessels may interact with congenital structural defects to augment fusiform dilatation. A genetic deficiency in α-glucosidase was found in patients with fusiform BA aneurysms [50].

In the dilated vessel, blood flow is slowed, which predisposes to thrombus formation. Artery -to-artery embolism or branch occlusion may lead to infarction [51–53]. One study reported that vertebrobasilar dolichoectasia was present in 6.4% of patients with cerebral infarction [54]. Symptoms may occur due to compression and traction on posterior fossa structures [52, 55]. Occipital–nuchal pain may develop, and cranial nerve palsies, hemifacial spasms, tinnitus, deafness, vertigo, and trigeminal pain have been reported [48, 56, 57]. Large BA aneurysms can compress the cerebral peduncle leading to hydrocephalus [58] or may manifest as cerebellopontine angle masses [59]. Dolichoectasia should be differentiated from dissecting aneurysm. Intracranial dolichoectatic VAs may compress the medulla resulting in hemiparesis and other neurological deficits [60].

Arterial Compression

Spondylitic osteophytes that project from the vertebral joints adjacent to the transverse foramen can compress the VA, usually at C1,2 level on neck rotation, and lead to recurrent TIAs or even strokes. In many cases, the contralateral VA is hypoplastic, ends at PICA or previously occluded, rendering the compressed VA the main supply to the structures in the posterior fossa [61–66]. Symptoms are precipitated by turning or rotation of the neck, during which the VA may become temporarily occluded. According to the series of 21 patients with this "rotational VA occlusion" syndrome, all patients developed vertigo accompanied by tinnitus (38%), fainting (24%), or blurred vision (19%) [67]. The induced nystagmus was mostly downbeat with horizontal and torsional components beating toward the compressed vertebral artery side. Although artery-to-artery embolism arising from stenosed VA was proposed [66], more recent studies suggest that symptoms are attributed to asymmetrical excitation of the labyrinth induced by transient ischemia [67, 68]. The prognosis is benign than previously thought, and conservative treatment is usually sufficient.

Posterior fossa ischemic strokes may occur during or after surgical or interventional procedures, such as aneurysm clipping, stenting, or surgical removal of tumors. In patients with aneurysms, blockage of the orifice of tributary vessels secondary to clot within the aneurysm [69] may be responsible for ischemic stroke. Surgical operation or endovascular intervention on the posterior communicating artery or BA aneurysm may result in occlusion of the PCA, SCA, or thalamic perforators [70] (Fig. 14.7). Other mechanisms include (1) dissection or intimal tear due to forceful retraction of the artery or interventional procedure, (2) sudden decompression of the artery by tumor removal, which had been encased for a long time, resulting in turbulent blood flow and subsequent thrombus formation [71], and (3) vasospasm due to localized SAH secondary to vessel injury.

In addition, PCA infarction may develop at the time of transtentorial brain herniation. The

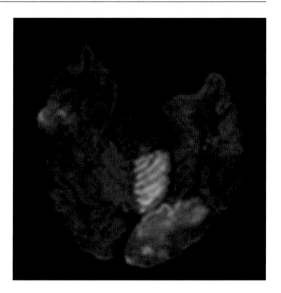

Fig. 14.7 A 56-year-old, previously healthy man developed dysarthria and left ataxia 1 day after coil embolization for basilar tip aneurysm. Diffusion-weighted MRI showed infarcts in the right superior cerebellar artery and posterior cerebral artery territories, which were probably related with the therapeutic procedure

PCA is usually compressed in its course around the midbrain between the herniated temporal lobe medially and the tentorium laterally [72, 73]. Compression may also occur contralateral to the herniation because of lateral displacement of the brainstem against the contralateral tentorium.

Fibromuscular Dysplasia

Fibromuscular dysplasia (FMD) is a vasculopathy of unknown cause characterized by hyperplasia of the intima and media of arteries, adventitial sclerosis, and breakdown of normal elastic tissue, without inflammation. Thickened septa and ridges protrude into the lumen [74]. The most common angiogram findings are a "string of beads" appearance: segments of constriction alternating with normal or dilated segments. Renal arteries and proximal carotid arteries are the two most commonly involved sites.

Extracranial VA involvement has been reported in 12–43% of affected patients. Majority of FMD are asymptomatic and found incidentally, but patients may develop ischemic stroke or TIA via artery-to-artery embolism, hemodynamic insufficiency, or their combination [75]. Branch occlusion can be the stroke mechanism when extracranial FMD extends to intracranial arteries [76] (Fig. 14.8). Hypertension secondary to renal involvement also contributes to the development of stroke in patients with FMD. FMD occurring in the intracranial arteries such as BA [77–79] or PCA [80] are rare and may result in TIA [78] and infarctions [77, 80]. In addition, some patients develop complications such as arterial dissection [81], aneurysms [82], and carotid-cavernous fistulas [83]. FMD may be associated with the moyamoya syndrome [84].

Moyamoya Disease

Moyamoya disease is characterized by progressive occlusion of the distal ICA or proximal MCA, with the development of fine meshworks of basal collateral vessels. Cerebral hypoperfusion is the predominant stroke mechanism in these patients, and repeated TIAs are observed when patients are dehydrated or hyperventilating. Less often, cerebral infarction due to thrombotic occlusion is encountered [85].

Posterior circulation stroke has been considered uncommon and appears in the late stage of moyamoya disease associated with more widespread vascular lesions including PCA involvement [86]. A study examining both pediatric and adult moyamoya disease patients showed that PCA involvement is present in 29% and 17%, respectively, suggesting that PCA involvement may be more common in young patients with moyamoya disease than previously recognized [87]. The occipital infarcts are the most common clinical presentation of posterior circulation moyamoya disease. The infarcts often include a part of the posterior MCA territory, probably because vascular collaterals from the PCA had supplied a part of the MCA territory in these patients with severe ICA steno-occlusive disease.

Migraine

Previous studies have described migraine as a cause of PCA infarction in 3–14% of the cases [88–90]. In the Lausanne Stroke Registry, migraine was the most common, usual cause of posterior circulation stroke [2]. However, there have been arguments as to the migraine as a real cause of PCA infarction. Angiograms in patients with migrainous stroke often show thrombotic arterial occlusion [88, 91], and more extensive investigations occasionally reveal hidden embolic sources such as patent foramen ovale (PFO) [92]. As discussed in Chap. 3, posterior fossa is a prediction side of embolism in patients with PFO. Therefore, the diagnosis of migraine stroke should be made cautiously, and thorough etiological workup should be performed even when infarcts develop along with migraine attack.

Reversible Cerebral Vasoconstriction Syndrome

Reversible cerebral vasoconstriction syndrome (RCVS) is characterized by the association of severe headaches with or without additional neurological symptoms and a "string and beads" appearance on cerebral arteries, which resolves spontaneously in 1–3 months [93]. Cerebral infarction occurs in 4–31% of the cases, usually later than hemorrhagic events (e.g., during the second week) [93]. The spasm usually involves both anterior and posterior circulations, and ischemic and hemorrhagic strokes are more often observed in the anterior circulation. However, it may predominantly occur in the posterior circulation and present with strokes in the PCA territory (Fig. 14.9).

Mitochondrial Disease

Mitochondrial encephalomyopathy, lactic acidosis, and stroke-like episodes (MELAS) present with infarction-like lesion most frequently in the occipital area [94, 95]. In one study [96], among 38 young (≤45 year old) patients who presented with

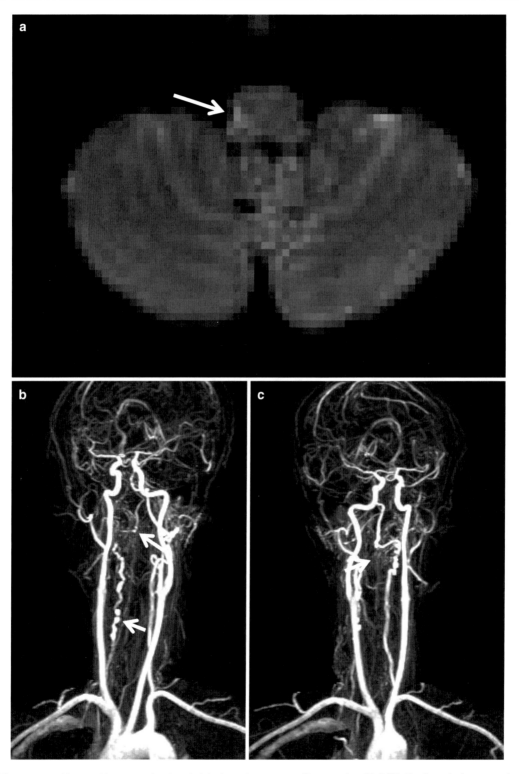

Fig. 14.8 A 56-year-old woman developed right lateral medullary infarction (**a**, arrow). MRA showed beaded appearance of right proximal vertebral artery (VA) and V3 segment (**b**, arrows) and left VA distal cervical segment (**c**, arrow). These findings are consistent with fibromuscular dysplasia

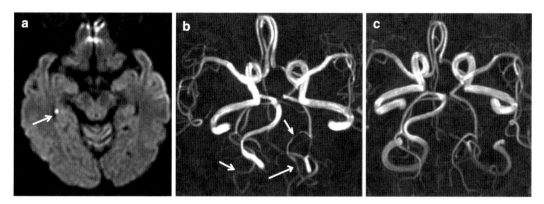

Fig. 14.9 A 65-year-old woman developed sudden severe, generalized headache. Diffusion-weighted MRI showed a small, asymptomatic infarct in the right hippocampal area (**a**, arrow). MRA showed multiple stenosis (**b**, arrows) and sausage-like dilation in both posterior cerebral arteries, which improved 1 month later (**c**). These findings are consistent with reversible cerebral vasoconstriction syndrome

occipital infarction, 4 patients (10%) had clinical or molecular diagnosis of mitochondrial disorder; two of them had mitochondrial DNA mutation, A3243G. Therefore, MELAS should be considered an etiology of young age occipital infarction. The pathogenesis of stroke-like lesions seems to be related with endothelial damage of small arteries associated with mitochondrial dysfunction [97] and metabolic derangement [98] rather than large artery occlusion. Therefore, the stroke-like lesion often does not exactly conform to the usual PCA territory [99, 100]. Patients generally have other features of MELAS such as short stature, hearing impairment, seizures, and maternal family history.

Takayasu's Disease

Takayasu's disease primarily involves the aorta and its branches, such as the innominate artery, subclavian arteries, and common carotid arteries. It mainly occurs in young (10–49 year) women (female: male, 7:1) in East Asia such as Korea and Japan. Pathologically, there are granulomatous inflammation, intimal proliferation, and scarring of adventitia that lead to vascular stenosis. Destruction of muscular media may lead to aneurysmal dilatation. Systemic symptoms include low-grade fever, fatigue, weight loss, arthralgia, and myalgia. Vascular symptoms include cool, painful extremities, limb claudication, dizziness, syncope, headache, and visual impairment. TIA or ischemic stroke is usually attributed to common carotid artery involvement and perfusion impairment (Fig. 14.10). Ischemic or hemorrhagic stroke may be attributed to concomitant renovascular hypertension.

Because VAs do not directly branch out from the aorta, the VA involvement is uncommon. Rather, intact VAs often play a role in supplying cerebral blood flow in the presence of bilateral occlusion of carotid arteries. Nevertheless, asymptomatic (Fig. 14.10) or symptomatic [101, 102] extracranial VA involvement is often observed.

Giant Cell (Temporal) Arteritis

Giant cell arteritis is a systemic vasculitis characterized by subacute granulomatous inflammation of the aorta and its major branches (large and medium vessels) with particular tropism for the extracranial carotid artery branches. Headache and visual loss, the most common clinical manifestations, are caused by involvement of the superficial temporal arteries and ophthalmic branches/central retinal arteries, respectively. Stroke is a rare complication of giant cell arteritis, occurring in about 3% of patients [103, 104]. Giant cell arteritis may involve extracranial VA and produce TIAs or brainstem/cerebellar infarctions [105–107]. Occasionally, the subclavian arteries become occluded. Because this condition is treatable, and the prognosis is poor if untreated, this possibility should be suspected in old patients with extensive VA steno-occlusive disease when

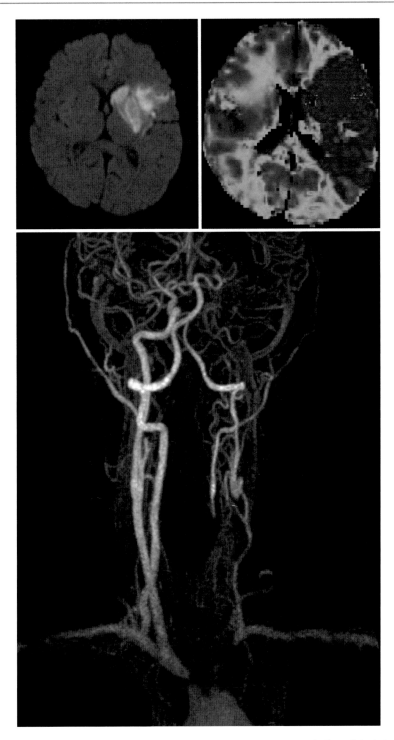

Fig. 14.10 A 39-year-old woman without vascular risk factors developed global aphasia and right hemiparesis. DWI showed left middle cerebral artery (MCA) territory infarction (upper left). Perfusion MRI showed decreased perfusion in the whole left MCA territory (upper right). MRA showed steno-occlusion of the left subclavian and common carotid artery, which was responsible for the present infarction. In addition, asymptomatic, proximal vertebral artery occlusion was found. The patient was treated under the diagnosis of Takayasu's arteritis

they have prolonged unexplained fever, headache, malaise, anemia, and ESR and/or CRP elevation.

Other Infectious or Immunologic Vasculitis

Vasculitis may be caused by infectious (e.g., bacterial, tuberculosis, spirochetal, fungal, viral) and immunologic (e.g., lupus, polyarteritis nodosa) disorders. Vasculitis more often involves the anterior circulation, but involvement of posterior circulation is not an exception [108].

Cerebral Autosomal Dominant Arteriopathy with Subcortical Infarcts and Leukoencephalopathy (CADASIL)

Cerebral autosomal dominant arteriopathy with subcortical infarcts and leukoencephalopathy (CADASIL) is a monogenetic stroke syndrome. The main pathological finding is the deposition of granular osmophilic material (GOM) in the small penetrating cerebral arteries, and clinical manifestations are characterized by recurrent

small vessel infarcts that ultimately lead to dementia and depression [109]. Small vessel diseases occur in both anterior and posterior circulation. Recently, involvement of large cerebral arteries has been reported in CADASIL patients [110, 111], suggesting that pathologic involvement may occur beyond the small cerebral vessels. One study described two patients with AICA territory infarction associated with AICA occlusion [111].

Persistent Anastomotic Links

A persistent trigeminal artery (PTA) is the most common embryonic carotid-basilar anastomosis, occurring in 0.1–1.0% of the general population. It usually forms a connection between the cavernous part of the ICA and the upper third of the BA [112]. A high incidence (85%) of VA hypoplasia or atresia is associated. Although the majority of the cases remain asymptomatic, the severe VA hypoplasia may lead to vertebrobasilar ischemic symptoms when collaterals are insufficient. In addition, brainstem TIA or infarction may occur due to emboli that originate from an ICA plaque [113] or diseased heart [114] and migrate through the PTA (Fig. 14.11).

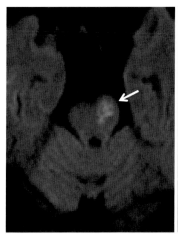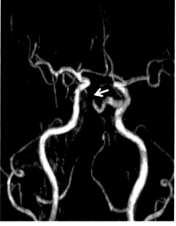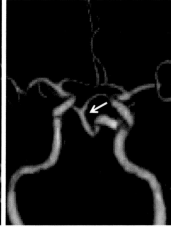

Fig. 14.11 A 70-year-old man with atrial fibrillation developed dysarthria and right hemiparesis. Brain CT did not show hemorrhages. While he received intravenous rt-PA, diffusion-weighted MRI and MRA were performed that showed a left pontine infarction (arrow, left image) and embolic occlusion of the persistent trigeminal artery (PTA) (arrow, middle image). Basilar artery (BA) and distal vertebral arteries (VAs) were not well visualized. His neurological deficits rapidly improved, and CT angiography 7 h after showed reperfused upper BA through the PTA (arrow, right image). Lower BA and VAs were considered hypoplastic in this patient. (Modified from Kwon et al. Brainstem Infarction Secondary to Persistent Trigeminal Artery Occlusion: Successful Treatment with Intravenous rt-PA. Eur Neurol 2010 2010;64:311)

References

1. Giroud M, Fayolle H, Andre N, Dumas R, Becker F, Martin D, et al. Incidence of internal carotid artery dissection in the community of Dijon. J Neurol Neurosurg Psychiatry. 1994;57(11):1443.
2. Bogousslavsky J, Van Melle G, Regli F. The Lausanne Stroke Registry: analysis of 1,000 consecutive patients with first stroke. Stroke. 1988;19(9):1083–92.
3. Schievink WI, Mokri B, O'Fallon WM. Recurrent spontaneous cervical-artery dissection. N Engl J Med. 1994;330(6):393–7.
4. Bogousslavsky J, Pierre P. Ischemic stroke in patients under age 45. Neurol Clin. 1992;10(1):113–24.
5. Lee TH, Hsu WC, Chen CJ, Chen ST. Etiologic study of young ischemic stroke in Taiwan. Stroke. 2002;33(8):1950–5.
6. Schievink WI, Mokri B, Whisnant JP. Internal carotid artery dissection in a community. Rochester, Minnesota, 1987-1992. Stroke. 1993;24(11):1678–80.
7. Lee VH, Brown RD Jr, Mandrekar JN, Mokri B. Incidence and outcome of cervical artery dissection: a population-based study. Neurology. 2006;67(10):1809–12.
8. Arnold M, Kappeler L, Georgiadis D, Berthet K, Keserue B, Bousser MG, et al. Gender differences in spontaneous cervical artery dissection. Neurology. 2006;67(6):1050–2.
9. Metso TM, Metso AJ, Helenius J, Haapaniemi E, Salonen O, Porras M, et al. Prognosis and safety of anticoagulation in intracranial artery dissections in adults. Stroke. 2007;38(6):1837–42.
10. Rubinstein SM, Peerdeman SM, van Tulder MW, Riphagen I, Haldeman S. A systematic review of the risk factors for cervical artery dissection. Stroke. 2005;36(7):1575–80.
11. Hausser I, Muller U, Engelter S, Lyrer P, Pezzini A, Padovani A, et al. Different types of connective tissue alterations associated with cervical artery dissections. Acta Neuropathol. 2004;107(6):509–14.
12. Kim BJ, Yang E, Kim NY, Kim MJ, Kang DW, Kwon SU, et al. Vascular tortuosity may be associated with cervical artery dissection. Stroke. 2016;47(10):2548–52.
13. Kobayashi J, Ohara T, Shiozawa M, Minematsu K, Nagatsuka K, Toyoda K. Isolated posterior inferior cerebellar artery dissection as a cause of ischemic stroke: clinical features and prognosis. Cerebrovasc Dis. 2015;40(5–6):215–21.
14. Choi YJ, Jung SC, Lee DH. Vessel wall imaging of the intracranial and cervical carotid arteries. J Stroke. 2015;17(3):238–55.
15. Park KJ, Jung SC, Kim HS, Choi CG, Kim SJ, Lee DH, et al. Multi-contrast high-resolution magnetic resonance findings of spontaneous and unruptured intracranial vertebral artery dissection: qualitative and quantitative analysis according to stages. Cerebrovasc Dis. 2016;42(1–2):23–31.
16. Kwon JY, Kim NY, Suh DC, Kang DW, Kwon SU, Kim JS. Intracranial and extracranial arterial dissection presenting with ischemic stroke: lesion location and stroke mechanism. J Neurol Sci. 2015;358(1–2):371–6.
17. Wilkinson IM. The vertebral artery. Extracranial and intracranial structure. Arch Neurol. 1972;27(5):392–6.
18. Yonas H, Agamanolis D, Takaoka Y, White RJ. Dissecting intracranial aneurysms. Surg Neurol. 1977;8(6):407–15.
19. Day AL, Gaposchkin CG, Yu CJ, Rivet DJ, Dacey RG Jr. Spontaneous fusiform middle cerebral artery aneurysms: characteristics and a proposed mechanism of formation. J Neurosurg. 2003;99(2):228–40.
20. Endo S, Nishijima M, Nomura H, Takaku A, Okada E. A pathological study of intracranial posterior circulation dissecting aneurysms with subarachnoid hemorrhage: report of three autopsied cases and review of the literature. Neurosurgery. 1993;33(4):732–8.
21. Kim JS. Pure lateral medullary infarction: clinical-radiological correlation of 130 acute, consecutive patients. Brain. 2003;126(Pt 8):1864–72.
22. Lin CH, Jeng JS, Yip PK. Middle cerebral artery dissections: differences between isolated and extended dissections of internal carotid artery. J Neurol Sci. 2005;235(1–2):37–44.
23. Piepgras DG, Mcgrail KM, Tazelaar HD. Intracranial dissection of the distal middle cerebral-artery as an uncommon cause of distal cerebral-artery aneurysm. J Neurosurg. 1994;80(5):909–13.
24. Kim JS, Lee HB, Kwon HS. RNF213 polymorphism in intracranial artery dissection. J Stroke. 2018;20(3):404–6.
25. Ohkuma H, Suzuki S, Kikkawa T, Shimamura N. Neuroradiologic and clinical features of arterial dissection of the anterior cerebral artery. AJNR Am J Neuroradiol. 2003;24(4):691–9.
26. Chiras J, Marciano S, Vega Molina J, Touboul J, Poirier B, Bories J. Spontaneous dissecting aneurysm of the extracranial vertebral artery (20 cases). Neuroradiology. 1985;27(4):327–33.
27. Mokri B, Houser OW, Sandok BA, Piepgras DG. Spontaneous dissections of the vertebral arteries. Neurology. 1988;38(6):880–5.
28. Huang YC, Chen YF, Wang YH, Tu YK, Jeng JS, Liu HM. Cervicocranial arterial dissection: experience of 73 patients in a single center. Surg Neurol. 2009;72(Suppl 2):S20–7; discussion S7
29. Frumkin LR, Baloh RW. Wallenberg's syndrome following neck manipulation. Neurology. 1990;40(4):611–5.
30. Easton JD, Sherman DG. Cervical manipulation and stroke. Stroke. 1977;8(5):594–7.
31. Goldstein SJ. Dissecting hematoma of the cervical vertebral artery. Case report. J Neurosurg. 1982;56(3):451–4.

32. Biousse V, Chabriat H, Amarenco P, Bousser MG. Roller-coaster-induced vertebral artery dissection. Lancet. 1995;346(8977):767.

33. Norris JW, Beletsky V, Nadareishvili ZG. Sudden neck movement and cervical artery dissection. The Canadian Stroke Consortium. CMAJ. 2000;163(1):38–40.

34. Caplan LR, Baquis GD, Pessin MS, D'Alton J, Adelman LS, DeWitt LD, et al. Dissection of the intracranial vertebral artery. Neurology. 1988;38(6):868–77.

35. Hosoya T, Adachi M, Yamaguchi K, Haku T, Kayama T, Kato T. Clinical and neuroradiological features of intracranial vertebrobasilar artery dissection. Stroke. 1999;30(5):1083–90.

36. Alexander CB, Burger PC, Goree JA. Dissecting aneurysms of the basilar artery in 2 patients. Stroke. 1979;10(3):294–9.

37. Masson C, Krespy Y, Masson M, Colombani JM. Magnetic resonance imaging in basilar artery dissection. Stroke. 1993;24(8):1264–6.

38. Ruecker M, Furtner M, Knoflach M, Werner P, Gotwald T, Chemelli A, et al. Basilar artery dissection: series of 12 consecutive cases and review of the literature. Cerebrovasc Dis. 2010;30(3):267–76.

39. Caplan LR, Estol CJ, Massaro AR. Dissection of the posterior cerebral arteries. Arch Neurol. 2005;62(7):1138–43.

40. Inoue T, Nishimura S, Hayashi N, Numagami Y, Takazawa H, Nishijima M. Postpartum dissecting aneurysm of the posterior cerebral artery. J Clin Neurosci. 2007;14(6):576–81.

41. Wetjen NM, Link MJ, Reimer R, Nichols DA, Giannini C. Clinical presentation and surgical management of dissecting posterior inferior cerebellar artery aneurysms: 2 case reports. Surg Neurol. 2005;64(5):462–7; discussion 7

42. Sedat J, Chau Y, Mahagne MH, Bourg V, Lonjon M, Paquis P. Dissection of the posteroinferior cerebellar artery: clinical characteristics and long-term follow-up in five cases. Cerebrovasc Dis. 2007;24(2–3):183–90.

43. Kanou Y, Arita K, Kurisu K, Ikawa F, Eguchi K, Monden S, et al. Dissecting aneurysm of the peripheral posterior inferior cerebellar artery. Acta Neurochir. 2000;142(10):1151–6.

44. Gotoh H, Takahashi T, Shimizu H, Ezura M, Tominaga T. Dissection of the superior cerebellar artery: a report of two cases and review of the literature. J Clin Neurosci. 2004;11(2):196–9.

45. Chang FC, Yong CS, Huang HC, Tsai JY, Sheng WY, Hu HH, et al. Posterior circulation ischemic stroke caused by arterial dissection: characteristics and predictors of poor outcomes. Cerebrovasc Dis. 2015;40(3–4):144–50.

46. Kim BM, Kim SH, Kim DI, Shin YS, Suh SH, Kim DJ, et al. Outcomes and prognostic factors of intracranial unruptured vertebrobasilar artery dissection. Neurology. 2011;76(20):1735–41.

47. Little JR, St Louis P, Weinstein M, Dohn DF. Giant fusiform aneurysm of the cerebral arteries. Stroke. 1981;12(2):183–8.

48. Nishizaki T, Tamaki N, Takeda N, Shirakuni T, Kondoh T, Matsumoto S. Dolichoectatic basilar artery: a review of 23 cases. Stroke. 1986;17(6):1277–81.

49. Hirsch CS, Roessmann U. Arterial dysplasia with ruptured basilar artery aneurysm: report of a case. Hum Pathol. 1975;6(6):749–58.

50. Makos MM, McComb RD, Hart MN, Bennett DR. Alpha-glucosidase deficiency and basilar artery aneurysm: report of a sibship. Ann Neurol. 1987;22(5):629–33.

51. Kwon HM, Kim JH, Lim JS, Park JH, Lee SH, Lee YS. Basilar artery dolichoectasia is associated with paramedian pontine infarction. Cerebrovasc Dis. 2009;27(2):114–8.

52. Pessin MS, Chimowitz MI, Levine SR, Kwan ES, Adelman LS, Earnest MP, et al. Stroke in patients with fusiform vertebrobasilar aneurysms. Neurology. 1989;39(1):16–21.

53. Passero S, Filosomi G. Posterior circulation infarcts in patients with vertebrobasilar dolichoectasia. Stroke. 1998;29(3):653–9.

54. Nakamura Y, Hirayama T, Ikeda K. Clinicoradiologic features of vertebrobasilar dolichoectasia in stroke patients. J Stroke Cerebrovasc Dis. 2012;21(1):5–10.

55. Moseley IF, Holland IM. Ectasia of the basilar artery: the breadth of the clinical spectrum and the diagnostic value of computed tomography. Neuroradiology. 1979;18(2):83–91.

56. Kerber CW, Margolis MT, Newton TH. Tortuous vertebrobasilar system: a cause of cranial nerve signs. Neuroradiology. 1972;4(2):74–7.

57. Paulson G, Nashold BS Jr, Margolis G. Aneurysms of the vertebral artery: report of 5 cases. Neurology. 1959;9:590–8.

58. Ekbom K, Greitz T, Kugelberg E. Hydrocephalus due to ectasia of the basilar artery. J Neurol Sci. 1969;8(3):465–77.

59. Rao KG, Woodlief RM. CT simulation of cerebellopontine tumor by tortuous vertebrobasilar artery. AJR Am J Roentgenol. 1979;132(4):672–3.

60. Maruyama K, Tanaka M, Ikeda S, Tada T, Yanagisawa N. A case report of quadriparesis due to compression of the medulla oblongata by the elongated left vertebral artery. Rinsho Shinkeigaku. 1989;29(1):108–11.

61. Chin JH. Recurrent stroke caused by spondylotic compression of the vertebral artery. Ann Neurol. 1993;33(5):558–9.

62. Rosengart A, Hedges TR 3rd, Teal PA, DeWitt LD, Wu JK, Wolpert S, et al. Intermittent downbeat nystagmus due to vertebral artery compression. Neurology. 1993;43(1):216–8.

63. Dadsetan MR, Skerhut HE. Rotational vertebrobasilar insufficiency secondary to vertebral artery occlusion from fibrous band of the longus coli muscle. Neuroradiology. 1990;32(6):514–5.

64. George B, Laurian C. Impairment of vertebral artery flow caused by extrinsic lesions. Neurosurgery. 1989;24(2):206–14.

65. Mapstone T, Spetzler RF. Vertebrobasilar insufficiency secondary to vertebral artery occlusion froma fibrous band. Case report. J Neurosurg. 1982;56(4):581–3.

66. Kuether TA, Nesbit GM, Clark WM, Barnwell SL. Rotational vertebral artery occlusion: a mechanism of vertebrobasilar insufficiency. Neurosurgery. 1997;41(2):427–32; discussion 32-3

67. Choi KD, Choi JH, Kim JS, Kim HJ, Kim MJ, Lee TH, et al. Rotational vertebral artery occlusion: mechanisms and long-term outcome. Stroke. 2013;44(7):1817–24.

68. Strupp M, Planck JH, Arbusow V, Steiger HJ, Bruckmann H, Brandt T. Rotational vertebral artery occlusion syndrome with vertigo due to "labyrinthine excitation". Neurology. 2000;54(6):1376–9.

69. Barrows LJ, Kubik CS, Richardson EP Jr. Aneurysms of the basilar and vertebral arteries; a clinico-pathologic study. Trans Am Neurol Assoc. 1956(81st Meeting):181–3.

70. Inao S, Kuchiwaki H, Hirai N, Gonda T, Furuse M. Posterior communicating artery section during surgery for basilar tip aneurysm. Acta Neurochir. 1996;138(7):853–61.

71. Schellhas KP, Latchaw RE, Wendling LR, Gold LH. Vertebrobasilar injuries following cervical manipulation. JAMA. 1980;244(13):1450–3.

72. Sato M, Tanaka S, Kohama A, Fujii C. Occipital lobe infarction caused by tentorial herniation. Neurosurgery. 1986;18(3):300–5.

73. Ropper AH. Syndrome of transtentorial herniation: is vertical displacement necessary? J Neurol Neurosurg Psychiatry. 1993;56(8):932–5.

74. Slovut DP, Olin JW. Fibromuscular dysplasia. N Engl J Med. 2004;350(18):1862–71.

75. Perez-Higueras A, Alvarez-Ruiz F, Martinez-Bermejo A, Frutos R, Villar O, Diez-Tejedor E. Cerebellar infarction from fibromuscular dysplasia and dissecting aneurysm of the vertebral artery. Report of a child. Stroke. 1988;19(4):521–4.

76. Osborn AG, Anderson RE. Angiographic spectrum of cervical and intracranial fibromuscular dysplasia. Stroke. 1977;8(5):617–26.

77. Tashiro K, Shigeto H, Tanaka M, Kawajiri M, Taniwaki T, Kira J. Fibromuscular dysplasia of the basilar artery presenting as cerebral infarction in a young female. Rinsho Shinkeigaku. 2006;46(1):35–9.

78. Demirkaya S, Topcuoglu MA, Vural O. Fibromuscular dysplasia of the basilar artery: a case presenting with vertebrobasilar TIAs. Eur J Neurol. 2001;8(1):89–90.

79. Hegedus K, Nemeth G. Fibromuscular dysplasia of the basilar artery. Case report with autopsy verification. Arch Neurol. 1984;41(4):440–2.

80. Frens DB, Petajan JH, Anderson R, Deblanc JH Jr. Fibromuscular dysplasia of the posterior cerebral artery: report of a case and review of the literature. Stroke. 1974;5(2):161–6.

81. Ringel SP, Harrison SH, Norenberg MD, Austin JH. Fibromuscular dysplasia: multiple "spontaneous" dissecting aneurysms of the major cervical arteries. Ann Neurol. 1977;1(3):301–4.

82. Cloft HJ, Kallmes DF, Kallmes MH, Goldstein JH, Jensen ME, Dion JE. Prevalence of cerebral aneurysms in patients with fibromuscular dysplasia: a reassessment. J Neurosurg. 1998;88(3):436–40.

83. Zimmerman R, Leeds NE, Naidich TP. Carotid-cavernous fistula associated with intracranial fibromuscular dysplasia. Radiology. 1977;122(3):725–6.

84. Pilz P, Hartjes HJ. Fibromuscular dysplasia and multiple dissecting aneurysms of intracranial arteries. A further cause of Moyamoya syndrome. Stroke. 1976;7(4):393–8.

85. Horn P, Bueltmann E, Buch CV, Schmiedek P. Arterio-embolic ischemic stroke in children with moyamoya disease. Childs Nerv Syst. 2005;21(2):104–7.

86. Kim JM, Lee SH, Roh JK. Changing ischaemic lesion patterns in adult moyamoya disease. J Neurol Neurosurg Psychiatry. 2009;80(1):36–40.

87. Hishikawa T, Tokunaga K, Sugiu K, Date I. Assessment of the difference in posterior circulation involvement between pediatric and adult patients with moyamoya disease. J Neurosurg. 2013;119(4):961–5.

88. Pessin MS, Lathi ES, Cohen MB, Kwan ES, Hedges TR 3rd, Caplan LR. Clinical features and mechanism of occipital infarction. Ann Neurol. 1987;21(3):290–9.

89. Kumral E, Bayulkem G, Atac C, Alper Y. Spectrum of superficial posterior cerebral artery territory infarcts. Eur J Neurol. 2004;11(4):237–46.

90. Cals N, Devuyst G, Afsar N, Karapanayiotides T, Bogousslavsky J. Pure superficial posterior cerebral artery territory infarction in the Lausanne Stroke Registry. J Neurol. 2002;249(7):855–61.

91. Broderick JP, Swanson JW. Migraine-related strokes. Clinical profile and prognosis in 20 patients. Arch Neurol. 1987;44(8):868–71.

92. Ries S, Steinke W, Neff W, Schindlmayr C, Meairs S, Hennerici M. Ischemia-induced migraine from paradoxical cardioembolic stroke. Eur Neurol. 1996;36(2):76–8.

93. Ducros A, Boukobza M, Porcher R, Sarov M, Valade D, Bousser MG. The clinical and radiological spectrum of reversible cerebral vasoconstriction syndrome. A prospective series of 67 patients. Brain. 2007;130(Pt 12):3091–101.

94. Ciafaloni E, Ricci E, Shanske S, Moraes CT, Silvestri G, Hirano M, et al. MELAS: clinical features, biochemistry, and molecular genetics. Ann Neurol. 1992;31(4):391–8.

95. Goto Y, Horai S, Matsuoka T, Koga Y, Nihei K, Kobayashi M, et al. Mitochondrial myopathy, encephalopathy, lactic acidosis, and stroke-like episodes (MELAS): a correlative study of the

clinical features and mitochondrial DNA mutation. Neurology. 1992;42(3 Pt 1):545–50.

96. Majamaa K, Turkka J, Karppa M, Winqvist S, Hassinen IE. The common MELAS mutation A3243G in mitochondrial DNA among young patients with an occipital brain infarct. Neurology. 1997;49(5):1331–4.

97. Sakuta R, Nonaka I. Vascular involvement in mitochondrial myopathy. Ann Neurol. 1989;25(6):594–601.

98. Gropen TI, Prohovnik I, Tatemichi TK, Hirano M. Cerebral hyperemia in MELAS. Stroke. 1994;25(9):1873–6.

99. Castillo M, Kwock L, Green C. MELAS syndrome: imaging and proton MR spectroscopic findings. AJNR Am J Neuroradiol. 1995;16(2):233–9.

100. Barkovich AJ, Good WV, Koch TK, Berg BO. Mitochondrial disorders: analysis of their clinical and imaging characteristics. AJNR Am J Neuroradiol. 1993;14(5):1119–37.

101. Lupi-Herrera E, Sanchez-Torres G, Marcushamer J, Mispireta J, Horwitz S, Vela JE. Takayasu's arteritis. Clinical study of 107 cases. Am Heart J. 1977;93(1):94–103.

102. Kim HJ, Suh DC, Kim JK, Kim SJ, Lee JH, Choi CG, et al. Correlation of neurological manifestations of Takayasu's arteritis with cerebral angiographic findings. Clin Imaging. 2005;29(2):79–85.

103. Caselli RJ, Hunder GG, Whisnant JP. Neurologic disease in biopsy-proven giant cell (temporal) arteritis. Neurology. 1988;38(3):352–9.

104. Gonzalez-Gay MA, Vazquez-Rodriguez TR, Gomez-Acebo I, Pego-Reigosa R, Lopez-Diaz MJ, Vazquez-Trinanes MC, et al. Strokes at time of disease diagnosis in a series of 287 patients with biopsy-proven giant cell arteritis. Medicine (Baltimore). 2009;88(4):227–35.

105. Ruegg S, Engelter S, Jeanneret C, Hetzel A, Probst A, Steck AJ, et al. Bilateral vertebral artery occlusion resulting from giant cell arteritis: report of 3 cases and review of the literature. Medicine (Baltimore). 2003;82(1):1–12.

106. Garcia-Porrua C, Pego-Reigosa R, Martinez-Vazquez F, Armesto V, Gonzalez-Gay MA. Bilateral vertebral artery occlusion in giant cell arteritis. Clin Exp Rheumatol. 2006;24(2 Suppl 41):S101.

107. Zamarbide ID, Maxit MJ. Fisher's one and half syndrome with facial palsy as clinical presentation of giant cell temporal arteritis. Medicina (B Aires). 2000;60(2):245–8.

108. Amarenco P, Kase CS, Rosengart A, Pessin MS, Bousser MG, Caplan LR. Very small (border zone) cerebellar infarcts. Distribution, causes, mechanisms and clinical features. Brain. 1993;116(Pt 1):161–86.

109. Lindgren A. Stroke genetics: a review and update. J Stroke. 2014;16(3):114–23.

110. Choi EJ, Choi CG, Kim JS. Large cerebral artery involvement in CADASIL. Neurology. 2005;65(8):1322–4.

111. Kang HG, Kim JS. Intracranial arterial disease in CADASIL patients. J Neurol Sci. 2015;359(1–2):347–50.

112. Suttner N, Mura J, Tedeschi H, Ferreira MA, Wen HT, de Oliveira E, et al. Persistent trigeminal artery: a unique anatomic specimen--analysis and therapeutic implications. Neurosurgery. 2000;47(2):428–33; discussion 33-4

113. Momma F, Ohara S, Ohyama T. Persistent trigeminal artery associated with brainstem infarct--case report. Neurol Med Chir (Tokyo). 1992;32(5):289–91.

114. Kwon JY, Lee EJ, Kim JS. Brainstem infarction secondary to persistent trigeminal artery occlusion: successful treatment with intravenous rt-PA. Eur Neurol. 2010;64(5):311.

Outcomes and Prognosis

15

Nitish Kumar, Vamshi K. S. Balasetti, Farhan Siddiq,
Brandi R. French, Camilo R. Gomez,
and Adnan I. Qureshi

Introduction

Ischemic stroke (i.e., infarction) occurring as a result of disorders affecting the vertebrobasilar system, results in ischemic injury to the brainstem, the cerebellum, and/or the posterior portions of the cerebral hemispheres [1]. Historically, these types of cerebrovascular events account for approximately 30% of all ischemic strokes [2]. The recognition of posterior circulation transient ischemic attack or stroke is more difficult to make compared to anterior circulation, mostly because of the complexity of the vertebrobasilar system. Current guidelines for the management of posterior circulation are similar to anterior circulation stroke, although several differences exist in their presentations, disease mechanism, and their outcomes [3–7]. The prognosis of posterior circulation differs depending on stenosis/occlusion, and vertebrobasilar stenosis, for example, increases the risk by three times [8–10]. Moreover, the etiology of stroke also affects the

functional outcomes, as shown by Chung et al., where large artery atherosclerosis and cardioembolic etiologies carry worse functional outcome at discharge and 3 months, respectively, in a posterior circulation stroke [11].

Mechanism of Vertebrobasilar Ischemic Stroke

The most common causes of posterior circulation ischemia are cardioembolism, large artery atherosclerosis, and small artery disease. Atherosclerosis often occurs at or near the origin of the vertebral artery [3]. Caplan et al. in 2004 proposed that the mechanism of ischemic stroke in anterior and posterior circulation is different. The conclusion was based on a study of 407 patients between 1988 and 1996 from New England Medical Center-Posterior Circulation Registry. Patients with posterior circulation ischemic events had a lower frequency of cardioembolic etiology (24%) compared with large artery disease (32%). In patients with anterior circulation ischemic events, a higher frequency of cardioembolic etiology was detected (38%) compared with large artery disease (9%) [2].

Posterior circulation ischemic stroke incidence rates are different for asymptomatic and symptomatic vertebrobasilar disease. In New England Medical Center-Posterior Circulation Registry, 9% of the 407 patients had complete occlusion vertebral artery occlusion and 2.7%

N. Kumar (✉) · V. K. S. Balasetti · B. R. French
C. R. Gomez · A. I. Qureshi
The Department of Neurology, University of
Missouri Columbia School of Medicine,
Columbia, MO, USA
e-mail: vbzzn@health.missouri.edu; frenchb@health.missouri.edu; crgomez@missouri.edu

F. Siddiq
The Division of Neurosurgery, University of Missouri
Columbia School of Medicine, Columbia, MO, USA
e-mail: farhansiddiq@missouri.edu

© Springer Nature Singapore Pte Ltd. 2021
J. S. Kim (ed.), *Posterior Circulation Stroke*, https://doi.org/10.1007/978-981-15-6739-1_15

had bilateral vertebral artery occlusion [2]. Atherosclerotic stenosis ≥50% in either the vertebral artery is found in approximately 25% of the patients with vertebrobasilar transient ischemic attack or stroke. The stenosis is most frequently located in the proximal vertebral artery [10]. Patients with symptomatic vertebrobasilar stenosis are at risk of stroke occurrence despite the medical therapy occurring in 10–15% of the patients in 2 years [12]. In one study, 7.6% of the patients with asymptomatic vertebral artery stenosis >50% were followed for mean 4.6 years; posterior circulation stroke occurred in <0.1% of the patients. The risk of stroke was higher for patients with vertebral artery stenosis than in patients without vertebral artery stenosis [5]. A study from Taiwan analyzed 286 patients who presented with posterior circulation stroke and found that basilar artery branch occlusive disease (28%) and large artery dissection (25.9%) were the two most common etiologies, followed by large artery atherosclerotic stenosis or occlusion (26%), cardioembolism (18.5%), and small vessel disease (7%) [11].

Early Outcomes: First 90 Days

Recurrent Stroke

A meta-analysis published in 2003 demonstrated a higher risk of recurrent ischemic strokes in the posterior circulation in the first 7 days (acute phase) in patients with vertebrobasilar stenosis (odds ratio 1.47, 95% confidence interval (CI) 1.1–2.0, $p = 0.014$) [9]. Conversely, they also found that the risk of recurrent stroke was low (odds ratio 0.74, 95% confidence interval 0.7–0.8) after the first 7 days. This was further confirmed in recent studies: Oxford Vascular Study and 1 hospital register-based study (St. George's Study) [8]. Both studies demonstrated that vertebrobasilar stenosis was a major predictor of recurrent stroke, particularly in the first month. A pooled individual patient analysis from the Oxford Vascular Study and St. George's Study demonstrated that 90-day risk of stroke from the first event was 24.6% in patients with vertebro-

basilar stenosis versus 7.2% in patients without any stenosis. This was further supported by another study that showed that risk of recurrence stroke and the risk of any vertebrobasilar disease recurrence (including both transient ischemic stroke and stroke) at 90 days was up to 3 times higher in patients with stenosis compared with those without stenosis [12].

Schonewille et al. did a prospective, observational study from the "The Basilar Artery International Cooperative Study" registry of 619 consecutive patients who presented with an acute symptomatic and radiologically conformed basilar artery occlusion [13]. Patients were divided into three groups based on the treatment they received: (1) antithrombotic treatment only, which comprised antiplatelets or systemic anticoagulation; (2) primary intravenous therapy including subsequent intra-arterial thrombolysis; and (3) intra-arterial therapy including thrombolysis, mechanical thrombectomy, stenting, or a combination of these approaches. The outcome was assessed at 1 month, and poor outcome was defined as a modified Rankin scale score of 4 or 5, or death. They reported that overall, 68% (492/592) of analyzed patients had a poor outcome at 30 days. They also showed that compared to antiplatelet or anticoagulant therapy, patients with a severe deficit had a lower risk of poor outcomes when received intravenous therapy (adjusted relative risk 0.88, confidence interval 0.76–1.01) or when received intra-arterial therapy (adjusted relative risk 0.94, confidence interval 0.86–1.02).

A systematic analysis from Finland by Lindsberg et al. looked at the outcome of basilar artery occlusion patients treated with intra-arterial thrombolysis or intravenous thrombolysis. Modified Rankin scale score 0–2, Barthel Index 95 to 100, or Glasgow Outcome Scale 5 was considered as good outcomes [14]. Approximately 3-month outcome was provided. Of 420 patients, 76/420 were treated with intravenous therapy and 344/420 were treated with intra-arterial therapy. Death or dependency was similar in both groups ($p = 0.82$) reportedly in 78% (59/76) of patients treated with intravenous therapy and 76%

(260/344) of patients treated with intra-arterial therapy. Even though recanalization rate was higher in intra-arterial group (65%, 225/344) compared to intravenous group (53%,40/76, $p = 0.05$), survival rates (50% vs 45%, $p = 0.48$) were equal. A similar rate of good outcomes (24% vs 22%, $p = 0.82$) was seen in both groups. Without recanalization, the likelihood of good outcome was close to 2%.

A systematic review and meta-analysis were done by Schonewille et al. and colleagues to analyze the efficacy of different methods of acute basilar artery occlusion. They reviewed 102 articles to analyze the treatment options. The weighted pooled rate of mortality was 43.16% (95% confidence interval 38.35–48.03%) in the intravenous thrombolysis group, 45.56% (95% confidence interval 39.88–51.28%) in the intra-arterial thrombolysis group, and 31.40% (95% confidence interval 28.31–34.56%) in the endovascular thrombectomy group. The weighted pooled rate of modified Rankin score 0–2 at 3 months was 31.40% (95% confidence interval 28.31–34.56%) in the intravenous thrombolysis group, 28.29% (95% confidence interval 23.16–33.69%) in the intra-arterial thrombolysis group, and 35.22% (95% confidence interval 32.39–38.09%) in the endovascular thrombectomy group [13].

A study from Switzerland looked at the 106 patients treated between 1992 and 2010 with intra-arterial thrombolysis. At 3 months, clinical outcome was good (modified Rankin scale score, 0–2) in 33% of the patients and 11.3% had a moderate outcome (modified Rankin scale score, 3). Mortality was 40.6% [14].

Death or Disability

A Korean study looked at 7718 patients for minor anterior circulation and minor posterior circulation stroke and disability at 3-month follow-up. Disability (modified Rankin scale score 2–6) was seen in 32.3% of the patients with minor posterior circulation stroke (compared to 30.3% of minor anterior circulation stroke, $p = 0.07$) and death in 1.3% of the patients

(compared to 1.5% of minor anterior circulation stroke, $p = 0.82$) [15].

Prospective data of 116 patients with posterior circulation stroke who were admitted to a single Qatar hospital were collected from 2005 through 2008 with mean duration from symptom onset to presentation of 29 h reported the following: 71% of the patients were discharged home while 10% died, and modified Rankin scale score at discharge was ≤2 in 53% and ≥4% in 13% of the patients. The modified Rankin scale score was ≤2 in 68% of the patients at 30-day follow-up. Almost 90% of the patients were alive with a modified Rankin scale score of ≤2 seen in 73% of the patients [16].

Predictors of Outcome

Chung et al. looked at the etiologies of posterior circulation stroke and their association with outcome. They also suggested age >70 years, National Institute of Health Stroke Scale >9, and certain stroke etiologies (large artery atherosclerosis and cardioembolism) as predictors of poor functional outcomes (defined by modified Rankin scale score >5), which are associated with poor functional outcomes at the discharge and 3 months [11, 17].

Etiologies of posterior circulation stroke affecting the outcomes were further supported in a study by Glass et al., which found that outcomes of posterior circulation stroke differed depending on vascular occlusive lesion, brain infarct location, and stroke mechanism [18].

Occlusion of the basilar artery led to the worst outcome (>50% of the patients had poor outcomes at 30 days, defined by death or severe disability) [18]. Basilar artery occlusive disease was responsible for the greatest risk of mortality and disability followed by intracranial vertebral, extracranial vertebral, and posterior cerebral artery. Schonewille et al. reported outcomes in patients with posterior circulation stroke at 28 days: almost 80% of the basilar artery occlusion patients had poor outcomes with a case fatality rate of 40%, and 65% of the survivors had severe residual deficits. They also identified 3 potential predictors of outcomes in patients treated by conventional methods (antiplatelets or anticoagulants or both): age (young vs old), stroke severity, and presenting symptoms (fluctuating vs maximum deficits from the onset) with younger age (<60 years), less severe stroke and fluctuating symptoms favoring better outcomes [19]. One study looked at 87 patients with predominantly minor stroke and occlusive basilar disease documented based on transcranial Doppler, magnetic resonance angiography, or conventional angiography and found an overall case fatality rate of about 2.3%. The low case fatality rate in this study could be due to a higher number of patients with minor deficits being diagnosed with vertebrobasilar disease [20].

A Chinese study combined the National Institutes of Health stroke scale score and posterior circulation Alberta stroke program early computed tomography score through diffusion-weighted imaging in 125 patients with posterior circulation stroke. Patients with higher baseline National Institutes of Health stroke scale score (6.3±7.4) and lower posterior circulation Alberta stroke program early computed tomography score (≤7) in the first 36 h of stroke onset had unfavorable outcomes (modified Rankin scale score at 90 days 3–6). Age >70 years and the presence of diabetes mellitus were significant predictors of unfavorable outcomes [21].

Tsao et al. looked at 21 consecutive patients retrospectively who received either intravenous or intra-arterial tissue plasminogen activator for posterior circulation ischemic stroke at University of California between 1993 and 2001. Results showed that high presenting Glasgow coma scale score ≥ 9 was predictive of good patient outcome (modified Rankin scale score at 3 months =/<2) [22].

Another study looked at the correlation between the severity of the neurologic deficit and posterior circulation stroke. Almost 1200 patients with anterior circulation stroke and 400 with posterior circulation strokes were included with median National Institutes of Health stroke scale scores of 7 and 2, respectively. Of the patients analyzed, 70% of the posterior circulation stroke patients had National Institutes of Health stroke

scale score ≤4, and around 15% of them had a poor prognosis [23]. Sato et al. in his study of 100 patients showed that the National Institutes of Health stroke scale score appears to have limitations in predicting outcomes in posterior circulation stroke [24]. The cutoff score of the baseline National Institutes of Health stroke scale score for a favorable outcome was relatively low in patients with posterior circulation stroke compared to patients with anterior circulation stroke. The National Institutes of Health stroke scale score seems to be weighted toward anterior circulation stroke and tends to underestimate the severity of the posterior circulation stroke [23–25].

Adaptation of the National Institutes of Health stroke scale score for elements common to the posterior circulation stroke, such as vertigo, dizziness, or confusion, may increase its sensitivity [26].

Another study of 88 patients in Switzerland reported statistically significant association of certain admission clinical characteristics with an outcome in patients presenting with stroke or transient ischemic attacks in the basilar artery stenosis or occlusion. Dysarthria, pupillary disorders, lower cranial nerve involvement, and consciousness disorders at admission were strongly ($P < 0.001$) associated with poor outcomes, defined by severe disability or death. A multivariate analysis showed that the outcome was poor in 100% of cases with either consciousness disorders or other 3 clinical characteristics [27]. Interestingly, in the absence of these factors, a poor outcome (severe disability or death) was reported in only 11% of the patients.

Sommer et al. used propensity-score matching to balance patient characteristics and stroke severity between 4604 patients of posterior circulation and 4604 patients of anterior circulation stroke enrolled within the Austrian Stroke registry [28]. A total of 477 (10.3%) patients within the posterior circulation stroke group were treated with tissue plasminogen activator compared to 4433 (~19%) of anterior circulation stroke patients. Patients with posterior circulation stroke had 19% higher odds of poor functional outcome ($p < 0.0001$) as assessed by the modified Rankin scale at 3 months. Patients who got tissue plasminogen activator did not show a significant difference in the functional outcome irrespective of infarct localization. However, more deficits in the posterior circulation stroke group were found to be driven by patients who could not receive tissue plasminogen activator and had presented after 4.5 h of the symptom onset. These patients had 34% odds of poor functional outcomes compared to anterior circulation stroke patients. These results were independent of stroke severity tissue plasminogen activator treatment, demographic, and vascular risk factors. This observation supported the findings of other few studies that showed the effectiveness of tissue plasminogen activator for stroke irrespective of localization [29–31]. The effect of time delays on the therapeutic outcomes of tissue plasminogen activator in posterior circulation stroke is further supported by the retrospective study of 95 patients done in China, which demonstrated that for patients with an onset-to-treatment time of 0–90 min, the rate of favorable outcome (defined by modified Rankin Scale<2) was 100% as opposed to 73.7% of favorable outcome for patients with an onset-to-treatment time of 181–237 min [32].

Only a few studies have looked at the direct relationship between the initial Glasgow coma scale score and clinical outcomes in the patients with posterior circulation stroke [33–35]. Schwarz et al. described 45 patients with posterior circulation stroke and found that those who had lower presenting Glasgow coma scale scores had worse clinical outcomes [35]. A few studies found tetraparesis and coma as independent predictors of poor outcomes [20, 36].

Late Outcomes: Beyond the First Year

Qureshi et al. and the group did a cohort study looking at the risk of recurrent stroke and death associated with vertebrobasilar stenosis and occlusion in 10,515 patients, diagnosed either by computed tomography, magnetic resonance angiography, or catheter angiogram [37]. Patients were selected from the Taiwan Stroke registry.

They found 66% of the patients with none-to-mild stenosis and 29.8% with moderate-to-severe stenosis, and occlusion was identified in 3.8% of the patients. There was a significantly higher risk of recurrent stroke at 1 year (hazard ratio 1.21, 95% confidence interval 1.01–1.45) among the patients with moderate-to-severe vertebrobasilar stenosis. There was a nonsignificantly higher risk of recurrent stroke (hazard ratio 1.49, 95% confidence interval 0.99–2.22) and a significantly higher risk of death (hazard ratio 2.21, 95% CI 1.72–2.83), among the patients with vertebrobasilar occlusion.

Another retrospective study looked at 102 patients diagnosed with symptomatic vertebrobasilar stenosis and followed up with them for the development of stroke and disability/death for 15±15.9 months (range 1–60 months). Recurrent stroke and mortality were reported in 14% and 21% of the patients, respectively, during the follow-up period.

Stroke-free survival was 76% and 48% at 12 months (95% confidence interval, 66–83%) and at 60 months (95% confidence interval, 27–65%), respectively. The risk of recurrent stroke was 11% per year, and the risk of recurrent stroke and/or death was 24% per year. Older patients had decreased stroke-free survival. Treatment with either antiplatelet agents in 41% or coumadin in 32% improved stroke-free survival [38].

A study from Greece reported 10-year outcomes in posterior circulation stroke patients, and 185 patients were followed up during 1998–2009. They divided their patients into pure posterior cerebral artery infarction group (pure cortical and combined cortical and deep posterior cerebral artery infarct) and posterior cerebral artery infarction-plus group (including posterior cerebral artery stroke and ≥ 1 concomitant infarction outside posterior cerebral artery territory). Of them, 56% of the patients of cortical-only infarct had no or minor disability compared to 26–36% in the posterior cerebral artery-plus group at 6-month follow-up. The 10-year probability of death was 55% for the pure posterior cerebral artery group vs 73% for posterior cerebral artery-plus ($p = 0.001$), showing that posterior cerebral artery strokes with concomitant infarction out-side the posterior cerebral artery territory was associated with an increased risk of disability and long-term mortality [39].

In another study of 51 patients with posterior circulation stroke, 30-day and 3-year survival rates were found to be 96% and 73% for top of the basilar group vs 100% and 71% in the group with involvement of either single penetrating or branch artery involvement, respectively [40].

Ottomeyer et al. looked at the long-term func-tional outcome and quality of life of patients who presented with acute basilar artery occlusion and got multimodal recanalization therapy. Ninety-one patients were treated during December 2002 and December 2009 by such therapy that included intravenous thrombolysis with consecutive on-demand intra-arterial therapy or intra-arterial therapy alone. The overall recanalization rate was 89%. Long-term survival (median follow-up for 4.2 years) was achieved in approximately 41% of the patients. Among survivors, 74% of the patients had a favorable functional long-term outcome (defined as modified Rankin scale score $\leq$ 3) [41].

Lindsberg et al. studied 50 consecutive patients between 1995 and 2003 with proven bas-ilar artery occlusion who were treated with intra-venous thrombolysis with recombinant tissue plasminogen activator. Recanalization was stud-ied in 43 patients and was verified in 26 patients (52%). In the first 3 months, 40% [20] of the patients died and 11 patients had good outcomes (modified Rankin scale score, 0–2); 12 (24%) were independent of activities of daily living (Barthel Index score, 95–100), and 6 (16%) patients were severely disabled (Barthel Index score, 0–50). After a median follow-up for 2.8 years, 15 (30%) patients reached good out-comes (modified Rankin scale score, 0–2) while 23 (46%) patients died [42].

Jung et al. looked at 3-month and long-term outcomes and their predictors in acute basilar occlusion treated with intra-arterial thromboly-sis. Between 3-month and long-term follow-up, 40.8% survivors showed clinical improvement of at least 1 point on the modified Rankin scale score, 53.7% were functionally unchanged, and 5.7% showed functional worsening ($P < 0.0001$).

Low baseline National Institutes of Health stroke scale score was identified as a predictor of good or moderate outcome (modified Rankin scale score, 0–3, $p < 0.0001$) and survival ($p = 0.001$) at 3 months. Younger age was identified as an additional predictor of survival ($p = 0.012$). Age was also an independent predictor ($p = 0.018$) for long-term clinical outcome [43].

Cognitive and Functional Outcomes

The information regarding the neuropsychiatric outcomes in patients with vertebrobasilar terri-tory stroke is scarce, and patients with heteroge-nous arterial lesions were included [44–46].

A case–control study from Brazil compared the cognitive statuses of basilar artery occlusion disease survivors (28 patients) and healthy con-trols (27 patients). They also looked at the corre-lation of functional capacity outcomes (modified Rankin scale score) with the cognitive profiles of basilar artery occlusion disease patients. Functional capacity was moderately correlated with the presence of cognitive impairment, indi-cating that functional results were due to poorer scores on cognitive tests. They found that 75% of the patients (21/28) had no functional disability (modified Rankin scale score of 0–1) at 4.2 years after the stroke suggestive favorable outcomes. Only 25% (7/28) of the patients had mild-to-moderate functional disability (modified Rankin scale score 2–3). Compared to controls, basilar artery occlusion disease patients presented with impairments in selective, sustained, and set-shifting action, processing speed, visuospatial skills, mental flexibility, and monitoring rules. Significant deficits in verbal episodic memory (immediate and delayed recall) and visuospatial episodic memory (immediate and delayed recall and recognition) were noted [47].

Patients with posterior circulation infarctions were noted to have abnormal neuropsychiatric profiles. The impairments were noted in execu-tive function, attention, memory, visuospatial ability, and language [17, 48, 49]. Neural links connecting anterior and posterior regions of the brain may be attributed [45, 46].

References

1. Bogousslavsky J, Van Melle G, Regli F. The Lausanne stroke registry: analysis of 1,000 consecutive patients with first stroke. Stroke. 1988;19(9):1083–92.
2. Caplan LR, Wityk RJ, Glass TA, Tapia J, Pazdera L, Chang HM, et al. New England Medical Center posterior circulation registry. Ann Neurol. 2004;56(3):389–98.
3. Markus HS, van der Worp HB, Rothwell PM. Posterior circulation ischaemic stroke and transient ischaemic attack: diagnosis, investigation, and secondary prevention. Lancet Neurol. 2013;12(10):989–98.
4. Merwick A, Werring D. Posterior circulation ischaemic stroke. BMJ. 2014;348:g3175.
5. Kim JS, Nah HW, Park SM, Kim SK, Cho KH, Lee J, et al. Risk factors and stroke mechanisms in atherosclerotic stroke: intracranial compared with extracranial and anterior compared with posterior circulation disease. Stroke. 2012;43(12):3313–8.
6. Caplan L. Posterior circulation ischemia: then, now, and tomorrow. The Thomas Willis Lecture-2000. Stroke. 2000;31(8):2011–23.
7. Paul NL, Simoni M, Rothwell PM. Transient isolated brainstem symptoms preceding posterior circulation stroke: a population-based study. Lancet Neurol. 2013;12(1):65–71.
8. Gulli G, Khan S, Markus HS. Vertebrobasilar stenosis predicts high early recurrent stroke risk in posterior circulation stroke and TIA. Stroke. 2009;40(8):2732–7.
9. Flossmann E, Rothwell PM. Prognosis of vertebrobasilar transient ischaemic attack and minor stroke. Brain. 2003;126(Pt 9):1940–54.
10. Marquardt L, Kuker W, Chandratheva A, Geraghty O, Rothwell PM. Incidence and prognosis of > or = 50% symptomatic vertebral or basilar artery stenosis: prospective population-based study. Brain. 2009;132(Pt 4):982–8.
11. Chung CP, Yong CS, Chang FC, Sheng WY, Huang HC, Tsai JY, et al. Stroke etiology is associated with outcome in posterior circulation stroke. Ann Clin Transl Neurol. 2015;2(5):510–7.
12. Gulli G, Marquardt L, Rothwell PM, Markus HS. Stroke risk after posterior circulation stroke/transient ischemic attack and its relationship to site of vertebrobasilar stenosis: pooled data analysis from prospective studies. Stroke. 2013;44(3):598–604.
13. Schonewille WJ, Wijman CA, Michel P, Rueckert CM, Weimar C, Mattle HP, et al. Treatment and outcomes of acute basilar artery occlusion in the basilar artery international cooperation study (BASICS): a prospective registry study. Lancet Neurol. 2009;8(8):724–30.
14. Lindsberg PJ, Mattle HP. Therapy of basilar artery occlusion: a systematic analysis comparing intra-arterial and intravenous thrombolysis. Stroke. 2006;37(3):922–8.
15. Sheng K, Tong M. Therapy for acute basilar artery occlusion: a systematic review and meta-analysis. F1000Res. 2019;8:165.
16. Akhtar N, Kamran SI, Deleu D, D'Souza A, Miyares F, Elsotouhy A, et al. Ischaemic posterior circulation stroke in State of Qatar. Eur J Neurol. 2009;16(9):1004–9.
17. Park KC, Yoon SS, Rhee HY. Executive dysfunction associated with stroke in the posterior cerebral artery territory. J Clin Neurosci. 2011;18(2):203–8.
18. Glass TA, Hennessey PM, Pazdera L, Chang HM, Wityk RJ, Dewitt LD, et al. Outcome at 30 days in the new England Medical Center posterior circulation registry. Arch Neurol. 2002;59(3):369–76.
19. Schonewille WJ, Algra A, Serena J, Molina CA, Kappelle LJ. Outcome in patients with basilar artery occlusion treated conventionally. J Neurol Neurosurg Psychiatry. 2005;76(9):1238.
20. Voetsch B, DeWitt LD, Pessin MS, Caplan LR. Basilar artery occlusive disease in the new England Medical Center posterior circulation registry. Arch Neurol. 2004;61(4):496–504.
21. Lin SF, Chen CI, Hu HH, Bai CH. Predicting functional outcomes of posterior circulation acute ischemic stroke in first 36 h of stroke onset. J Neurol. 2018;265(4):926–32.
22. Tsao JW, Hemphill JC 3rd, Johnston SC, Smith WS, Bonovich DC. Initial Glasgow coma scale score predicts outcome following thrombolysis for posterior circulation stroke. Arch Neurol. 2005;62(7):1126–9.
23. Inoa V, Aron AW, Staff I, Fortunato G, Sansing LH. Lower NIH stroke scale scores are required to accurately predict a good prognosis in posterior circulation stroke. Cerebrovasc Dis. 2014;37(4):251–5.
24. Sato S, Toyoda K, Uehara T, Toratani N, Yokota C, Moriwaki H, et al. Baseline NIH stroke scale score predicting outcome in anterior and posterior circulation strokes. Neurology. 2008;70(24 Pt 2):2371–7.
25. Kasner SE. Clinical interpretation and use of stroke scales. Lancet Neurol. 2006;5(7):603–12.
26. Olivato S, Nizzoli S, Cavazzuti M, Casoni F, Nichelli PF, Zini A. E-NIHSS: an expanded National Institutes of Health stroke scale weighted for anterior and posterior circulation strokes. J Stroke Cerebrovasc Dis. 2016;25(12):2953–7.
27. Devuyst G, Bogousslavsky J, Meuli R, Moncayo J, de Freitas G, van Melle G. Stroke or transient ischemic attacks with basilar artery stenosis or occlusion: clinical patterns and outcome. Arch Neurol. 2002;59(4):567–73.
28. Sommer P, Posekany A, Serles W, Marko M, Scharer S, Fertl E, et al. Is functional outcome different in posterior and anterior circulation stroke? Stroke. 2018;49(11):2728–32.
29. Forster A, Gass A, Kern R, Griebe M, Hennerici MG, Szabo K. Thrombolysis in posterior circulation stroke: stroke subtypes and patterns, complications and outcome. Cerebrovasc Dis. 2011;32(4):349–53.
30. Sarikaya H, Arnold M, Engelter ST, Lyrer PA, Mattle HP, Georgiadis D, et al. Outcomes of intravenous thrombolysis in posterior versus anterior circulation stroke. Stroke. 2011;42(9):2498–502.
31. Dornak T, Kral M, Hazlinger M, Herzig R, Veverka T, Burval S, et al. Posterior vs. anterior circulation

infarction: demography, outcomes, and frequency of hemorrhage after thrombolysis. Int J Stroke. 2015;10(8):1224–8.

32. Huang Q, Song HQ, Ma QF, Song XW, Wu J. Effects of time delays on the therapeutic outcomes of intravenous thrombolysis for acute ischemic stroke in the posterior circulation: an observational study. Brain Behav. 2019;9(2):e01189.

33. Cross DT 3rd, Moran CJ, Akins PT, Angtuaco EE, Diringer MN. Relationship between clot location and outcome after basilar artery thrombolysis. AJNR Am J Neuroradiol. 1997;18(7):1221–8.

34. Cross DT 3rd, Moran CJ, Akins PT, Angtuaco EE, Derdeyn CP, Diringer MN. Collateral circulation and outcome after basilar artery thrombolysis. AJNR Am J Neuroradiol. 1998;19(8):1557–63.

35. Schwarz S, Egelhof T, Schwab S, Hacke W. Basilar artery embolism. Clinical syndrome and neuroradiologic patterns in patients without permanent occlusion of the basilar artery. Neurology. 1997;49(5):1346–52.

36. Grond M, Rudolf J, Schmulling S, Stenzel C, Neveling M, Heiss WD. Early intravenous thrombolysis with recombinant tissue-type plasminogen activator in vertebrobasilar ischemic stroke. Arch Neurol. 1998;55(4):466–9.

37. Qureshi AI, Qureshi MH, Lien LM, Lee JT, Jeng JS, Hu CJ, et al. One-year risk of recurrent stroke and death associated with vertebrobasilar artery stenosis and occlusion in a cohort of 10,515 patients. Cerebrovasc Dis. 2019;47(1–2):40–7.

38. Qureshi AI, Ziai WC, Yahia AM, Mohammad Y, Sen S, Agarwal P, et al. Stroke-free survival and its determinants in patients with symptomatic vertebrobasilar stenosis: a multicenter study. Neurosurgery. 2003;52(5):1033–9; discussion 9–40

39. Ntaios G, Spengos K, Vemmou AM, Savvari P, Koroboki E, Stranjalis G, et al. Long-term outcome in posterior cerebral artery stroke. Eur J Neurol. 2011;18(8):1074–80.

40. Nadeau S, Jordan J, Mishra S. Clinical presentation as a guide to early prognosis in vertebrobasilar stroke. Stroke. 1992;23(2):165–70.

41. Ottomeyer C, Zeller J, Fesl G, Holtmannspotter M, Opherk C, Bender A, et al. Multimodal recanalization therapy in acute basilar artery occlusion: long-term functional outcome and quality of life. Stroke. 2012;43(8):2130–5.

42. Lindsberg PJ, Soinne L, Tatlisumak T, Roine RO, Kallela M, Happola O, et al. Long-term outcome after intravenous thrombolysis of basilar artery occlusion. JAMA. 2004;292(15):1862–6.

43. Jung S, Mono ML, Fischer U, Galimanis A, Findling O, De Marchis GM, et al. Three-month and long-term outcomes and their predictors in acute basilar artery occlusion treated with intra-arterial thrombolysis. Stroke. 2011;42(7):1946–51.

44. Garrard P, Bradshaw D, Jager HR, Thompson AJ, Losseff N, Playford D. Cognitive dysfunction after isolated brain stem insult. An underdiagnosed cause of long term morbidity. J Neurol Neurosurg Psychiatry. 2002;73(2):191–4.

45. Hoffmann M, Schmitt F. Cognitive impairment in isolated subtentorial stroke. Acta Neurol Scand. 2004;109(1):14–24.

46. Hoffmann M, Cases LB. Etiology of frontal network syndromes in isolated subtentorial stroke. Behav Neurol. 2008;20(3):101–5.

47. Campanholo KR, Conforto AB, Rimkus CM, Miotto EC. Cognitive and functional impairment in stroke survivors with basilar artery occlusive disease. Behav Neurol. 2015;2015:971514.

48. Martinaud O, Pouliquen D, Gerardin E, Loubeyre M, Hirsbein D, Hannequin D, et al. Visual agnosia and posterior cerebral artery infarcts: an anatomical-clinical study. PLoS One. 2012;7(1):e30433.

49. Capitani E, Laiacona M, Pagani R, Capasso R, Zampetti P, Miceli G. Posterior cerebral artery infarcts and semantic category dissociations: a study of 28 patients. Brain. 2009;132(Pt 4):965–81.

Printed in the United States
by Baker & Taylor Publisher Services